MAN & WOMAN BOY & GIRL

MAN &
BOY &

THE DIFFERENTIATION
GENDER IDENTITY FROM

BY JOHN MONEY AND

THE JOHNS HOPKINS UNIVERSITY PRESS

MAN & WOMAN BOY & GIRL

THE DIFFERENTIATION AND DIMORPHISM OF GENDER IDENTITY FROM CONCEPTION TO MATURITY

JOHN MONEY & ANKE A. EHRHARDT

THE JOHNS HOPKINS UNIVERSITY PRESS BALTIMORE AND LONDON

Manufactured in the United States of America

The Johns Hopkins University Press, Baltimore, Maryland 21218
The Johns Hopkins University Press Ltd., London

Library of Congress Catalog Card Number 72-4012
ISBN 0-8018-1405-7 (cloth)
ISBN 0-8018-1406-5 (paper)

Library of Congress Cataloging in Publication data will be found on the last printed page of this book.

Originally published, 1972
Johns Hopkins Paperback, 1972
Second printing (cloth and paper), 1973
Third printing (cloth and paper), 1973
Fourth printing (cloth), 1973
Fourth printing (paper), 1974

TABLE OF CONTENTS

PREFACE

A scientific topic—the sexual differentiation of man and woman from conception to maturity—is presented in this book in such a way as to integrate experimental and clinical data and concepts from each of the scientific specialties that have something to contribute: genetics, embryology, neuroendocrinology, endocrinology, neurosurgery, social, medical and clinical psychology, and social anthropology. One goal of the book is to organize old and new knowledge into a theoretical formulation of the behavioral dimorphism and differentiation of male and female—into a theory not simply of psychosexual development but also of psychosexual differentiation, and into a theory encompassing all the determinants of human sexual behavior more comprehensively than is done by traditional developmental theories of masculinity and femininity. The goal of such a theoretical formulation cannot be achieved in the usual multidisciplinary book with each chapter by a different author, each written from the outlook of the author's particular specialty.

Because this book is designed to transcend several traditional specialties in order to integrate the pertinent available information relevant to psychosexual differentiation, some of the chapters are reviews of the work of others. Other chapters review original work in psychohormonal research and the medical psychology of sex by the authors and their collaborators.

The clinical material in all chapters of the book is drawn from the extensive file of longitudinal case and group studies assembled in the psychohormonal research unit of The Johns Hopkins Hospital and School of Medicine since 1951. These studies range over all the endocrinopathies, sexual and other, of childhood and adolescence, and over various other related and contrasting developmental conditions and pathologies, as follows:

Absent Genitalia

Penile agenesis or microphallus
- a) raised female 6
- b) raised male 11

Penile amputation 5
Vaginal atresia 10
Vulvectomy 2

Chromosome Anomalies

XXY syndrome 37
XYY syndrome 8
XXYY syndrome 1
Trichromosome X 6
Turner's syndrome 109

Gynecomastia

Adolescent boys 28

Hermaphroditism

Androgen insensitivity
- a) hypospadias, juvenile gonadectomy (reared female) 5
- b) partial, feminizing hypospadias
  - (i) reared female 2
  - (ii) reared male 8
- c) simulant female, testicular feminizing syndrome (reared female) 24

Female with phallus
- a) progestin-induced
  - (i) reared female 18
  - (ii) reared male 1
- b) spontaneously induced
  - (i) reared male 2
  - (ii) reared female 1

Hyperadrenocortical female
- a) reared female 81
- b) reared male 10

Hypospadiac male
- a) cryptorchid
  - (i) reared female 18
  - (ii) reared male 15
- b) not cryptorchid
  - (i) reared female 8
  - (ii) reared male 16

Males with mullerian organs
- a) reared male 7
- b) reared female 10

True hermaphroditism 7

Paraplegia

Male and female 15

Priapism

Male 8

Puberty, Delayed

All types, male 88
All types, female 29

Puberty, Precocious

Brain lesions 9
Hyperadrenocorticism, boys 20
Idiopathic
- a) boys 13
- b) girls
  - (i) mature $\leq$ 8 yrs 45
  - (ii) mature $\geq$ 8 yrs 17

Psychosexual Disorders

Exhibitionism 3
Homosexual, male (no other diagnosis) 35
Homosexual, female (no other diagnosis) 9
Incongruous gender role, prepubertal boys 36
Incongruous gender role, prepubertal girls 4
Incest 7
Miscellaneous other diagnoses 40
Pedophilia 5
Transexual reassignment, male-to-female 25
Transexual reassignment, female-to-male 11
Transexual reassignment applicants 20
Transvestite, male 28
Transvestite, female 6

Sex Reassignment[1]

Ablatio penis 2
Hermaphrodite 19
Hermaphrodite, neonates reannounced 16
Microphallus 3
Transexual 36

This book will be of interest especially to students of psychology, sociology, anthropology, ethology, genetics, neuroendocrinology, and medicine. In addition, it is a book for clinicians and, indeed, also for the general reader for whom especially the glossary of technical terms is provided. It is written at a time when rapid advances in research from various disciplines have opened new vistas against which to reexamine traditional behavioral opinions on masculinity and femininity. Therefore, it is hoped that the book will serve as a source of information and as a stimulus for new research. The theoretical implications may serve as a focus of fruitful controversy. In connection with the women's liberation movement they have, in fact, already engendered dispute. The advocates of male supremacy like to quote the findings of Chapter 6, about prenatal determinants of gender dimorphic behavior, while neglecting the findings of Chapter 7 and Chapter 8, regarding the dramatic importance of postnatal determinants. The advocates of women's liberation, by contrast, attend chiefly to Chapters 7 and 8, and neglect Chapter 6. The ultimate scientific resolution of the debate will lie in surpassing the traditional, now outdated dichotomy of heredity and environment, and in properly understanding the principle of interactionism between prenatal and postnatal determinants of psychosexual differentiation, especially in connection with the principle of the critical developmental period.

The history of this book dates back to a monograph on the psychology of hermaphroditism begun in 1949 (Money, 1952). Work on this monograph

[1]All the cases classified under **Sex Reassignment** are also included in one of the preceding diagnostic categories.

led to a contact with the late Lawson Wilkins who had recently established the first pediatric endocrine clinic in the world at The Johns Hopkins Hospital. The clinic became a magnet for referrals of children with birth defects of the sex organs, many of them genetic females with the adrenogenital syndrome, their symptoms including hermaphroditic, ambiguous-looking external sexual anatomy. Patients with this condition had formerly been attracted to this hospital because of the pioneering but unsuccessful attempt of Hugh H. Young, in urology, to control the developmental virilization typical of the syndrome by means of surgical removal of most of the cortex of each adrenal gland.

By the beginning of 1950, Lawson Wilkins in Baltimore, and Fuller Albright and Frederic C. Bartter in Boston, working competitively, had simultaneously demonstrated that the adrenocortical hormonal error responsible for hermaphrodization and virilization in the adrenogenital syndrome could be controlled by the administration of cortisone, a newly synthesized hormone of the adrenal cortex. Wilkins devoted a large part of the remainder of his life to the study and treatment of the adrenogenital syndrome. He took advantage of the opportunities and implications for psychologic research that the new treatment for the syndrome had opened up by obtaining a research grant from the Josiah Macy, Jr. Foundation, to provide a place in his clinic for a medical psychologist specializing in psychohormonal research.

Among the many clinical research projects in the psychohormonal research unit over the years, one grew to become a Ph.D. dissertation (Ehrhardt, 1969), and to have a special history in the planning and production of the present volume.

All told, some twenty years of research ranging over many clinical syndromes pertinent to psychosexual function and gender-identity differentiation are represented between these two covers, and this is the first time that all the information has been put together.

ACKNOWLEDGMENTS

Research grants and gifts were provided over the years from institutions and individuals, as follows, and are gratefully acknowledged.

—Erickson Educational Foundation. Research Grant, 1966-1972. Post-doctoral Fellowship Award, 1969-1970, to Dr. Ehrhardt for the initial work on this book.
—United States Public Health Service, National Institutes of Health. Research Grant #R01-HD00325, 1957—. Research Career Development Award #K03-HD18635, 1962-1972.
—The Henry Foundation.
—Mrs. Marion Colwill and the Stiles E. Tuttle Trust
—Dr. and Mrs. Hershel Herzog
—The Josiah Macy, Jr., Foundation, Research Grant, 1951-1960.

The following members of the psychohormonal research unit have contributed to the work of producing this book: Viola G. Lewis, Nanci A. Bobrow, Florence C. Clarke, Georg Wolff, Charles Annecillo, Richard Clopper, Kate Rollo-Black, Mary Kerber and, from the Office of Psychoendocrinology in Buffalo, Susan W. Baker.

The authors wish to express their gratitude to their close colleagues, Robert M. Blizzard, M.D., and Claude J. Migeon, M.D., and members of their Pediatric Endocrine Clinic, for their collaboration in a productive and very congenial working relationship; and likewise to Howard W. Jones, Jr., M.D., and William W. Scott, Ph.D. M.D., and members of their Departments of Gynecology and Urology, respectively; and to Digamber S. Borgaonkar, Ph.D., in the Division of Medical Genetics.

The Chairmen of the two departments under whose aegis the work of this book has been carried out are Joel Elkes, M.D., Henry Phipps Professor of Psychiatry and Behavioral Sciences, and Robert E. Cooke, M.D., Given Foundation Professor of Pediatrics.

Figure 2.1 is reproduced with permission from E. Witschi, Hormones and Embryonic Induction, Archives d'Anatomie Microscopique et de Morphologie Experimentale, 54:601-611, 1965 (Masson & Cie, Paris).

Figure 10.1 is reproduced with permission from J. M. Tanner, Growth at Adolescence, Blackwell Scientific Publications, Ltd., Oxford, England, 1962.

Photographs for other figures were generously supplied with permission to reproduce them as follows: Figure 2.2 by Dr. Toki-o Yamomoto, Nagoya University; Figures 5.1 and 5.2 by Dr. Friedmund Neumann, Schering A. G. Laboratories, Berlin; Figures 5.3, 5.4, and 5.5 by Drs. Robert Goy and Charles Phoenix, Oregon Regional Primate Center; Figures 12.1 and 12.2 by Dr. Paul MacLean, N. I. M. H.; and Figures 12.3 and 12.4 by Dr. M. W. Schein, Pennsylvania State University.

MAN & WOMAN
BOY & GIRL

1

SYNOPSIS

Introduction

In developmental psychosexual theory, it is no longer satisfactory to utilize only the concept of psychosexual development. Psychosexual (or gender-identity) differentiation is the preferential concept, for the psychodevelopment of sex is a continuation of the embryodevelopment of sex. Alone among the divers functional systems of embryonic development, the reproductive system is sexually dimorphic. So also in subsequent behavioral and psychic development, there is sexual dimorphism.

In the theory of psychosexual differentiation, it is now outmoded to juxtapose nature versus nurture, the genetic versus the environmental, the innate versus the acquired, the biological versus the psychological, or the instinctive versus the learned. Modern genetic theory avoids these antiquated dichotomies, and postulates a genetic norm of reaction which, for its proper expression, requires phyletically prescribed environmental boundaries. If these boundaries are either too constricted, or too diffuse, then the environment is lethal, and the genetic code cannot express itself, for the cells carrying it are nonviable.

The basic proposition should be not a dichotomization of genetics and environment, but their interaction. Interactionism as applied to the dif-

NOTE: For literature supporting statements in this Synopsis, see references given in the context of the chapters that follow.

ferentiation of gender identity can be best expressed by using the concept of a program. There are phyletically written parts of the program. They exert their determining influence particularly before birth, and leave a permanent *imprimatur* (see Glossary). Even at that early time, however, the phyletic program may be altered by idiosyncrasies of personal history, such as the loss or gain of a chromosome during cell division, a deficiency or excess of maternal hormone, viral invasion, intrauterine trauma, nutritional deficiency or toxicity, and so forth. Other idiosyncratic modifications may be added by the biographical events of birth. All may impose their own imprimatur on the genetic program of sexual dimorphism that is normally expected on the basis of XX or XY chromosomal dimorphism.

Postnatally, the programing of psychosexual differentiation is, by phyletic decree, a function of biographical history, especially social biography. There is a close parallel here with the programing of language development. The social-biography program is not written independently of the phyletic program, but in conjunction with it, though on occasions there may be dysjunction between the two. Once written, the social-biography program leaves its imprimatur as surely as does the phyletic. The long-term effects of the two are equally fixed and enduring, and their different origins not easily recognizable. Aspects of human psychosexual differentiation attributable to the social-biography program are often mistakenly attributed to the phyletic program.

In the history of the egg from fertilization to birth, the sequence of developmental events can be likened to a relay race (Figure 1.1). The program of sexual dimorphism is carried first by either the X or the Y sex chromosome, supplied by the male parent to pair with the X chromosome from the female parent. The XX or XY chromosomal combination will pass the program to the undifferentiated gonad, to determine its destiny as testis or ovary. Thereafter, the sex chromosomes will have no known direct influence on subsequent sexual and psychosexual differentiation.

The undifferentiated gonad differentiates and passes the program to the hormonal secretions of its own cells. More accurately, the program is passed to the secretions of the testis. In the total absence of fetal gonadal hormones, the fetus always continues to differentiate the reproductive anatomy of a female. Ovarian hormones are, according to present evidence, irrelevant at this early stage. Testicular hormones are imperative for the continuing differentiation of the reproductive structures of a male.

Testicular secretions, their presence or absence or their intrusion from exogenous sources, account not only for the shape of the external genitals but also for certain patterns of organization in the brain, especially, by inference, in the hypothalamic pathways that will subsequently influence

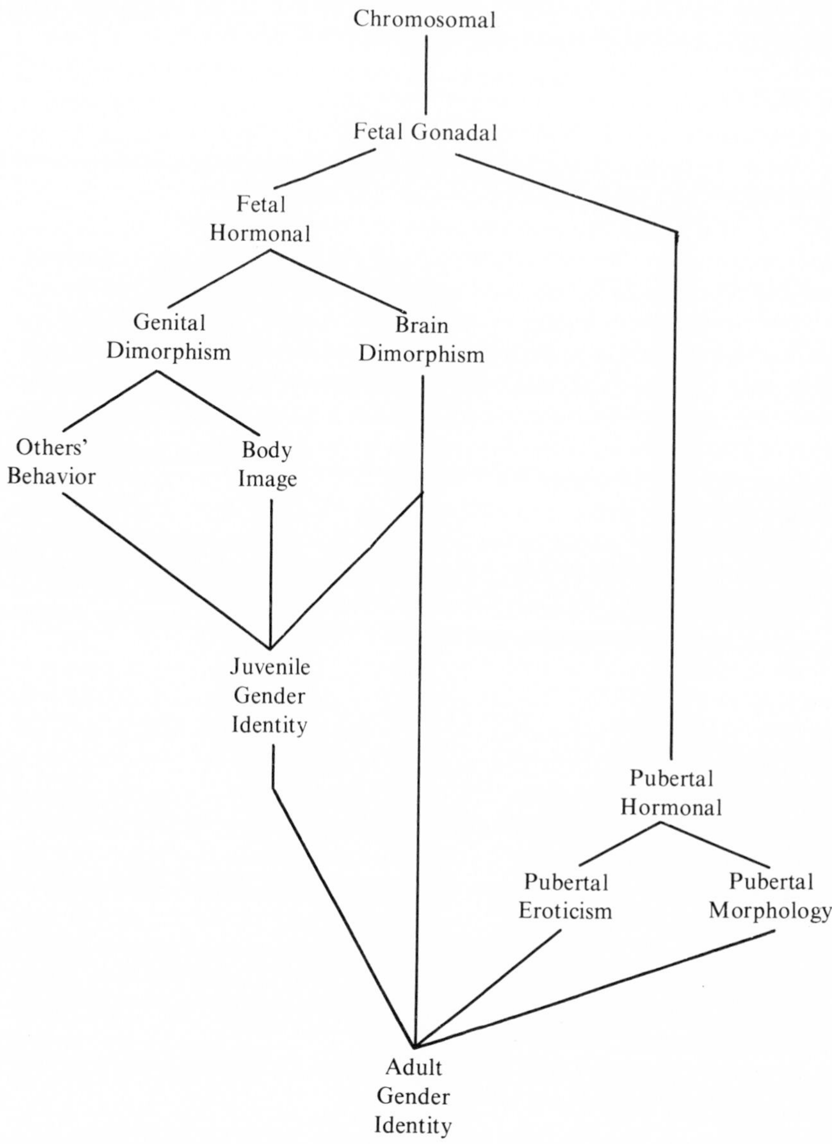

Figure 1.1. Diagram to illustrate the sequential and interactional components of gender-identity differentiation.

certain aspects of sexual behavior. Thus they pass on the program, dividing it between two carriers, namely, the genital morphology and that part of the central nervous system, peripheral and intracranial, which serves the genital morphology.

Genital morphology completes its program-bearing work by passing the program on, first to those adult individuals who are responsible for sex assignment and rearing the child as a boy or girl, and later to the child in person as he, or she, perceives the genital organs.

The central nervous system, insofar as prenatal hormonal factors made it sexually dimorphic, passes on its program in the form of behavioral traits which influence other people, and which are traditionally and culturally classified as predominantly boyish or girlish. These traits do not automatically determine the dimorphism of gender identity, but they exert some influence on the ultimate pattern of gender identity, for instance in tomboyish feminine identity in girls, and its opposite in boys.

The predominant part of gender-identity differentiation receives its program by way of social transmission from those responsible for the reconfirmation of the sex of assignment in the daily practices of rearing. Once differentiated, gender identity receives further confirmation from the hormonal changes of puberty, or lack of confirmation in instances of incongruous identity.

With the initiation of parenthood, the whole program is set in motion yet once again, as a new generation comes into being.

Definitions

Gender Identity: The sameness, unity, and persistence of one's individuality as male, female, or ambivalent, in greater or lesser degree, especially as it is experienced in self-awareness and behavior; gender identity is the private experience of gender role, and gender role is the public expression of gender identity.

Gender Role: Everything that a person says and does, to indicate to others or to the self the degree that one is either male, or female, or ambivalent; it includes but is not restricted to sexual arousal and response; gender role is the public expression of gender identity, and gender identity is the private experience of gender role.

Terminology and Nature of Hermaphroditism

Hermaphroditism can be induced at will in experimental animals for the purpose of investigating the effects of genetic, hormonal and morphologic sexual dimorphism on sexual behavior. Ethical considerations forbid parallel experiments in human beings. Therefore, the spontaneous occurrence of human hermaphroditism is of special value for psychologists of sexual behavior as well as for the students of that specifically human variable—verbal report. From the combined sources of information—behavior and verbal report—one constructs a conception of gender role and gender identity of another human being—or possibly of one's own. This conception usually agrees with dimorphism of sexual appearance, though the match is not always, nor of necessity, concordant.

As ordinarily defined, hermaphroditism or intersexuality in human beings is a condition of prenatal origin in which embryonic and/or fetal differentiation of the reproductive system fails to reach completion as either entirely female or entirely male. In the very strictest sense, one could speak of chromosomal hermaphroditism, as in individuals with a 47,XXY chromosome count, namely Klinefelter's syndrome, or one of its variants such as 48,XXXY. In such individuals, the reproductive system passes as male, except for infertility of the testes. In ordinary usage, they are not classified as hermaphrodites. The same is true of rare cases of chromosomal mosaicism in which the pattern is 46,XX/46,XY, and the gonads dysgenetic—provided the external genitals are not ambiguously formed, which they may be.

As ordinarily defined, hermaphroditism means that a baby is born with the sexual anatomy improperly differentiated. The baby is, in other words, sexually unfinished. If the external genitalia are involved, then they look ambiguous, for an incompletely differentiated penis may be indistinguishable from an incompletely differentiated clitoris, irrespective of genetic and gonadal sex. Moreover, a genetic female may be prenatally androgenized to such a degree that the baby is born looking like a boy with undescended testes. Conversely, a genetic male may be born with a genital appearance indistinguishable from that of a normal female.

The terms hermaphroditism and intersexuality may today be used interchangeably, even though some earlier writers tended to apply hermaphroditism to cases of known hormonal etiology, whether genetic or other, and intersexuality to cases of unknown, but ostensible genetic etiology. These writers contrasted true hermaphroditism with pseudohermaphroditism, in the mistaken belief that only the gonads revealed the truth. Thus, a true hermaphrodite was defined as possessing both ovarian and testicular tissue, either separately or in the form of ovotestis, whereas a pseudohermaphrodite was defined as having only ovarian or testicular tissue, both types showing ambiguity of the internal and/or external reproductive structures also. There was no place in this scheme for the hermaphrodite with gonadal tissue that was incompletely differentiated as either male or female. In current usage, a male or a female pseudohermaphrodite is the same as, respectively, a male or a female hermaphrodite, the shorter term being preferable. A hermaphrodite with vestigial or undifferentiated ovaries or testes is said to be gonadally dysgenetic.

Chromosomal and Gonadal Sex

In normal differentiation of sexual morphology in the embryo and fetus, one expects that the dimorphism of the sex chromosomes will determine dimorphism of the gonads. This expectancy is reasonably fulfilled in hermaphroditism, insofar as the discordance of bilateral ovaries and a 46,XY chromosomal pattern does not occur, nor does the discordance of bilateral testes and a 46,XX chromosomal pattern, except for questionable cases.

Female hermaphrodites characteristically possess bilateral ovaries, along with the 46,XX chromosomal pattern of the normal female. The 46,XX pattern does not, however, guarantee that two ovaries will differentiate, for the 46,XX pattern is the one most commonly found in true hermaphrodites who possess either one or two ovotestes, or one ovary and one testis, or in very rare cases two ovaries and two testes. The 46,XX pattern may also be found in cases of dysgenetic gonads, neither of them clearly ovarian nor clearly testicular.

Possession of testes bilaterally is not necessarily characteristic of male hermaphrodites. One of the pair may be either missing, vestigial, or dysgenetic. The chromosomal pattern is usually 46,XY, as expected in a male, but chromosomal mosaicism, such as 45,X/46,XY, or some other chromosomal anomaly may also be found. The same anomalies of the sex chromosomes may be associated with the gonadal anomalies of true hermaphroditism and also when both gonads are dysgenetic.

Gonadal, Hormonal, and Morphologic Sex

In normal fetal development, sexual dimorphism of the gonads can be expected to be paralleled by dimorphism of the sexual anatomy. This expectancy is not upheld in hermaphroditism. The reason is that the gonads do not, of and by themselves alone, dictate the developmental fate of the anlagen of the genital structures, but only by way of the hormones they release. Errors, excesses, or deficiencies of these hormones, even if they are of extra-gonadal origin, are critical in hermaphroditism, and are responsible for the anatomical incongruencies that constitute the hermaphroditic condition.

The normal rule in embryonic development is that the primordial gonad begins its differentiation as a testis, if that is to be its fate, after the sixth week of gestation, and about six weeks ahead of the timing of ovarian differentiation, according to Jost (*1972*). This priority of the appearance of typical testicular tissue is perhaps related to another embryologic fact, namely, that if both embryonic gonads are removed prior to the critical period when the other sexual anatomy is formed, then the embryo will proceed to differentiate as a morphologic female, regardless of genetic sex. Nature's rule is, it would appear, that to masculinize, something must be added. There are two additive principles. Both are governed by the developing testes. One is known only inferentially and is called the mullerian-inhibiting substance, by reason of its function, namely to suppress all further development of the primitive mullerian ducts which in the female form the uterus, fallopian tubes, and upper segment of the vagina. When this substance fails in a genetic male embryo, a boy is born with a uterus and fallopian tubes in addition to normal male internal organs. The external organs may be normally male, except for cryptorchidism.

The second additive principle is testosterone, the male sex hormone. In early embryonic life, testosterone released by the testes has a localized, bilateral influence, namely in promoting proliferation of the wolffian ducts to form the internal male reproductive structures. Subsequently, testosterone has a more distant influence: by circulating in the blood stream, it reaches the anlagen of the external sexual organs and dictates their developmental program. The genital tubercle becomes a penis instead of a clitoris. The skin-folds wrap around the penis on both sides of the genital slit and fuse in the midline, forming the urethral tube and foreskin, in place of the bilateral minor labia and the clitoral hood. The outer swellings, on either side of the genital slit, fuse in the midline to form the scrotum to receive the testes, instead of remaining in place as the bilateral labia majora of the female.

If testosterone is added to the bloodstream of a genetic-female fetus during a critical period in development, the girl will be born with either a grossly enlarged clitoris or, in rare instances, a normal-looking penis and empty scrotum. In human beings, such masculinization occurs in the adrenogenital syndrome of female hermaphroditism, in which the source of excess androgen is the fetus's own abnormally functioning adrenocortical glands. It may also occur should the mother, while pregnant, have a male-hormone producing tumor or should she be given a now-obsolete synthetic pregnancy-saving hormone that in some rare instances has masculinized the daughter fetus (progestin-induced hermaphroditism).

The obverse of masculinization of the external genitalia of the genetic female is failure of masculinization of the genetic male. In human beings, such failure has been known to occur as the result of a genetically induced metabolic error (17 α-hydroxylase deficiency) which prohibits the normal synthesis of hormonal steroids, in particular androgen, in the testes or adrenal cortices. Affected babies rarely survive. Failure of external masculinization of the genitalia is total and complete also in the testicular feminizing syndrome of androgen insensitivity. The fault lies not in the testes, but in a genetically transmitted defect that blocks at the cellular level the uptake of androgen by the target organs. Affected individuals are born looking like females.

The androgen-insensitivity syndrome may occur in partial form, so that a genetic-male baby is born with external genitalia that are incompletely masculinized and ambiguous-looking. It is more common, however, that such ambiguity (whereby the phallus cannot be distinguished upon inspection as either an enlarged clitoris or an imperfectly formed penis lacking fusion of the urethral tube) is the end result not of androgen insensitivity, but of the fetal testes' failing to produce sufficient androgen at the critical period of external genital differentiation.

Ambiguity of the external genital appearance is the rule in true hermaphroditism, and may represent the end product of rivalry between masculinizing and feminizing tendencies, that is to say, of too much androgen to permit perfect feminization, but not enough to induce perfect masculinization.

Fetal Hormonal Sex, the Nervous System, and Behavior

Normal differentiation of genital morphology entails a dimorphic sex difference in the arrangement of the peripheral nerves of sex which, in turn, entails some degree of dimorphism in the representation of the periphery at the centrum of the central nervous system, that is to say, in the structures and pathways of the brain.

The concept of central nervous system dimorphism of sex was neglected until it was brought into focus by the contemporary surge of research on the influence of prenatal hormones, by way of the brain, on subsequent dimorphism of sexual behavior. This surge of research was initiated by William C. Young, partly in response to early clinical studies on human hermaphroditism showing that individuals of the same hermaphroditic diagnosis would, if reared oppositely, differentiate a gender identity in agreement with their biography, irrespective of chromosomal, gonadal, or hormonal sex, and even, perhaps, of uncorrected morphologic appearance.

Human hermaphroditic studies have, meanwhile, benefited from the new experimental findings on animals, which suggest that the prenatal hormonal environment does exercise, during a few critical days of brain development, a determining influence on neural pathways that will subsequently mediate sexually dimorphic behavior. In human beings, the pathways have not yet been anatomically identified. The lower an animal in the phyletic scale, the more likely is its prenatally determined behavior to be stereotypic and uninfluenced by later history. The higher primates, and man especially, are more subject to the influence of postnatal biographical history. Thus, individuals of the same hermaphroditic diagnosis, oppositely reared, differentiate opposite-sexed gender identities postnatally, but they have in common certain traits of temperament or personality, presumably in consequence of their similar prenatal hormonal environment. These traits are generally classified as sexually dimorphic. They are not, however, exclusively the property of either sex. They may be incorporated into either a male or a female gender identity pattern, if not in conformity with the cultural norm, then as a culturally acceptable variant of it.

Illustrations of the general principle can be found in both male and female hermaphroditism. In the case of female hermaphroditism, one assumes that the excess of male hormone which brings about masculinization of the external genitalia will be present in sufficient quantity, and at the critical developmental period, to influence the brain. To establish a relationship between a prenatal hormonal masculinizing influence and subsequent behavioral traits, the preferred cases are those in which hormonal masculinization ceases at birth. This condition is met in progestin-induced hermaphroditism, since the masculinizing agent was synthetic progestin administered to the mother. It also is met in adrenogenital hermaphroditism, if the excess of adrenocortical androgen is kept suppressed by cortisone therapy from birth onward.

In either syndrome, it is more likely that the baby will have been assigned and reared as a girl than as a boy, though the latter does sometimes occur. Those reared as girls are more instructive for present purposes, as the possible sequelae of prenatal hormonal masculinization on behavior are not masked by social masculinization.

It is a handicap in the study of sexually dimorphic behavior that, for all the millennia in which men and women have existed, no one yet has an exhaustive list of what to look for. Today's information is not, therefore, final or absolute. With the safeguard of this proviso, one may sum up current findings by saying that genetic females masculinized in utero and reared as girls have a high chance of being tomboys in their behavior. The elements of tomboyism are as follows.

1. The ratio of athletic to sedentary energy expenditure is weighted in favor of vigorous activity, especially outdoors. Tomboyish girls like to join with boys in outdoor sports, specifically ball games. Groups of girls do not offer equivalent alternatives, nor do their toys. Tomboyish girls prefer the toys that boys usually play with.

2. Self-assertiveness in competition for position in the dominance hierarchy of childhood is strong enough to permit successful rivalry with boys. Tomboyish girls do not, however, usually compete for top-echelon dominance among boys, possibly because their acceptance among boys is conditional on their not doing so. Rivalry for dominance may require fighting, but aggressiveness is not a primary trait of tomboyism. In fact, aggressiveness per se is probably not a primary trait of boyishness either, except as a shibboleth of shoddy popular psychology and the news media. Tomboyish girls are relatively indifferent to establishing a dominance position in the hierarchy of girlhood, possibly because they are not sufficiently interested in all the activities of other girls. They are more likely to establish a position of leadership among younger children who follow them as hero worshippers.

3. Self-adornment is spurned in favor of functionalism and utility in clothing, hairstyle, jewelry, and cosmetics. Tomboyish girls generally prefer slacks and shorts to frills and furbelows, though they do not have an aversion to dressing up for special occasions. Their cosmetic of choice is perfume.

4. Rehearsal of maternalism in childhood dollplay is negligible. Dolls get relegated to permanent storage. Later in childhood, there is no great enthusiasm for baby-sitting or any caretaker activities with small children. The prospect of motherhood is not ruled out, but is viewed in a perfunctory way as something to be postponed rather than hastened. The preference, in anticipation, is for one or two children, not a large family.

5. Romance and marriage are given second place to achievement and career. Priority of career over marriage, preferably combining both, is already evident in the fantasies and expectancies of childhood. The tomboyish girl reaches the boyfriend stage in adolescence later than most of her compeers. Priority assigned to career is typically based on high achievement in school and on high IQ. There is some preliminary evidence to suggest that an abnormally elevated prenatal androgen level, whether in genetic males or females, enhances IQ. Once sexual life begins, there is no evidence of lack of erotic response—rather the opposite. There is no special likelihood of lesbianism.

6. In adulthood, according to preliminary evidence, responsiveness to the visual (or narrative) erotic image may resemble that of men rather than women. That is to say, the viewer objectifies the opposite-sexed

figure in the picture as a sexual partner, as men typically do. Men objectify the female figure. Tomboyish women objectify the male figure. Ordinary women generally do not objectify. They project themselves into the figure of the stimulus woman and fantasy themselves in a parallel situation, but with the romantic partner of their own desire.

Further evidence is needed to know whether the tomboyish response to erotic imagery is contingent on elevated androgen levels in adulthood, or only on a delayed prenatal androgen effect.

The traits that make for tomboyishness in a prenatally androgenized chromosomal and gonadal female assigned and reared as a girl are readily assimilated into a purely boyish gender identity differentiation, should the baby have been assigned and reared as a boy. For the boy, there may be special problems of adjustment that the growing child must solve with respect to phallic repair, implantation of prosthetic testes, and, eventually, fatherhood by means either of the sperm bank or adoption. But these problems are no different than those encountered in the genetic-male hermaphrodite with a hypospadiac phallus and dystrophic, undescended gonads. The genetic male may actually be confronted with a more distressing problem if he happens to be afflicted with androgen insensitivity, a condition which does not occur in the genetic female.

For chromosomal hermaphrodites with the complete and totally feminizing form of the androgen-insensitivity syndrome, the behavioral findings are the obverse of tomboyism in chromosomal females. In such chromosomal males, however, the prenatal hormonal effect cannot be distinguished from the postnatal cultural effect, since the baby is born with female morphology and is assigned and reared as a girl. The more pertinent cases are those of a forme fruste of the androgen-insensitivity syndrome (that is, partial prenatal androgen failure with ambiguous genitalia at birth) followed by rearing as a boy. Such cases are rare and sufficient data have yet to be collected; but present impressions fit in well enough with the thesis that they represent the obverse of tomboyism. There is no name for the opposite of tomboyism. It is not sissyness, as ordinarily defined and understood.

External Morphologic Sex and Assigned Sex

To return to the metaphor of a relay race, the fetal sex-hormonal determinant or precursor of gender-identity differentiation passes on the developmental program that was handed to it successively by way of the gonads from the sex chromosomes. The new program-bearer is the morphology of the external genitals which exercise their initial influence by way of the parents' responses to them.

Parents wait for nine months to see whether the mother gives birth to a boy or a girl. They feel themselves so incapable of influencing what nature ordains that it simply never occurs to them that they are also waiting for the first cue as how to behave toward the new baby. Yet, as soon as the shape of the external genitals is perceived, it sets in motion a chain of communication: It's a daughter! It's a son! This communication itself sets in motion a chain of sexually dimorphic responses, beginning with pink and blue, pronominal use, and name choice, that will be transmitted from person to person to encompass all persons the baby ever encounters, day by day, year in and year out, from birth to death. Dimorphism of response on the basis of the shape of the sex organs is one of the most universal and pervasive aspects of human social interaction. It is so ingrained and habitual in most people, that they lose awareness of themselves as shapers of a child's gender-dimorphic behavior, and take for granted their own behavior as a no-option reaction to the signals of their child's behavior which they assume to have preordained by some eternal verity to be gender-dimorphic.

There are some parents who are so culturally imbued with parental ideals of juridical fair play that they have a blind spot even for the fact that their behavior toward a daughter is, by certain criteria, different from that toward a son. They insist that they treat all siblings alike, and mean, by implication, that they are impartial in the distribution of rewards and punishments. A videotape would rapidly show, however, that these same parents do indeed have a dimorphism of expectancy built into their interactions with daughters as compared with sons. For other parents, a videotape is not necessary. They are more articulate observers of their own behavior, and can report ways in which they differentially treat sons and daughters.

No parents encounter a more dramatic illustration of the son-daughter dimorphism of their own behavior than do those parents of a hermaphroditic child whose announced sex is reassigned after the period of earliest infancy. Ideally, the clinical evaluation of a hermaphroditic baby should be exhaustive and complete at the time of birth, so that the criteria governing the sex of assignment can be properly weighted and the announcement made unequivocally once and for ever.

The ideal is not always met, because few people are prepared ahead of time to know how to react when a baby is delivered and found to have ambiguous genitalia. All too often, a decision as to the sex of announcement is improvised. Subsequently, after a detailed evaluation, a revision of the announcement may be decided upon. If the revision is made neonatally, one speaks simply of a sex reannouncement. Later, after the baby has begun to absorb the gender dimorphism of the language into the development of his or her sense of gender identity, one speaks more accurately not of a sex reannouncement, but reassignment. A reassignment requires a change in responses from the baby. A reannouncement requires changes in the behavior only of other people. It is ill-advised to impose a sex reassignment on a child in contradiction of a gender identity already well advanced in its differentiation—which means that the age ceiling for an imposed reassignment is, in the majority of cases, around eighteen months.

For a sex reassignment, the age of eighteen months—or the few months preceding it—is quite late enough to make parents overtly cognizant of the gender difference in their behavior when they take a son to the hospital and bring home a daughter, or vice versa. By way of illustration (more fully reported in Chapter 7), one father related a story of his romper-room activities with his two young children, upon arrival home from work in the evenings, after the younger one, a genetic male hermaphrodite with a phallus the size of a clitoris and otherwise ambiguous genitalia, had been reassigned as a girl at age 15 months. The older child, a boy, liked a rather rowdy kind of solo dancing, rock-and-roll type. The younger one liked to follow suit, but the father's impulse was to bring her close to himself, to dance as a couple. Though initially she preferred to copy her big brother, the girl soon learned to enjoy her privileged daughter-role with her father.

This anecdote illustrates very well the principle of complementation in the experiences of rearing which shape the differentiation of gender role and gender identity. Traditionally in psychology, especially social psychology, this principle has passed unrecognized, and attention has been directed exclusively to the principle of identification. The fact is that children differentiate a gender role and identity by way of complementation to members of the opposite sex, and identification with members of the same sex.

It is prerequisite to the effective developmental manifestation of both complementation and identification that the sexes be distinguishable from one another, regardless of how great or small the amount of overlap in appearance and behavior culturally prescribed or permitted in any place or period of history. It is a popular pastime, nowadays, to talk and write about the American male's loss of masculinity, thereby misinterpreting what should more accurately be interpreted simply as an accommodation of certain traditional facets of gender role, male and female, to changing times and circumstances. Nature herself supplies the basic irreducible elements of sex difference which no culture can eradicate, at least not on a large scale: women can menstruate, gestate, and lactate, and men cannot. The secondary sexual characteristics of adulthood are reminders of this dichotomy, but the external sex organs are, of course, the primary visible evidence of the different reproductive role of male and female.

Provided that a child grows up to know that sex differences are primarily defined by the reproductive capacity of the sex organs, and to have a positive feeling of pride in his or her own genitalia and their ultimate reproductive use, then it does not much matter whether various child-care, domestic, and vocational activities are or are not interchangeable between mother and father. It does not even matter if mother is a bus driver and daddy a cook. It does not even matter if the father (by adoption) is a female-to-male transexual, provided his hormonal and surgical masculinization have given him the outward appearance and voice of a man, and provided he relates to the child's mother as her lover and husband—irrespective of how they actually perform coitally.

What is difficult—and very difficult indeed—for a young child, is to have a father (or a mother) who switches roles. Some cases have been recorded of a transexual father who naively believed that he could, after reassignment, return to his family, playing the role of aunt to his own children. In other cases, the transexual father knows that it is in his young children's best interest if he separates from them and does not burden them with his gender problem. Those parents most likely to burden their children with blurring of gender differences are transvestite fathers. Their compulsion to impersonate a woman may be so overpowering that they may not effectively hide it from their children. In some cases, the children may be obliged to play elaborate deceits, addressing their father in public as a woman. His impersonation may be so effective that a younger child will have no way of ascribing male sexual status to his father in female dress, unless he knows that the penis, though covered by the clothing, is still the final arbiter.

For all their rarity, and indeed because of it, parental transexualism and transvestism draw one's attention to the child's knowledge of comparative sexual anatomy as a basis for the secure differentiation of his or her own gender identity. Simply seeing the nudity of his own age mates, without seeing the changes of pubescence and the appearance of adulthood, may not be enough. There are, indeed, some inventive young children who come up with the idea that just as breasts and pubic hair grow later, so also may a penis grow out on a girl, or drop off from a boy. Children who hold to such theories are likely to be the ones whose sense of gender identity differentiates insecurely.

Valuable as it is, knowledge of visible sexual anatomy is incomplete. The ideal is for children to be reared to know also the reproductive roles of the sex organs, and to be able to look forward with approval to the proper use of their own, when the time is right. They then are secure in being able to distinguish between the imperative and the optional elements of gender-dimorphic behavior. Their own gender identity then becomes differentiated the more securely.

The significance of a style of rearing that allows ordinary boys and girls to become acquainted, unostentatiously, with the facts of nudity and reproduction is even more evident by its absence in the rare case of a hermaphroditic child raised in secrecy, prudery, and without early corrective surgery. When physicians fail to schedule first-stage corrective genital surgery for a hermaphroditic infant, it usually means that they have covertly postponed a fixed commitment to the sex of rearing because they do not feel secure in committing themselves to one decision or the other. The experts' uncertainty is rapidly conveyed to the parents whose own equivocation is then covertly transmitted to the child, as contagiously as though it were rubella. Small wonder, then, that the child may reach the stage of wondering whether older people are all knaves and fools. By the laws of binary arithmetic, if one claim is wrong, then perhaps the other is correct. The dilemma of uncertainty may thus lead to a child's growing conviction that this uncertainty can be resolved only by changing to live as a member of the other sex. A child so affected may become a good candidate for sex reassignment, whether chromosomal and gonadal sex agree with the reassigned sex or not.

Other hermaphrodites whose sex assignment and anatomical status are left ambiguous, and whose ultimate surgical prognosis is not disclosed to them, may adapt to the sex of ostensible assignment, though handicapped by a sense of shame and mortification. The only other option is for the child to swing on a boy-girl pendulum, alternating the one role with the other. This is a theoretical option only, fraught with too much cognitive dissonance to be found in the histories of hermaphrodites, except the very rare history of a hermaphrodite who qualifies secondarily as a transvestite. Most human beings cannot tolerate such a biographical inconsistency.

Differentiation of Gender Identity

Assignment of sex is not synonymous with the registration of sex on the birth certificate. Registration is a discrete act, whereas assignment becomes synonymous with rearing, insofar as a child is daily confronted with his boyhood, or her girlhood, in innumerable reaffirmations of assignment, including the gender forms of personal reference embedded in the nouns and pronouns of the language.

Gender identity does not always differentiate in conformity with registered sex. A self-evident example is that of a hermaphrodite child whose name, first registered as that of a boy, is changed to that of a girl, without change of the birth certificate. If the parents are consistently unequivocal in their rearing of their child as a girl, then the chances are high that the child will differentiate a girl's gender identity. Parents who neglect to change a birth certificate are, however, thereby indicating the likelihood that they have no conviction that their child is a daughter instead of a son (especially if masculinized external genitalia remain surgically uncorrected). Consequently, they are likely to be ambiguous in the gender-dimorphic signals and expectancies that they transmit to the child. For example, if the child should show a tomboyish level of athletic energy expenditure, they might respond as though such behavior is an expected (and maybe dreaded) confirmation of masculinity, and not as though it is an acceptable variant of a female personality.

When an hermaphroditic child with uncorrected genital ambiguity manifests early in life the signs of differentiating an ambiguous gender identity, or one contradictory of the assigned sex, then it is probable that the child has been responding developmentally to the evidence of the ambiguous and uncorrected sex organs. The evidence of the body may be even more ambiguous in the special case of a genetic female with the adrenogenital syndrome, surgically uncorrected and hormonally untreated, being raised ambiguously as a female. For this child the body will be accelerated in pubertal development, though virilizing as for a male, beginning as early as the age of three. Such early virilization is due to the fact that the same excess of prenatal adrenal androgens that created the hermaphroditic sex organs continues unchecked by cortisone therapy.

Yet, even such a premature excess of body masculinization does not inexorably preordain that a hermaphroditic child living as a girl will differentiate either an ambivalent or a masculine gender identity. The variable that holds the balance of power would seem to be the consistency of the experiences of being reared as feminine, especially in the early years. The noteworthy years are from the onset of language acquisition, at around eighteen months, until between age three and four. A child upon whom a sex reassignment is imposed during this formative period does not, as a rule, fare well in psychosexual differentiation, and may never differentiate the appropriate new gender identity so as eventually to fall in love in agreement with it. Forced changes of sex at a later age, without consideration of gender-identity status, are likely to result in iatrogenic psychopathology.

Further testimony to the importance of the early years in gender-identity differentiation may be found in young children of normal genital anatomy who manifest behavior and express desires appropriate to the opposite sex. In some, though not all such cases, one can identify insidious ambiguity in the gender-appropriate signals transmitted from the parents to the child. The diversity of parent-child interaction in such cases, together with the fact that other siblings differ from the index case, requires one to consider the possibility that the boy who becomes an extreme sissy, or the girl who becomes an extreme amazon do, in fact, get born into the family with some degree of prenatally determined disposition that makes them easily vulnerable to postnatal disorders of gender-identity differentiation.

In support of this thesis, one may take the case of boys with the XXY (Klinefelter's) syndrome. They constitute a high-risk group for psychopathology in general, including psychosexual pathology, which itself includes bisexuality. By contrast 45,X (Turner's syndrome) girls constitute a low-risk group for homosexuality or bisexuality. The same is true of either boys or girls with physical sexual precocity.

Genetic females with a prenatal hermaphroditic history of exposure to androgens differentiate psychosexually as boys if they are assigned and reared as boys and treated with congruent surgical and hormonal therapy, as indicated. The same individuals, if assigned as girls, but raised ambivalently, might easily differentiate a gender identity as lesbians—more easily than girls not known to be subject to intrauterine androgens.

No one knows how many genetic females born with normal female genitalia might, in fact, have been subject to prenatal androgen excess insufficient to influence the external anatomy, though perhaps sufficient to influence the brain. A hitherto unsuspected example of such a prenatal influence was recently reported by Lynwood G. Clemens (personal communication) from Michigan State University. He found that the larger the number of brothers in a litter of rats, the greater the likelihood that the sisters would display masculine mounting behavior when hormonally primed with androgen in adulthood.

The converse of the prenatally androgenized genetic female with normal genital anatomy would be the genetic male with normal genitalia but a prenatal history of androgen deficit. In the male fetus, the influence of its own testicular androgen can be suppressed by injections of antiandrogen, e.g., cyproterone acetate, into the pregnant mother. There is another recent discovery by Ingeborg Ward (1972) that points in the direction of an androgen-deficit effect on the brain of genitally normal males. Pregnant female rats were exposed to the extreme stress of constraint under glaring light, in order to test the effect of the mother's hormonal response to stress on the offspring. The result was that the sons grew up to be deficient in male mating behavior when tested with receptive females.

In experiments with animals, other ways have been discovered to counteract the influence of androgen on the fetus. Gorski's experiments at UCLA demonstrated that if a pregnant animal is injected with androgen in order to have her give birth to daughters with a penis and, at the same time, is injected with sleeping pill medication (phenobarbital or pentobarbital) then the masculinizing influence of the androgen injection will be cancelled. The same cancellation can be achieved with injections of the experimental antibiotics, puromycin and actinomycin-D.

In human beings, no one yet knows the influence on pregnancy of drugs or foods, or even the mother's own, perhaps anomalous placental hormones, or anomalous hormones or hormone deficiency from another maternal source, on the central nervous system of the fetus and the subsequent gender-dimorphic behavior of the child, boy or girl. This paragraph, therefore, has to be left incomplete, except by way of a warning, namely, that it is premature to attribute all aspects of gender-identity to the postnatal period of gender-identity differentiation.

Nonetheless, the evidence of human hermaphroditism makes it abundantly clear that nature has ordained a major part of human gender-identity differentiation to be accomplished in the postnatal period. It then takes place, as does the development of native language, when a prenatally programed disposition comes in contact with postnatal, socially programed signals. The test cases are matched pairs or hermaphrodites, chromosomally, gonadally and otherwise diagnostically the same, but antithetical in sex assignment, biographical history, and gender identity. The contrast between two such young adult individuals in gender role and gender identity is so complete that the ordinary person meeting them socially or vocationally has no clues as to the remarkable contents of their medical histories.

A similar extraordinary contrast has been observed even when a child born as a normal male was surgically reassigned as a female, following an accidental burn in circumcision by cautery. The burn totally ablated the penis. The child is not yet postpubertal and erotically mature, so that the final word remains to be written. Meanwhile, in gender behavior, she is quite gender-different from her identical twin brother (see further details in Chapter 7).

Gender-identity differentiation resembles bilingual differentiation in the child who has two native languages. Bilingualism is confusing for an infant if both languages are spoken to him interchangeably by all people in his linguistic environment. He is then likely to be slower than unilingual children in mastering either language. The child's bilingual learning is unconfused if clearly delineated according to the principle of one person, one language, and always the same language, exclusively. Thus a child may delineate Chinese, say, as the language of exclusive communication with the persons at home, whereas English is the language of persons in the neighborhood and school. Then the complete separateness of the persons who talk and understand only the one language, or the other, allows the demarcation of boundaries around what would otherwise be a chaotic confusion of sound waves. The separateness of the language models defines the separateness of the languages.

The same principle applies to the models of gender role from whom a child establishes his or her own gender-identity differentiation. It is preferable if the irreducible elements of the male gender role are exhibited by males, and of the female gender role by females. Then children learn by identification with persons of the same sex, and by complementation to persons of the opposite sex. Confusion arises when an important person, like a parent, of either sex, gives equivocal or negative signals, either of identification or of complementation, regarding the irreducible elements of either gender role. Such a signal would be a covert one from a mother who despises her son's father's penis and, therefore, her son's also, or resents her own capacity for pregnancy and, therefore, her daughter's prospects of pregnancy also. Parallel messages may be transmitted covertly by a father.

Clear demarcation of the boundaries of the masculine and the feminine gender roles, as above-indicated, is important to the child differentiating a gender identity, because he or she actually learns both. The parallel with bilingualism is closer than it seems, if one thinks of those bilingual children who despise the outmoded language of their immigrant elders in favor of the prestige language of their new community. These children may learn to understand the language they hear at home, but may never utter a word of it, provided the parents understand what they say in the new language. They are ashamed of the old peoples' language, and subject it to a heavy veto of inhibition. In the brain it is coded with a negative sign, meaning unfit for use.

For the ordinary little boy growing up, everything pertaining to the female gender role is brain-coded as negative and unfit for use. The opposite holds for little girls. The negatively coded system in both instances is not a void, however. It serves as a template, so to speak, of what not to do, and also as a guide of what to expect in the behavior of the opposite sex, when one's own behavior must be complemental.

The positively coded system is the one in which the individual becomes truly proficient in all minor details. The negatively coded system may never manifest itself throughout an entire lifetime. There is always a possibility, however, that in senility, when inhibitions weaken, the old man or woman may show some traits, even erotic traits, of opposite-sexed gender identity, unthinkable in earlier years. The key in the lock of inhibition may also be turned by a brain lesion, as in the rare case of a temporal lobe epileptic focus that induces not only seizures but compulsive transvestism. Both have been known to disappear when successful temporal lobe surgery turned the lock of inhibition metaphorically into position again.

There are some children who do not differentiate the initial dualistic potential of gender identity into an exclusively monistic realization of gender identity. Rarely, the child may have a genital deformity, hermaphroditic or otherwise, which in adulthood prevents effective copulation in agreement with the sex of ostensible assignment. Such a child may leave the door ajar, metaphorically speaking, especially in imagination, as though to guarantee an exit into a sex reassignment, should the original assignment prove utterly untenable. In a hormonal male, after puberty, the imagery of sex reassignment, either way, may appear vividly in masturbation fantasies. The hormonal female is less likely to masturbate or have erotic orgasm-dreams.

A more frequent example of retained dualism of gender identity, however, is that found in the adult transvestite, especially the genetic male transvestite. It is characteristic of this condition that, in the dissociative manner of Dr. Jekyll and Mr. Hyde, the classic literary example of multiple personality, the two gender identities may be expressed in alternation. The transvestite's two personalities each has its own wardrobe, male and female, and each its own name. The degree to which each personality will appear publicly convincing will depend, for the most part, on the extent of its experience in public, eliciting gender-appropriate reactions from other people, until its own responses, in turn, become habitual and artless. Of course, this usually means that the male transvestite becomes publicly convincing as a male first, this usually being the way he is required to dress. But he may practice cross-dressing from early boyhood, and in consequence become able to present himself very convincingly in the female role in adolescence. It is possible for impersonation to be so effective that one is hard pressed to believe that the person whom men feel erotically attracted toward as, say, Brenda, is the same person whom women fall for as Bob.

A full-time cross dresser may eventually achieve the goal of his lifetime's longing and quit changing back to his masculine clothes and role. Some such people have for so long felt so utterly out of place in the role of their external genitalia that they demand the body, as well as the clothing of the other sex. Properly speaking, they are not transvestites but transexuals. Their compelling desire is for hormonal and surgical sex reassignment so that they can live full-time in the gender role for which, they feel, they themselves always have had the matching gender identity.

The etiology of the unresolved dualism of transvestism, or of the resolution of transvestic dualism paradoxically into transexualism, is imperfectly understood. There may well be an as yet undiscovered fetal metabolic or hormonal component which acts to induce a predisposition to ambiguity or incongruity of postnatal gender identity differentiation. There may be a special disposition in the organization of the brain toward the acquisition of roles and their dissociation in the manner of multiple personality or fugue state. In either case, a prenatal disposition is probably insufficient in itself, and needs to be augmented by postnatal social history. In some families, it is relatively easy to implicate familial interaction as a component factor in gender-identity maldifferentiation in one of the offspring, but this is not always so. This same statement applies to obligative homosexuality (as contrasted with facultative homosexuality), as well as to transvestism and transexualism or related psychosexual malfunctions.

Gender Identity and Pubertal Hormones

The postnatal phenomena of hermaphroditic gender-identity differentiation, with and without sex reannouncement or reassignment, define the early postnatal years as the critical ones for the establishment of gender identity. They are critical for the establishment of gender identity as male, female, ambiguous, or incongruous. The same applies to children of normal sexual anatomy in whom the beginning signs of incongruous gender identity have been observed as early as the third or fourth year, particularly in boys.

It is highly probable that these early years are of critical significance for the laying down of the precursors of all the paraphilias, though it is still not possible to be explicit and definite as to the long-term effect of erotic and erotically related experiences during the middle and later years of childhood on ultimate psychosexual and erotic function. Clinical data can be marshaled to suit both sides of the argument. Thus, children on whom sexual experience is imposed by an older playmate or adult need not manifest deleterious long-term effects, especially if the aftermath of the experience is wisely managed by adults. By contrast, teenagers and young adults often enough trace an aberration of their own psychosexual expression to earlier childhood exposure. Such an example is that of a teenaged boy who had a recurrent obsessive fantasy to rediscover in actual experience what had happened to him at age six, when he was awakened by his teenaged baby-sitter, a frotteur, rubbing his penis on him.

The theory of a period of complete psychosexual latency in the middle to prepubertal years of childhood is now outmoded. Given the necessary privacy, children of this age do play normally at copulation and other sexual activities, rehearsing in play what will become serious business later. At the same time, the sexes tend to segregate for most of their play, as if to keep themselves away from the contamination of the gender role of the opposite sex while consolidating their own. This is also the age for spontaneously establishing and consolidating the concepts and practices of modesty, privacy, and selective inhibition, in relationship to love and sex.

Love, in the sense of falling in love or having a love affair, typically does not occur until after the onset of hormonal puberty, though the correlation between the two is not perfect. Children whose hormonal puberty is precocious, perhaps as early as the age of three, do not fall in love at the same early age; aged ten for a girl and twelve for a boy are the earliest ages yet observed. The biological clocks for hormonal puberty and for falling in love are, apparently, differently set. The difference is apparent not only in hormonal pubertal precocity, but also its delay. In some cases of delayed hormonal puberty, falling in love can precede the onset of hormonal puberty.

Isolated precocity of falling in love, or its delay, relative to normal onset of hormonal puberty, is a phenomenon that needs further study. There is some preliminary evidence to suggest that an abnormally early and perhaps intense prepubertal love affair is a precursor or augury of adolescent psychosexual malfunction.

All things considered, it seems feasible as a working hypothesis to say that the anlagen of behavioral normalcy, anomaly, ambiguity, or incongruity of gender identity are laid down long before hormonal puberty. The same applies, in all probability, to the anlagen of partial or complete adjunctive paraphiliac complications, for example, sado-masochism or exhibitionism-voyeurism. The change that comes about with the advent of hormonal puberty is not one that determines the relationship between erotic image and erotic arousal. It determines only the degree of arousal to an image already predetermined to have some degree of arousal power. In other words, the pubertal hormones regulate the strength of libido, but not the stimulus to which libido responds.

Hermaphroditism is of particular pertinence in relationship to pubertal hormones and the stimulus to erotic responsivity: matched pairs of hermaphrodites, concordant for diagnosis and pubertal hormonal output but discordant for sex of rearing, typically are discordant also for sex of erotic-stimulus arousal. Their love affairs and erotic responsiveness may emerge concordant with the sex of rearing, and this is possible even if the hormonal sex and body development of puberty have not been therapeutically corrected to agree with the sex of rearing.

This finding of concordance between sex of rearing and postpubertal erotic stimulus image, even when pubertal hormonal sex is discordant, is all the more surprising, since estrogen given to a genetic and hormonal male has a functional castrating and antiandrogenizing effect. By contrast, androgen given to a genetic and hormonal female has a libido-enhancing effect. A likely resolution of this seemingly contradictory confusion lies in the proposition that androgen is the libido hormone for both men and women. It has long been known that both sexes produce both hormones, though in different proportions. Hormonal sex differences are a matter of ratios, not absolutes. Clinical evidence of iatrogenic changes in the androgen/estrogen ratio of human males and females, as reflected in behavior, has long been observed. Quantitative experimental evidence has recently been demonstrated in the rhesus monkey by Herbert (1967; 1970) and Everitt and Herbert (1969; 1970). They proved that, without ovaries and without androgens from the adrenal cortex, the rhesus female lost interest in the male. Her nonodiferous vagina then also no longer attracted his interest. Michael, in London (Michael, Keverne, and Bonsall, 1971), has shown that the odiferous substance is constituted of short-chain aliphatic acids.

The majority of human beings have a gender identity, plus or minus paraphiliac complications, that is so firmly set by the time of puberty that it cannot be changed. In consequence, one cannot force or dictate any adolescent hermaphrodite into a successful sex reassignment, even if the reassignment would permit a guarantee of fertility. Only a hermaphrodite with an ambivalent gender identity will be able to negotiate the change. By the same token, one cannot expect every individual of normal anatomy but with discordant gender identity to be susceptible to psychotherapeutic change of gender identity. Such individuals whose gender identity is not ambivalent but clearly incongruously monosexual are best helped by being rehabilitated according to the sex of their gender identity. Those individuals with an ambiguity problem most likely to respond to psychotherapy are, for example, bisexuals as compared with exclusive homo- or hetero-monosexuals.

2

GENETIC DIMORPHISM

X and Y Chromosomes

The dimorphism which will eventually appear in the differentiation of gender identity and behavior is represented at the very beginning of life in the dimorphism of the sex-determining chromosomes, X and Y. The presence of two X chromosomes (XX) in the egg fertilized by the sperm heralds the differentiation of a female, if all goes well, and if the developmental program proceeds according to Nature's preferred plan. Alternatively, an X chromosome plus a Y (XY) herald that a male will be differentiated, if all goes well.

It is not invariable that all does go well in Nature. There are deviations from the preferred plan—of divers types and for various and sundry reasons. Extra X or Y chromosomes may be added, or one taken away. A chromosome may be broken or otherwise distorted. Even without such a mishap, the conditions in which the earliest stages of cellular and embryonic differentiation take place may be altered and atypical, so that the normal masculine or feminine course of differentiation is interfered with, ending up with an individual whose sexual differentiation is paradoxical or discordant with the XX or XY chromosomal pattern in the cells.

All the occasions when Nature's preferred chromosomal plan for sexual differentiation is deviated from are extremely important for the theory of gender identity, for they give one a chance to investigate the relationship between genetics and the sexual dimorphism of behavior—that is to say, they provide a glimpse into the genetics of masculinity and femininity of behavior.

In the case of human development, the glimpse cannot be created at will, as in planned breeding experiments, because of the ethical limitations that we human beings place on our unwarranted interference with one another's lives. One must rely instead on Nature's own experiments—the quirks and errors of chromosome sorting that occur spontaneously. In the case of animals, planned experiments can be designed.

Animal Experiments

Witschi and his coworkers in Switzerland and the U.S., and Yamamoto and his coworkers in Japan have produced a line of genetic experiments in frogs and fish, respectively, that, in a way, are quite unnerving for the traditionalist in the genetics of sexual dimorphism of either anatomy or behavior. Both investigators learned with success the interventionist art of completely reversing the program of sexual differentiation that should have been dictated by the chromosomal pattern.

Witschi's group worked with the frog, Xenopus laevis. In this species, males are identified chromosomally as ZZ, and females as ZW. Thus, ZW larvae or tadpoles normally develop into females. Under the condition of Witschi's experiment, however, they developed as males (Witschi, 1965). To bring about this discordant development, the experimenters performed the extremely delicate task of grafting a differentiated testis from a developing ZZ tadpole into a ZW tadpole still young enough to be sexually neutral (Mikamo and Witschi, 1963). The implanted graft antagonized ovarian differentiation of the ZW tadpole's undifferentiated gonadal structures and influenced them to differentiate as testicles instead. The testicles continued their development after removal of the graft.

It was even easier to do the converse experiment of promoting paradoxical feminine differentiation in the ZZ tadpole (Witschi, 1950; Gallien, 1956; Witschi and Dale, 1962). All that is required is to add estrogen, the female sex hormone, to the swimming water in which the eggs have hatched. Then the ZZ tadpoles all differentiate as females, with ovaries. When they turn into frogs, these ZZ animals behave sexually as females and lay eggs that hatch into tadpoles. Thus their sexual behavior and reproductive capability is totally discordant with their ZZ genetic status as males. The converse holds true with respect to the masculinized ZW animals. As frogs, their sexual behavior and reproductive capacity is as males, and is totally discordant with their ZW genetic status as females.

Mikamo and Witschi (1964) took the experimental step of interbreeding their altered frogs, whose bodily and behavioral phenotype was discordant with their genotype, and of breeding them with regular ZZ males and ZW females. The results are illustrated in Figure 2.1. The pairing of regular ZW females and experimental ZW males (both of each pair having the same ZW genotype), produced a completely new genotype, WW, not known to occur in nature, which differentiates corporeally and behaviorally as a female. Here, then, is evidence that it is possible by environmental intervention to change the very fabric of heredity itself—evidence of a type completely unthought of by the great polemicists of heredity versus environment, in an earlier, now outmoded era of science.

Whereas in the frog it is the female that has divergent sex chromosomes (ZW), in the fish, as in man, it is the male (XY). Working with a species of killifish, Oryzias latipes, also known as medaka, Yamamoto (1955; 1962) did experiments that parallel those of Witschi on the frog. By adding female sex hormone (either estrone or stilbestrol) to the water in which the hatchlings lived, Yamamoto produced individuals that were male (XY) in genetic type, but female in body type and behavior. Conversely, by adding male sex hormone to the water, he produced fish of the XX (female) genotype that were male in body and behavior type.

By mating experimentally produced XY fish of feminized body type with normal XYs with male body type, Yamamoto obtained progeny that were genetically and morphologically XX and female (25 per cent), XY and male (50 per cent), and YY and male (25 per cent) respectively, as illustrated in Figure 2.2. These YY fish, like Witschi's WW frogs represent a new phenotype, not known to occur in nature. Whereas WW frogs have not been specially studied with respect to behavior, YY killifish have been subject to detailed experimental observation, behaviorally.

Hamilton, Walter, Daniel, and Mestler (1969) tested YY and XY fish, both with male body type, in competition with one another. They compared 14 matched pairs, serially, in competitive mating for a lone normal (XX) female. The YY fish were clearly dominant over the XY. They induced 137 of 155 spawnings—88 per cent versus 12 per cent, clearly a significant difference, statistically ($p \leq .01$). In addition, cumulative counts showed significantly higher mean values for the YYs in several aspects of dominance behavior. The YY fish had a higher number of contacts with females. They spent more time chasing the XYs than vice versa. When one male would chase another and catch up with him, he would bite the pursued, and the biting was done almost exclusively by the YYs. Hamilton and his

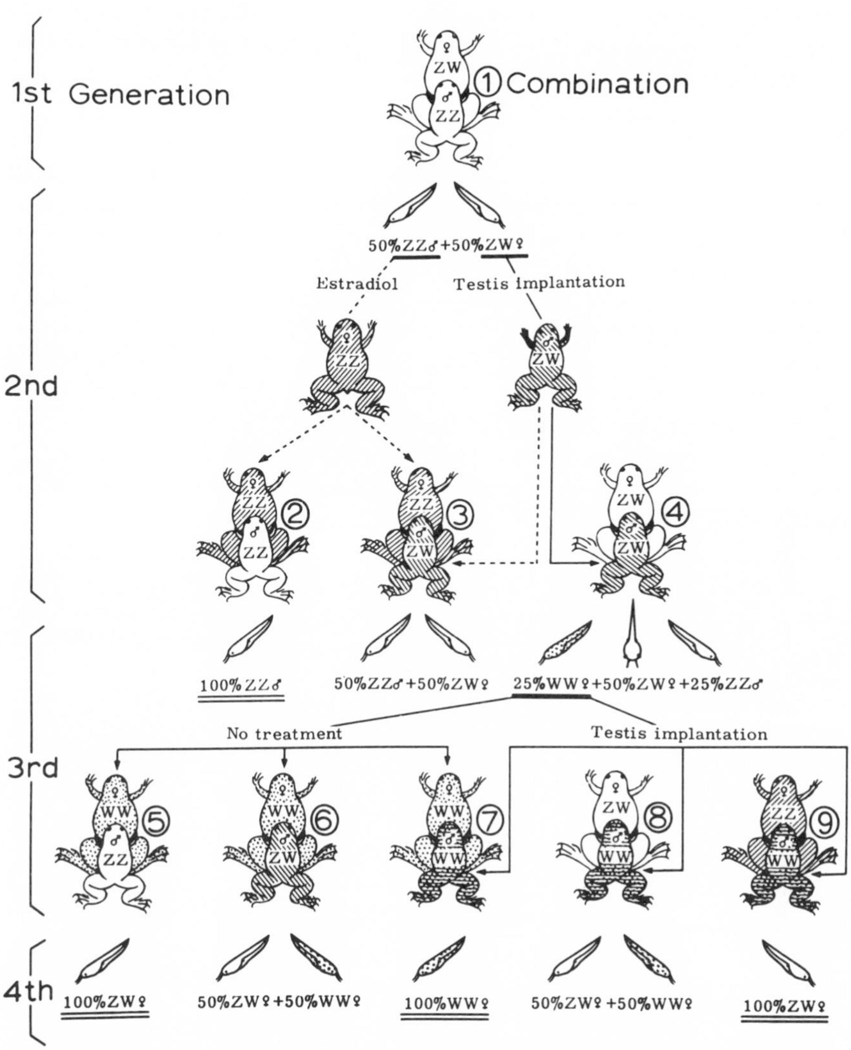

Figure 2.1. Diagram to illustrate hormonal induction of sex reversal in the frog, Xenopus laevis, and interbreeding with sex-reversed genetic males and females. White: normal animal; hatched down left: male feminized with estradiol; hatched down right: female masculinized by testis graft; hatched horizontally: WW animals masculinized by testis graft. Stippling indicates WW constitution (reproduced by courtesy of Emil Witschi).

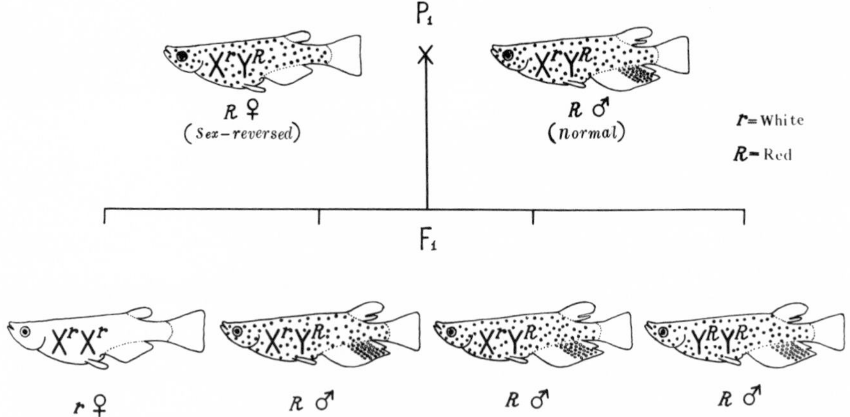

Figure 2.2. Diagram to illustrate the result of interbreeding a normal XY male with a sex-reversed XY male, to produce a YY male of the killifish, Orizias latipes (photo courtesy of Toki-o Yamamoto).

colleagues suggested that the extra Y chromosome, rather than the absence of the X was responsible for the YYs' increase in mating dominance. Be that as it may. The primary significance of the experiments is that one can quantitatively alter sexually dimorphic adult behavior, by initial experimental intervention prior to fertilization, so as to alter the very genotype itself.

Frogs and fish both lay eggs to be fertilized in water, thus rendering the embryo, right from the moment of fertilization, easily accessible to man's experimental intervention. In mammals, it goes without saying, the task of experimental intervention is vastly more complicated. It has not yet been possible to bring about in a mammal a complete contradiction between the genotype and the body type, so that the sex glands themselves will be altered and fertile in the sex contradictory of the genotype. More loosely said, it is not yet possible to bring about a sex reversal in a mammal with resultant fertility. It is possible, however, by experimentally manipulating the hormonal environment of the embryo at an early, critical period in utero, to produce a female body type (minus fertility) discordant with an XY genotype, and a male body type (also minus fertility) discordant with an XX genotype. In other words, and oversimplifying somewhat, it is possible experimentally to produce a genetic male with a female body, or a genetic female with a male body. This phenomenon, loosely referred to as sex reversal (or partial sex reversal), is dealt with in Chapter 3.

Human Cytogenetic Syndromes

The occurrence of atypical genotypes in human beings is not the result of a planned experiment, as in animals, but of Nature's own caprice—one resorts to the concept of caprice, because there is not yet a systematic and coherent explanation of what, in the very basic sense, causes the phenomenon of abnormal genotypes. The mechanism of how a particular chromosomal anomaly occurs in the course of cell division and reproduction, at the very beginning of life, has been spelled out in many texts (for example, Bartalos and Baramki [1967]), but the stimulus of its occurrence is not yet well understood.

With respect to the X and the Y chromosome in human beings, the anomalies that have so far been discovered involve either the loss of one chromosome or the addition of one or more too many. Concerning chromosomal loss, it is possible for one of the X chromosomes from the XX pair, or for the Y from the XY pair, to be lost without a lethal effect—the fertilized X cell divides and grows through embryonic life to produce always the body type of a female, though minus fertility. By contrast, the loss of an X chromosome from an XY combination, leaving only a Y (45,Y) is lethal. No human beings have been found with a 45,Y chromosomal pattern. In the case not of chromosome loss but addition, it is not lethal if either one or more than one of the X or Y chromosomes gets incorporated into the fertilized cell. Among the viable genetic possibilities so far discovered are XXX, XXY and XYY, and there are others also, including mosaicism, the condition in which some of the cells of a given individual have one or more supernumerary chromosomes, or a missing chromosome, while the others do not. One may infer with confidence from today's accumulated cytogenetic information that, in the absence of a single Y chromosome, the body type differentiates as female. When at least one Y chromosome is present, the body type will differentiate as male, unless some special genetic or intrauterine biochemical factor intervenes to inhibit masculinity.

It first became possible to spell out the relationship between a missing or extra X or Y chromosome and the sexual dimorphism of body type after Tjio and Levan (1956), working with a new technique for counting chromosomes, proved that the number of human chromosomes is 46 and not 48, as had until then been thought (Figure 2.3). They opened the way for the first time in history to the accurate counting of human chromosomes as a routine, albeit still tedious and expensive, laboratory test. In 1959, the first reports came in of abnormal numbers of chromosomes in certain clinical cases, for example, Turner's (45,X) syndrome and Kline-

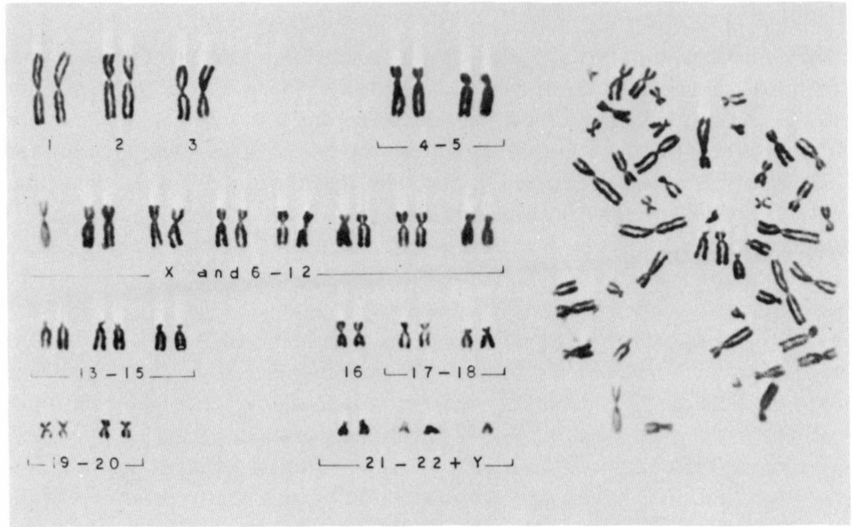

Figure 2.3. A spread of human chromosomes from the nucleus of a single cell, and their classified arrangement or karyotype. The presence of the X and Y chromosomes signifies the male genotype.

felter's (47,XXY) syndrome. Thus, it is only as recently as 1959 that the science of clinical cytogenetics began—and also its offshoot, clinical behavior cytogenetics, with its special bearing on psychosexual dimorphism.

Prior to the era of chromosome counting, there had been ten years, dating from the 1949 discovery of Barr and Bertram, in which a useful, though less detailed test for sexual dimorphism at the genetic level could be applied (Barr and Bertram, 1949; Moore, 1966). This is the sex-chromatin test (Figure 2.4). It is a simple and rapid staining test which shows a distinctive spot of color (the Barr body) in the nuclei of cells taken from a normal female, but absent in cells taken from a normal male. The cells may be easily obtained by lightly scraping the buccal mucosa of the cheeks inside the mouth. They are used to prepare a buccal smear for staining and viewing on a microscopic slide. The sex chromatin spot is now believed to be an X chromosome in a dormant "curled up" state.

The special value of the Barr-body test today is in screening large populations. Applied to the screening of morphologic females, it permits rapid

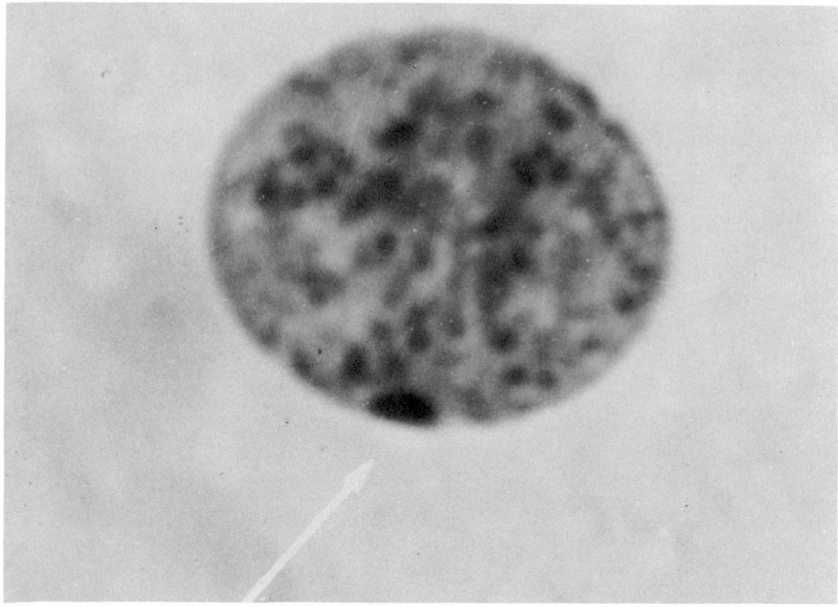

Figure 2.4. The nuclear sex chromatin or Barr body of the nucleus of a human cell. Its presence signifies a duplicate X chromosome and is expected in cells from a female. It is found also in the 47,XXY condition.

identification of those who have an X chromosome missing (Turner's syndrome) or those who have one X too many (triple-X syndrome). Applied to the screening of morphologic males, it permits rapid identification of those who have a supernumerary X chromosome (XXY, Klinefelter's syndrome). When there is more than one supernumerary X, whether in a person of male or female body type, there is a sex chromatin spot for each extra X chromosome. The Barr-body test does not tell anything about the Y chromosome and so is not applicable to screening morphologic males for the presence of a supernumerary Y. The screening test used for this purpose is one based on a quinacrine staining technique which produces a fluorescent patch on a Y chromosome not seen on others, thus signaling the presence or absence of a Y chromosome, or the presence of more than one (Pearson, Bobrow, and Vosa, 1970).

There are four clinical syndromes in which the number of sex chromosomes deviates from the expected dimorphic patterns, XX and XY. The four have already been alluded to in the foregoing. They are the 45,X (Turner's) syndrome and its cytogenetic variants, the XXX syndrome, the XYY syndrome and the XXY (Klinefelter's) syndrome, each with its cytogenetic variants. In this chapter, the significance of the syndromes lies in their relationship to developmental psychosexual dimorphism.

In the 45,X syndrome, the single X chromosome may have been provided by the mother. Then the missing chromosome would be the Y which should have been provided by the father. However, if the father's sperm carried not a Y but an X, then the missing X would be the one the mother should have provided. In some cases, if the parents differ for X^g blood-antigen type, or for color blindness, it can be ascertained whether it is the father's Y, or the mother's X chromosome that is missing in the child. Until the evidence of further investigative surveys has been accumulated, there is nothing definitive that can be said with respect to father-daughter versus mother-daughter behavioral correlations, dependent on whether the daughter got her sole X chromosome from her father or from her mother.

The 45,X condition and its chromosomal variants is characterized by a female body type (Figure 2.5), but with ovaries represented only by dysgenetic streaks. Rarely, the clitoris is slightly enlarged. Ovarian deficiency is responsible for lack of puberty, for which hormonal replacement is necessary. Stature is deficient, usually between 4½ to 5 feet. The risk of several congenital organ-defects is increased, but some individuals escape them entirely. Intellectually, there may be a relative specific disability for space-form intelligence; and a relative inertia of emotional arousal, which proves to be advantageous.

Unless rare and exceptional sociodevelopmental influences between parents and child should intervene, a female psychosexual differentiation invariably ensues. At the expected age of puberty, there may (or may not) be a protracted period of psychosexual infantilism, dependent chiefly on the timing of the hormonal induction of puberty by the administration of estrogen, the female sex hormone. Sometimes, in the strategy of treatment, the ultimate gain of possibly an extra, much-needed inch in stature is traded off against an earlier gain in breast development and earlier menstrual onset. Provided a girl is herself, in person, given counseling and permitted to help in the decision, then psychosexual infantilism can be largely avoided, in the long run.

The XXX condition is compatible with a normal female body type (Figure 2.6), and with fertility which may, however, be diminished. There may be accompanying mental retardation, but not invariably so. Gender-identity differentiation is as a female, there being apparently no difference from females with the 46,XX chromosome constitution, in this respect.

The XYY body type is male, possibly with increased height to over six feet (Figure 2.7). Spermatogenesis in the adult testes may be reduced, to the point of actual sterility. Various other anomalies, congenital or developmental, may occur selectively, affecting some individuals and not others. Behavior disorder is also a possibility, and is presumed secondary to a primary defect of excessive impulsiveness. Weak control of impulse may lead to bisexuality, casual or consistent, perhaps partly determined by social circumstances, place of abode, and availability of partners. At least some XYY men appear weak in the capacity to fall in love and establish an enduring affectional relationship.

As compared with Turner's syndrome and the XXX and XYY syndromes, the XXY (Klinefelter's) syndrome alone may lay claim to represent cytogenetic hermaphroditism, for XXY may be considered as either X+XY or XX+Y. The claim is even stronger in the case of the XXXY variant of the syndrome. There is no corresponding morphologic hermaphroditism, however. XXY individuals are masculine in body type (Figure 2.8). The penis is commonly small. The adult testes are shrunken on account of degeneration of the spermatic tubules with resultant infertility. The level of testicular androgen output varies from case to case. Typically it is low, with deficient postpubertal virilization as a result. The deficiency applies also to libido, which may be increased by supplementary injections of fairly high levels of long-acting testosterone, on a regular basis.

Individuals with Klinefelter's syndrome constitute a population at risk with respect to psychopathology which may be of almost any type, including severe mental retardation. The sexual psychopathologies are included, and among them gender-identity anomalies, for example, transvestism, transexualism and various manifestations of homosexuality and bisexuality. The occurrence of gender-identiy anomalies is sporadic, however, and not a consistent concomitant of the supernumerary X chromosome. Therefore, one is not entitled to speculate on a correlation or concordance of psychic hermaphroditism with cytogenetic hermaphroditism. Rather, one may conjecture that the extra X chromosome introduces an element of instability into brain functioning which may manifest itself as a vulnerability to developmental psychologic deficit or impairment. Impairment of gender-identity differentiation may be included.

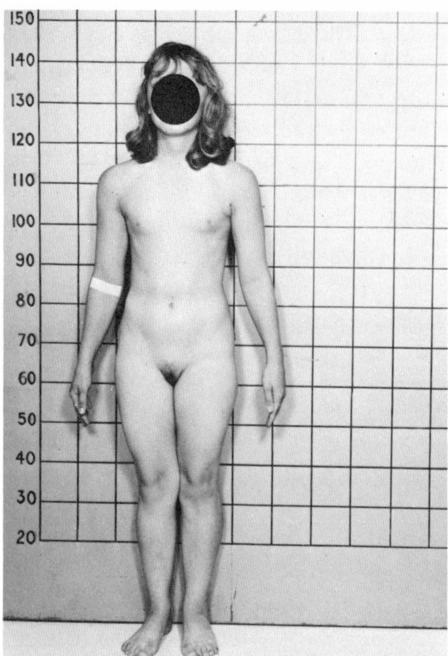

Figure 2.5. A young woman aged 21 years, with Turner's syndrome (45,X karyotype). Note the short stature and the absence of pubertal development pending substitution therapy with estrogen. Other possible anatomical anomalies are, in this case, missing.

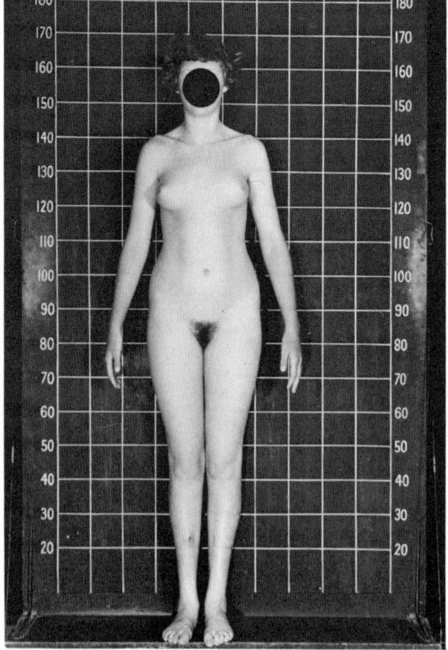

Figure 2.6. A young adult woman with a 47,XXX karyotype, of normal sexual physique, but severely mentally retarded.

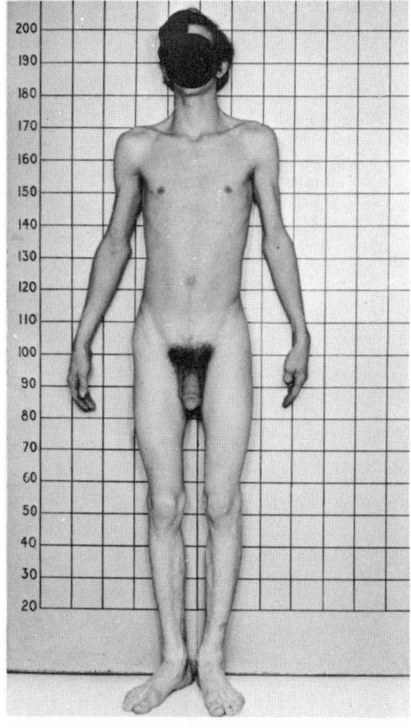

Figure 2.7. A young adult male with a 47,XYY karyotype, 6 feet, 11 inches tall. Tallness is a common characteristic of this syndrome.

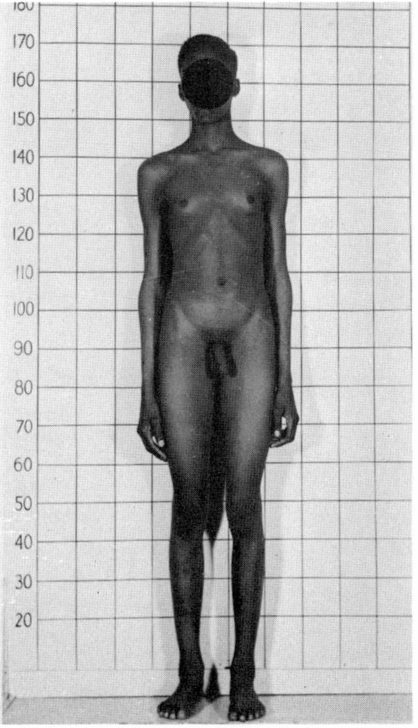

Figure 2.8. A 18-year-old male with a 47,XXY karyotype. Note the disproportionately long arms and legs, breast enlargement, small penis and small testes.

3

FETAL GONADS, GENITAL DUCTS, AND EXTERNAL GENITALIA

Differentiation of the Indifferent Gonad

Until about the sixth week after conception, the embryo does not begin to differentiate sexually. The genetic male and the genetic female look alike. Differentiation begins with the gonads, then proceeds to the internal reproductive structures, and is completed with differentiation of the external genitals as male or female.

The importance of these embryonic and fetal events for psychosexual differentiation is indirect. There is no automatic cause-and-effect relationship between the masculinity or femininity of the gonads and gender identity. Likewise, there is no preordained, cause-effect relationship between the differentiation of either the internal duct structures or the external genitals and gender identity.

Despite the absence of a direct cause-and-effect relationship between the events or products of embryonic and fetal differentiation of the organs of generation and the ultimate gender identity, the indirect effects and long-term repercussions are enormously important. To spell out the complexities and details of these effects and repercussions is part of the purpose of the chapters which follow. To begin, it is necessary to summarize how embryonic development actually takes place.

The ovary and the testis have their common beginning in a primitive, bipotential structure. At this indifferent or bipotential stage, the gonad can differentiate in either direction, as male or female. In structure, it may develop either of two portions. One is the inner or core portion, the medulla. The other is the outer or rind portion, the cortex.

If the medullary portion of the primitive gonad proliferates, under the influence of directives programed in the genetic code of the XY (male) pair of chromosomes, then a testis is formed. This proliferation begins after the sixth week of gestation. At the same time, the cortical portion of the indifferent gonad begins to regress or vestigiate, and soon largely disappears, though microscopic evidence of its erstwhile existence can be found even in adulthood.

Once the testicles have been formed, they remain in the abdominal cavity until approximately the seventh month of pregnancy. Then they migrate down the inguinal canals, in the groins, and eventually reach the scrotum. In the normal male, descent of the testes is usually finished before birth, but may be delayed until four to six weeks of extrauterine life. In rare cases, testicular descent may be delayed until puberty, or may require surgical intervention.

In the differentiation of the ovary, it is not the cortical but the medullary portion of the indifferent gonad that vestigiates. The process commences later than in the differentiation of the testis, as late as the twelfth week (Jost, 1972). The cortical structure undergoes a wave of rapid proliferation at 3 to 4 months of gestation, while the medullary component disappears, except for microscopic traces. Cortical proliferation is complete at around the sixth month of gestation. At birth, the normal pair of ovaries is said to have between 300,000 and 400,000 ova, of which approximately 300 to 400 will eventually go through the process of ovulation. The billions of sperms produced by the testes are not all present at birth, as ova are believed to be, but are produced anew throughout life.

The cortex of the undifferentiated gonad is programed to differentiate into an ovary by the genetic code of the XX (female) pair of chromosomes. Without a second X chromosome, ovaries cannot develop, though with more than two Xs, they can. The mechanism by which the X and Y chromosomes regulate gonadal differentiation has not yet been empirically demonstrated. It is assumed that there are gonad-determining genes on the XY and XX chromosome pair which program the secretion of inductor substances from the primitive gonadal medulla or cortex. These hypothetical substances presumably control cell proliferation and vestigiation respectively, according to sex.

Experimental Anomalies of Gonadal Differentiation

Among creatures as low in the phyletic scale as the garden worm, hermaphroditism represents a condition of simultaneous bisexuality. A worm makes both eggs and sperms. It provides its eggs with new genetic material, however, by fertilizing them with sperms from another member of the species while transferring its own sperms to fertilize the eggs of the partner. Higher in the phyletic scale, among the fishes, especially species of serranids, sparids, maenids, and monopteri, and in the well-known member of the family poecillidae, the Mexican swordtail (Xiphophorus helleri), hermaphroditism represents a condition of sequential bisexuality (Chan, 1970). Such an hermaphroditic fish spends part of its life as a male making sperms, and part of its life as a female making eggs, or vice versa. Still higher in the phyletic scale, among birds, bisexuality of breeding capacity does not normally occur, though occasionally the adult gonads may change their secretions, as is the case when a hen takes some of the behavioral traits of a cock.

Among mammals, hermaphroditism of reproductive capacity does not occur as a phyletic trait either simultaneously or sequentially, nor does it occur as a pathologic anomaly. The reproductive system of mammals is not capable of postnatal reversal in fertility or sexual anatomy. Prenatally, experimental sex reversal in mammals does not extend to total reversal of gonadal differentiation of the type presented in Chapter 2 with respect to fish and amphibians. Partial reversal of gonadal differentiation was achieved experimentally in a marsupial, the opossum, by Burns (1955; 1961). The opossum is a particularly suitable experimental animal, as the gonads are, at birth, still at the beginning of differentiation. Burns was successful in arresting testicular development by treating the newborn male opossum with estrogen (estradiol dipropionate). As a result, the incompletely differentiated gonads became not testes, but ovotestes with ovocytes in the ovarian component.

Turner and Asakawa (1964), employed the method of several predecessors whereby not synthetic hormones, but the hormonal secretions of one gonad are used to influence another gonad transplanted adjacent to it. With the mouse as experimental animal, they castrated adult males and then transplanted under their kidney capsules a pair of gonads taken from two-week old mouse fetuses. One of the fetal gonads was a testis, the other an ovary. As the transplanted gonads grew in close proximity, the testis so influenced the ovary that the latter became an ovotestis. The ovarian (cortical) component produced ovocytes; and the testicular (medullary) component produced spermatogonia and primary spermatocytes. Thus, germ cells originally destined to be eggs were induced to develop as sperms, under the influence of secretions from the neighboring testis.

Clinical Anomalies of Gonadal Differentiation

In human beings, there is generally a consistent relationship between the XX or the XY sex-chromosome pattern and, respectively, the female or male direction of gonadal differentiation. Exceptions are rare. One of them occurs in association with true hermaphroditism which is no more and no less genuine than male or female hermaphroditism. It is called true hermaphroditism because it is, by definition, that condition of incomplete or unfinished external sexual differentiation at birth in which both testicular and ovarian structures are represented internally in the gonads. There may be one ovary and one testis, or a pair of each, though most frequently both gonads are of mixed structure. That is, they are ovotestes. The sex-chromosome pattern is most commonly XX, or possibly a mosaic variation, like X/XY or XX/XY. In embryonic differentiation, the relationship between sex-chromosomal constitution and gonadal structure in true hermaphroditism has not yet been explained. The morphology of the internal organs, on the left side and the right, may be controlled by the fetal gonadal hormones released on the same side; and the morphology of the external organs depends on the total amount of masculinizing androgens released and circulated in the blood stream. The less the amount of androgens, the more feminine the external genital appearance.

The mixture of ovarian and testicular structure in true hermaphroditism may result in ambiguity of secondary sexual features at puberty, though most often either the masculine or the feminine dominates. The gonadal ambiguity also does not automatically dictate ambiguity in the differentiation of gender identity, which is usually either masculine or feminine.

Whereas gonadal differentiation is ambiguous in true hermaphroditism, in another rare condition, anorchia, the gonads differentiate as testes and then degenerate. In true anorchia, degeneration is complete; in hyporchia it is partial. Since the testes did, before degenerating, actually exist during the critical embryonic period of sex-organ formation, the boys are otherwise anatomically sexually normal. The testicular defect precludes fertility and, dependent on severity, creates a need for sex-hormone replacement therapy at puberty and throughout adult life. Silicone testes, soft to the feel, can be surgically implanted for cosmetic appearance. The cause of testicular degeneration may, in such cases, have been due to a little understood condition in which the body becomes immunized against one of its own organs.

When the testes do not disappear completely, one or both of them may remain undescended or cryptorchid. An undescended testis may be an imperfect, and perhaps sterile one, and also subject to increased risk of cancer in adult life. A testis that remains in the abdomen is always infertile, as the temperature there is too warm to permit spermatogenesis. Testicular nondescent most typically occurs in boys who are otherwise sexually normal. If the organ does not descend of its own accord, it may be encouraged to do so by means of hormonal (gonadotropin) treatment, or may be brought down surgically.

In the presence of embryonic testes, provided they function correctly, the remainder of the sexual anatomy differentiates as male. If the testes themselves fail to differentiate, then in their place there is usually only a streak of undifferentiated tissue. From inspection of the dysgenetic streak alone, it is not possible to know whether it is a testis that failed, or an ovary. The sexual anatomy of the body gives no clue, for it always differentiates as female, except when a testis is present. Thus, an embryo becomes anatomically female when either ovaries or testes fail to differentiate, as well as when ovaries appear.

When gonads are missing in a morphologic female, it is exceptionally rare to find that the chromosomal pattern or karyotype is of the male type, 46,XY, signifying, that the missing gonads should have been testes. It is also rare to find that the karyotype is normally female, 46,XX, and that ovaries have failed to develop, though the condition does exist. When the gonads of a morphologic female are only streaks, the most common genetic finding is that one sex chromosome is missing, as in the 45,X karyotypic sex. Alternatively, the second X chromosome may be abnormal in size and in the genes it carries. Another alternative is mosaicism. In chromosomal mosaicism some cells of the body carry one or more chromosomes than others, for example, 45,X/46,XX or 45,X/46,XX/47,XXX, and such like. These various possibilities occur in Turner's syndrome, the clinical condition which is described in Chapter 2.

Differentiation of the Ducts of the Internal Genitalia

At the seventh week of intrauterine life, when the gonadal structures have still not completely differentiated into either testes or ovaries, the fetus is equipped with primordia of both male and female genital ducts (Figure 3.1). In normal female development, the mullerian ducts serve as the anlagen for uterus, fallopian tubes and the upper part of the vagina. In normal male development, the wolffian ducts have the potentiality of dif-

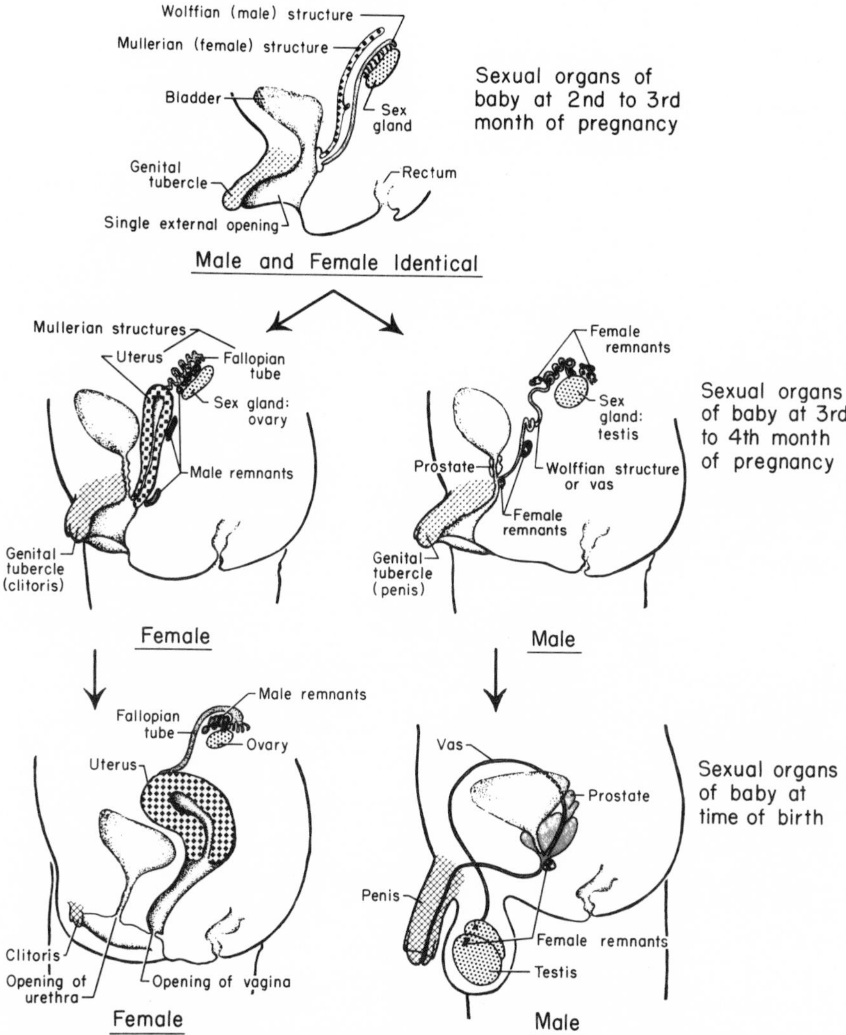

Figure 3.1. Three stages in the differentiation of the sexual system, internal and external. Note the early parallelism of the mullerian and wolffian ducts, with the ultimate vestigation of one and the development of the other.

ferentiating into the vas deferens, seminal vesicles, and the ejaculatory ducts. During the third fetal month, either the mullerian or the wolffian ducts proliferate, while the opposite structures vestigiate and disappear, except for small remnants.

The mechanism responsible for the differentiation of one or the other sex of the genital ducts is not yet understood in complete detail. In experiments on the rabbit, Jost (1947, 1958) was the first to demonstrate conclusively that secretions from the fetal testes play a decisive role. If functional testes are present, and the body's ability to react adequately to their secretions is not impaired, the mullerian ducts involute, while the wolffian ducts develop. In the absence of functional testes, the wolffian ducts involute and the mullerian ducts differentiate. The influence of a testis on mullerian regression is local and unilateral; its influence on wolffian proliferation is local at first, but later can spread to both sides. Absence or early removal of one testis leads to mullerian development on that side, while the male duct develops normally on the other side with a testis present. Female duct differentiation is apparently not dependent on the presence of an ovary, since equally good development of uterus and tubes occurs with no gonads present as when both ovaries are present.

It is generally agreed (Federman, 1967; Williams, 1968) that the fetal testis secretes two duct-organizing substances. One, the effect of which can be copied experimentally, is androgen, the male sex hormone. Androgen from the testis induces growth and differentiation of the adjacent wolffian duct, initially, and later of the contralateral one also, should the other testis be missing. The other substance causes the adjacent mullerian duct to atrophy, its effect being unilateral only. Since its chemical structure is not known, this substance is referred to simply as the mullerian inhibiting substance.

Clinical studies on various forms of hermaphroditism have shown that the differentiation of male genital ducts is linked to the presence of a fetal testis. In true hermaphrodites who have a testis on one side and an ovary on the other, wolffian duct differentiation will probably predominate on the side of the testis and mullerian duct differentiation on the side of the ovary. If, instead of an ovary, there is an undifferentiated gonadal streak on one side, then again it is mullerian duct differentiation that predominates on that side. If, on the other side, the only gonadal tissue is testicular in structure, then the mullerian duct vestigiates on that side, and the masculine (wolffian) structures predominate. Such a case will be, by nosological convention, one of male hermaphroditism (since no ovarian tissue is present).

There is another type of male hermaphroditism in which the mullerian ducts develop into a normal uterus and fallopian tubes, despite the fact that both testes are present. The penis and scrotum are normal, at birth. The only external sign that something is amiss may be simply the undescent of one or both testes; or there may be a congenital hernia in the groin where one testis is attempting to descend, dragging the mullerian organs with it. This hernia need not be evident at birth. Its appearance may be delayed until puberty or later. In such cases, it is inferred that the mullerian inhibiting substance failed to be secreted on schedule in embryonic life as it should have been in a genetic male embryo, whereas the masculinizing hormone was released. The resultant anomaly is the very rare one of a male with a uterus. The fertility of the testes in such males is questionable. Otherwise they live and develop as normal males. The superfluous internal female structures, discordant with genetic, gonadal and external morphologic sex, can safely be removed surgically.

The principle manifested in the foregoing example is that the secretions of the embryonic testes add the extra factor that will determine whether the internal duct system will differentiate as male instead of female. There is no condition of the persistence of internal wolffian structures in an otherwise normal female. The mullerian structures themselves, however, may be missing or malformed in a chromosomally normal female with two ovaries. One such malformation is a bicornate uterus, in which the arms of the fallopian tubes branch-off wrongly, like the arms of a Y instead of a T. A more extensive malformation is that in which the uterus has no cavity, being cord-like in structure, and the vagina is not a cavity connecting with the uterus, but a shallow dimple (vaginal atresia). Like most congenital malformations, these deformities of the female reproductive organs are obscure in etiology. Deformity of the uterus may or may not be compatible with pregnancy. Vaginal atresia can be corrected surgically to permit normal sexual intercourse, but without the possibility of pregnancy unless the uterus is well formed, which usually is not the case.

Malformations of the female that preclude pregnancy do not affect the normal differentiation of a feminine gender identity in childhood. Typically, they are not discovered until after a feminine gender identity has been well established. Then, in teenage, gynecologic advice may be sought because menstruation has failed to begin or, even later in life, because of failure to get pregnant or carry a pregnancy.

Differentiation of the External Genitalia

Embryologically, differentiation of the external genitalia is the final step in the development of sexual morphology. Whereas the female and male internal genital structures differentiate from two separate primordia, the external genitalia develop from the same primordia (Figure 3.2). Until

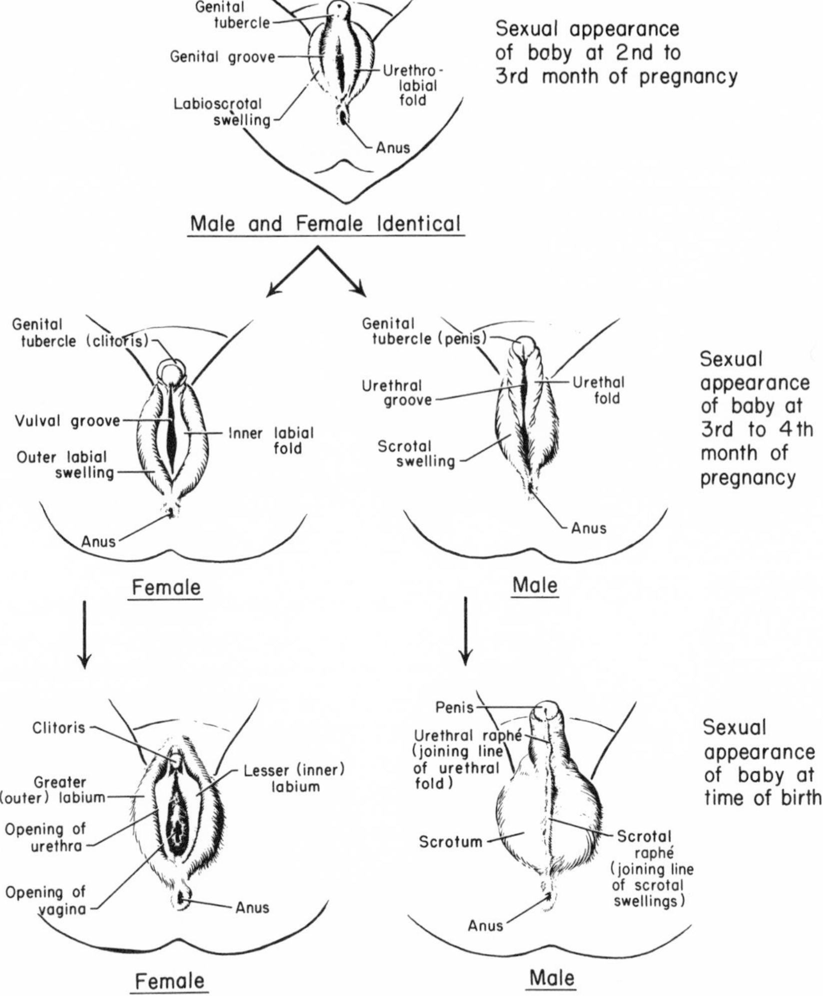

Figure 3.2. Three stages in the differentiation of the external genital organs. The male and the female organs have the same beginnings and are homologous with one another.

the eighth week of fetal life, the anlagen of the external genitalia of both sexes are identical, and have the capacity to differentiate in either direction. They consist of a genital tubercle above a urogenital slit. Nearest each side of the slit are urethral folds and, adjacent to them, labioscrotal swellings. The genital tubercle forms the corpora cavernosa and glans of either the penis or the clitoris. In the female, the urethral folds remain separate and become the labia minora. In the male, the urethral folds fuse to enclose the urethral tube of the penis. In the female, the labioscrotal swellings remain separate and form the labia majora; in the male, they fuse in the midline and form the scrotum. The genital tubercle expands to become a penis, and diminishes to become a clitoris.

Experimental proof of the hormonal control of dimorphic differentiation of the external genitalia (Lillie, 1917; Dantchakoff, 1936, 1937) had its final confirmation in the rabbit experiments of Jost (1947, 1958), already mentioned. Jost demonstrated that there is a critical period in fetal life when the presence of testes is essential if the bipotential anlagen of the external sexual organs are to develop as male instead of female. The critical period is marvelously short. In the rabbit, castration on embryonic day 19 was early enough to ensure complete feminization of genital ducts and external genitalia in the genetic male. Castration on day 24 was already too late to interfere with masculine differentiation in favor of resumption of feminine differentiation, with resulting hermaphroditic ambiguity of appearance. Castration did not interfere with female differentiation in the genetic female: castrated female fetuses developed completely female genital ducts and external genitalia; castrated male fetuses developed also completely as females unless the missing testicular hormones were artificially replaced.

The principle shown in these experiments is this: mammalian female differentiation of the genital ducts and external genitalia is independent of the presence of ovaries; male differentiation, however, is dependent on androgenic substances, normally produced by the testes.

Prenatal testicular substances can be eliminated not only by the delicate task of surgically castrating a mammal in utero, but also by hormonal suppression. Neumann and his colleagues (Neumann and Hamada, 1964; Neumann and Elger, 1965) discovered the action of an antiandrogenically active steroid, cyproterone acetate (1,2α-methylene-6-chloro-$\Delta^{4,6}$-pregnadien-17α-ol-3,20-dione 17α-acetate) as a new method to inhibit the effect of androgen from the fetal testes on morphologic differentiation. They demonstrated experimentally that gravid rats, treated with cyproterone acetate during gestation, gave birth to genetic male offspring that had the external genital appearance of a female. Since the genital development of a rat is not complete at birth, further development of the vagina was induced by continued treatment with cyproterone acetate after birth. The end result was a genetic male rat with a vagina similar to a genetic female, though not as wide and long. The internal genital organs were neither fully male nor female. The male wolffian duct system was not differentiated, since it is dependent on androgens which were cancelled out by cyproterone acetate. However, antiandrogen was not able to promote the development of uterus and tubes, the mullerian structures. They regressed as expected in normal differentiation, so that the feminized animal ended up with agenesis of the internal mullerian reproductive structures (Elger, Berswordt-Wallrabe, and Neumann, 1967). Antiandrogen was able to antagonize the action only of testosterone but not of the inhibiting substance responsible for regression of the mullerian ducts (Elger, 1966).

Whereas cyproterone acetate is a newly synthesized antiandrogenic substance, estrogen, the female sex hormone, has been available in synthetic form for nearly 40 years, and also is a powerful antiandrogenic substance. When given to adult males, estrogen suppresses the secretion of male sex hormone from the testes, thus acting as a functional castrating agent. It has this effect because it takes the place of androgen in relaying a feedback message to the pituitary, telling it to inhibit the secretion of gonadotropic hormones that activate testicular secretion of androgen.

For demasculinization of the fetus, cyproterone acetate has an advantage over estrogen (specifically estrodial benzoate) since it does not interfere with gestation in the way that injected estrogen does. When the pregnant mother animal is experimentally injected with estrogen for the purpose of hermaphroditizing the young, the excess of the hormone above that normally produced by the pregnant mother is likely to kill the developing fetus which is then resorbed. It is also likely to delay parturition, bringing about the death of the babies instead of their live birth. If they are to survive, they must be delivered by Caesarian section. The mortality rate is high: Jean (1968a) obtained only 433 offspring that survived into adulthood from 1,186 fetuses in 244 mother mice.

Early experiments on the effects of prenatal estrogen on sexual differentiation of the embryo and fetus were done on the rat by Greene, Burrill and Ivy (1940), and on various other species, including the mouse, hamster, and opossum, by Raynaud, Moore, Burns, Dantchakoff and others (see review by Burns, 1961; Jean, 1968a, 1968b). These different experiments demonstrated an antimasculinizing effect of estradiol benzoate, the estrogen typically used, on genetic male fetuses. The effect is consistent with that more recently demonstrated with cyproterone acetate. Failure of masculinization was particularly noticeable with respect to the external genitalia, which were feminized, instead. In some instances, internal differentiation of the wolffian ducts was partially suppressed. Normal masculine vestigiation of the mullerian ducts was not affected. Behavioral studies in adulthood were not undertaken.

Genetic females that survived in the litters of mothers injected with estradiol benzoate showed various malformations of the female genital tract, including failure of the clitoris to fuse and form a urinary canal (the clitorine urethra) which is normal in the female rat and mouse. Some females also showed a paradoxical persistence of parts of the wolffian ducts that should have vestigiated. This interference with normal feminine differentiation had also a delayed effect, namely on ovarian function in adulthood, including persistent estrus and ovulatory failure. The persistent estrus syndrome can be produced by prenatal treatment of the female with androgen (see Chapters 4 and 5). Insofar as estradiol benzoate partially mimics androgen in its effect on the unborn female, it may be because the huge doses used had a toxic effect, or because estradiol benzoate is an exogenous and not a naturally occurring form of estradiol.

Experimentally produced hermaphroditic animals have their clinical counterparts in human beings who are born with various spontaneously occurring discrepancies of external genitalia and internal sex organs. The human counterpart of the cyproterone effect is the spontaneously occurring syndrome of androgen insensitivity, also known as testicular feminization (see Chapter 6). Girls or women with this syndrome have a 46,XY chromosomal karyotype, but they appear externally the same as 46,XX females (Figures 3.3 and 3.4). Though the gonads do not have the histological structure of ovaries, but of testes (with immature tubular development and no spermatogenesis), they feminize the body as though they were ovaries. They do so with the normal amount of estrogen secreted by testes in the normal male, and are able to do so because there is, throughout the body, a cellular insensitivity to testicular androgens, also secreted in the normal male amount.

Insensitivity to androgen accounts for the feminine body morphology and development found in this syndrome, but it leaves unexplained the failure of the mullerian ducts to develop into a uterus and fallopian tubes. This failure is attributable to the fact that the embryonic gonads did produce the mullerian inhibiting substance, on schedule, before androgenic masculinization was due to take place in fetal life.

The androgen-insensitivity syndrome represents the most extreme degree, in human beings, of nonmasculinization in a genetic, 46,XY male. There are lesser degrees of imperfect fetal masculinization that constitute the various types of male hermaphroditism. From the point of view of embryonic etiology, the least complicated form of male hermaphroditism is that in which the early stages of masculinization take place, but the later ones fail. Then the baby is born with an unfinished phallic organ that could be an oversized clitoris, or an undersized penis with an uncovered gutter instead of a urethral tube on the underside (Figure 3.5). The urinary opening, in more or less the female position, may be through a large and funnel-shaped urogenital sinus that represents an incompletely formed vaginal cavity.

The type of birth defect depicted in Figure 3.5 may be found in either a genetic male or female. Visual appearance alone gives no clue as to the genetic or gonadal sex. Therefore, the condition is usually classified as sexually ambiguous, that is, as hermaphroditism. If the gonads are descended, however, they are usually assumed to be testes (though they may be ovotestes) and the diagnosis is then declared to be severe (third degree) hypospadias in a male.

On the basis of this declaration, the sex of rearing may mistakenly be assigned as male. The mistake is tragic when the phallus is only an enlarged clitoris in size, for it cannot be repaired surgically into a functional penis. It is preferable, in such cases, to assign the baby as a girl and to direct surgical correction and pubertal hormonal therapy as for a female. The wisdom of such a decision is reinforced if the case proves to be one of androgen insensitivity, and unable to respond to injections of male sex hormone, at the time of puberty. Such cases are doubly tragic, in adulthood, when the person has been reared as a male and has differentiated the gender identity of a male, for he is not only incapable of functioning sexually, but also of maturing and aging physically as a male so as to look his age.

Defective masculinization may occur not only as a micropenis with hypospadias, but also as agenesis of the penis (see Chapter 8). In extreme cases, there is literally no penis at all, and the urethra may open into the rectum. In other cases, a micropenis is no more than a tiny glans attached to a skinny tube without the thickness and structure of the corpora cavernosa, or with an extreme deficit of this structure (Figure 3.6). The testes are likely to be small and infertile. In some, but not all cases, the body is androgen insensitive. When it applies, androgen insensitivity may be invoked to explain the agenesis of the penis. In other cases, embryonic failure of the penis to grow to its proper size cannot, at present, be explained.

Experimental feminization of the genetic male fetus has its antithesis in experimental masculinization of the genetic female fetus. This can be achieved by injecting the pregnant mother animal with male sex hormone. (Dantchakoff, 1937; Phoenix, Goy, Gerall, and Young, 1959). Experiments on rats (Whalen, Peck, and LoPiccolo, 1966), guinea pigs (Young, Goy, and Phoenix, 1964) and rhesus monkeys (Phoenix, Goy, and Young, 1967) have demonstrated that the fetally masculinized genetic females are usually born with a uterus and tubes, and with a more or less developed prostate as well. Externally there is a penis, with an empty scrotum. Dependent on the amount of male sex hormone injected into the mother, the penis may be either perfectly formed, or hypospadiac, with the urinary opening wrongly placed.

The human counterpart in genetic females occurs in two syndromes. One is the andrenogenital syndrome (see Chapter 6), in which the masculinizing hormone is produced by overactive, erroneously working adrenocortical glands. In this condition, the adrenal cortex makes the wrong hormone—an androgen instead of cortisol.

The other syndrome of masculinization of a genetic female is produced by abnormal amounts of androgen from the mother (see Chapter 6). The mother may have had an androgen-producing tumor while pregnant. The greatest likelihood, however, is that she had a prescription for synthetic progestin to prevent a threatened miscarriage. In a few cases, there has been an untoward androgenic side-effect of the pregnancy-preserving hormone, producing unexpected masculinization of a female fetus.

Like female rhesus monkeys treated with testosterone in fetal life, genetic human females masculinized in utero are born with varying degrees of masculinization of the external genitalia, dependent on the amount and timing of androgenic exposure. There is hypertrophy of the clitoris and a degree of labioscrotal fusion, the appearance being the same as shown in Figure 3.5. In rare cases, the clitoris becomes a normal penis and the labia fuse to become a normal scrotum (Figure 3.7). The scrotum is always empty as the gonads, like the uterus and other internal structures, are female.

One of the newest advances in sex research has been the discovery that fetal hormones have not only an organizing influence on the genital morphology, but also on the central nervous system mediating sex-related behavior. Experimental evidence to this effect in animals, and clinical findings in human beings, is the subject matter of the next chapter.

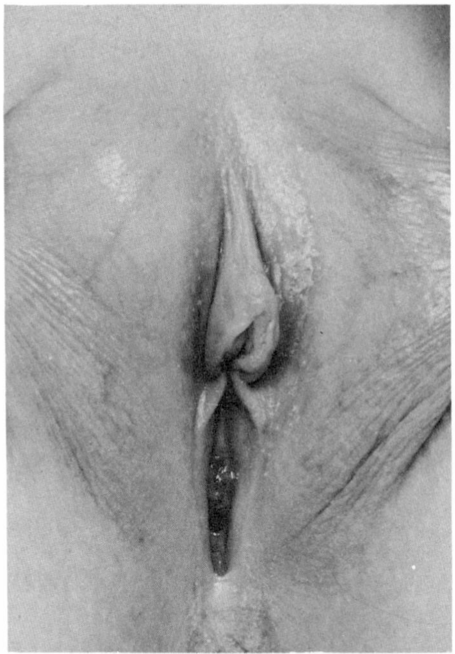

Figure 3.3. Female sexual appearance in a child with the androgen-insensitivity, testicular feminizing syndrome. The karyotype is 46,XY and the gonads are testicular in histology though totally sterile.

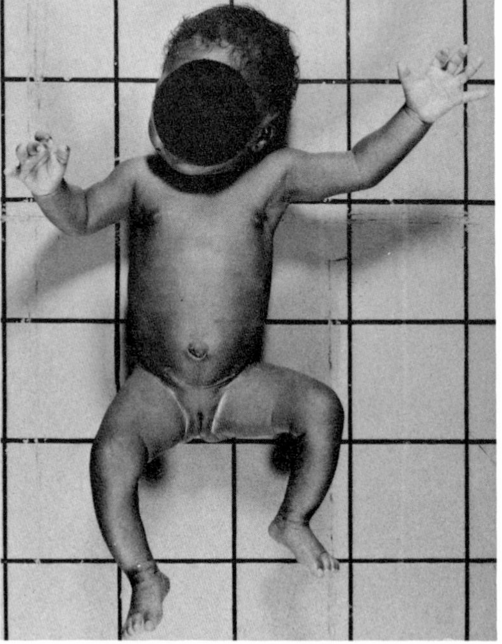

Figure 3.4. A newborn baby with the androgen-insensitivity, testicular feminizing syndrome, indistinguishable in appearance from a normal female.

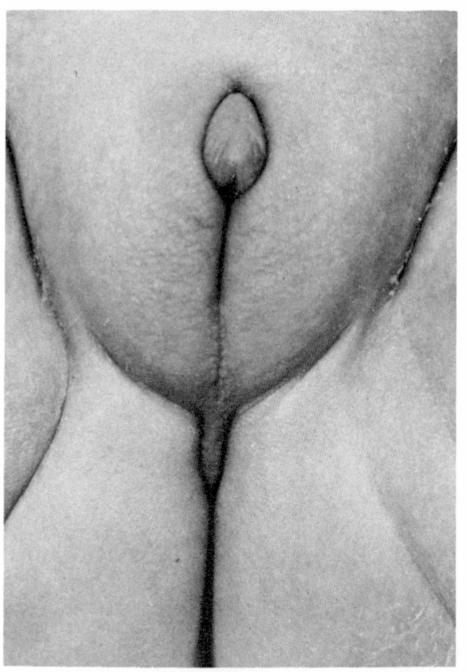

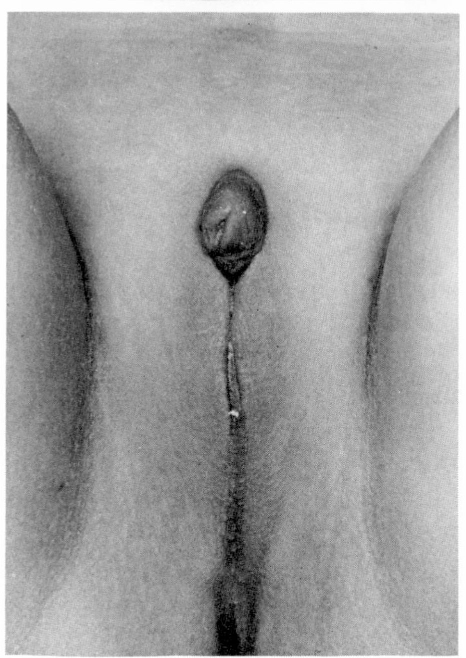

Figure 3.5. Genital appearance of a genetic male baby born with a micropenis. The urethral tube is present within the skin of the penis, but the inner body of the penis is mostly missing. The baby was assigned and corrected as a girl.

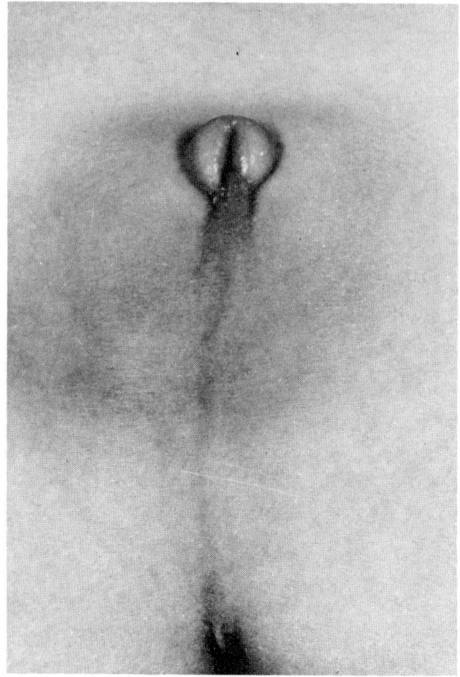

Figure 3.6. Genital appearance of a genetic male born with a micropenis that has no urethral tube and is, in fact, little more than a glans penis with a large, funnel-shaped opening. The baby was assigned and corrected as a girl.

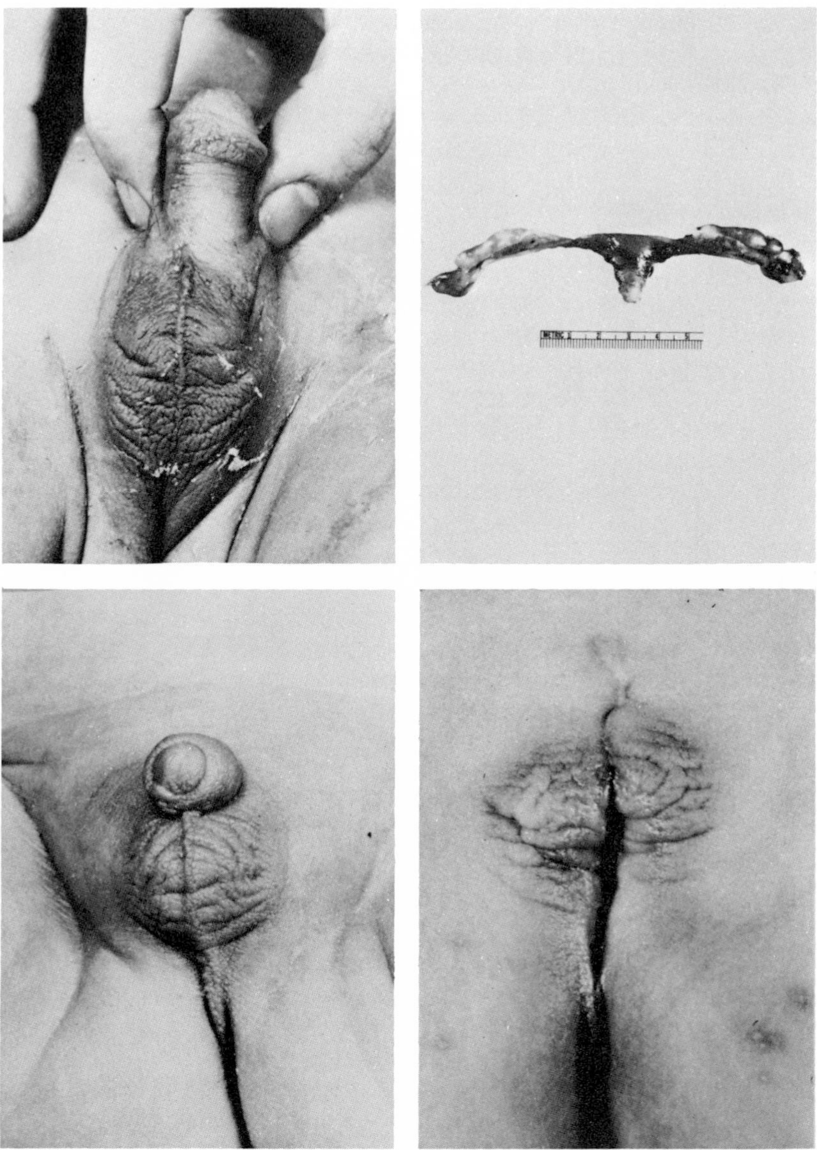

Figure 3.7. Two examples of phallic differentiation into a penis instead of a clitoris in genetic female (46,XX) babies born with the masculinizing adrenogenital syndrome. One was assigned and corrected as a girl (bottom) and the other as a boy (top).

4

FETAL HORMONES AND THE BRAIN: EFFECT ON PITUITARY GONADOTROPIN CYCLES

Cyclic Versus Acyclic Secretion of Gonadotropins

Among the nonseasonal animals, one of the principal distinctions between male and female is that the female has a cyclic pattern of ovarian hormone (estrogen and progestin) release, with a resultant estrous cycle—or in the primates, menstrual cycle. Cyclic ovarian function is regulated by cyclic release of gonadotropic hormones from the pituitary gland.[1] Gonadotropin release is, in turn, regulated by neurohumoral secretions from nuclei that lie in close proximity to the pituitary in the adjacent hypothalamic structures of the brain (see reviews by Bogdanove, 1964; Everett, 1964, 1969; Harris, 1964; Jacobsohn, 1965; Gorski, 1966, 1971; Barraclough, 1967; Flerkó, 1967; Saunders, 1968; Whalen, 1968; Neumann, Steinbeck, and Hahn, 1970). In the male, gonadotropin release is noncyclic.

[1]The gonadotropic hormones, or gonadotropins, are FSH, LH and LTH. LTH is alternatively named prolactin. FSH (follicle stimulating hormone) in the female stimulates the growth of a new egg follicle on the cortex of the ovary. At this phase of its cycle, the ovary secretes a predominance of estrogen. LH (luteinizing hormone) increases proportionately and becomes dominant over FSH when the egg follicle ruptures allowing the egg to escape. Under the influence of LH, the empty follicle turns into a corpus luteum (yellow body) which secretes progestin or pregnancy hormone. At this phase of the cycle, the total output of progestin predominates over that of estrogen. If the egg does not get fertilized, then the cycle starts over again. If the egg does get fertilized, then the pituitary releases increasing amounts of LTH

The release of gonadotropins is a biochemical and not a behavioral event. Since, however, gonadotropin release is sexually dimorphic (cyclic in the female and noncyclic in the male), it rather obviously is pertinent, even though indirectly, to matters of psychosexual and behavioral dimorphism.

Recognition of a sex difference in gonadotropin release from the pituitary dates back to the experiments of the endocrinologist, Pfeiffer (1936), working in the laboratory of Witschi. Pfeiffer was able to demonstrate that sexual differentiation as applied to the pituitary occurs neonatally, in the rat, and not at the time of maturity, though he erroneously conjectured the site of differentiation to be the pituitary itself, and not the hypothalamus.

Pfeiffer's findings parallel in principle those outlined in Chapter 3, concerning the influence of fetal androgen on the differentiation of external genital morphology. In 1936, however, there was no method by which to prove that androgen was the responsible substance. Pfeiffer's method was to make a surgical transplant of gonadal tissue of the opposite sex into the neck region of newborn rats. A few rats were allowed to keep their own gonads, but the majority were first castrated. Some of the castrated animals received no gonadal transplant. In all cases, when the animal reached the age of puberty, a piece of ovarian tissue was transplanted into the anterior chamber of the eye. The lens of the eye acted as a window through which to see whether ovulatory cycles, as marked by the presence of ovarian follicles, were being induced by the animal's own pituitary in the ovarian transplant. The findings were consistent: with a history of neonatal testicular tissue, even when the testicular tissue was transplanted into a genetic female, the characteristic female cycling pattern did not appear at puberty. By contrast, a genetic male, neonatally castrated, failed to develop the acyclic pattern of the male, but manifested the cyclic pattern of the female instead: the female pattern appeared with or without an implant of ovarian tissue neonatally, but not if the animal had been castrated and implanted with a replacement of testicular tissue.

(luteotropic hormone, or prolactin; see review by Meites and Nicoll, 1966) to prolong the release of progestin from the corpus luteum until the placenta is sufficiently developed to release its own placental progestin in amounts necessary to maintain the pregnancy. LTH again becomes active in the wake of childbirth in its role as prolactin, the milk-producing hormone.

FSH and LH were named for their stimulating action on the ovarian follicle of the female, before it was known that the hormones are also released by the pituitary of the male. In the male, FSH stimulates sperm production in the seminiferous tubules of the testes. LH stimulates the other cells of the testes, the interstitial or Leydig cells, to secrete androgen—for which reason it is also known as ICSH (interstitial cell stimulating hormone). There is no known function of LTH in the male.

It is today no longer necessary to go through the elaborate procedure of transplanting gonadal tissue, for parallel effects can be now achieved by the injection of readily available synthetic hormone, androgenic or estrogenic, respectively.

Techniques of Hypothalamic-Pituitary Investigation

Proof that the hypothalamus and not the pituitary is the site where neonatal hormones exert their influence on subsequent ovulatory cycling was obtained by means of the technique of exchange transplants of the pituitary (Harris and Jacobsohn, 1952; Martinez and Bittner, 1956). If a female has her own pituitary replaced by that of a male, it is only when the transplant is precisely located in contiguity with her hypothalamus that it will be able to secrete gonadotropic hormones. Then her own hypothalamic releaser-program cycles the release of gonadotropins from the transplanted male gland, the same as it did from her own. Likewise, there is no change in his acyclic release pattern, if a male has his own pituitary gland replaced by that of a female, the transplant being contiguous with the male's hypothalamus. Segal and Johnson (1959) proved the same point with respect to female animals that had been androgen-injected at birth and rendered incapable of cycling: replacement of the pituitary did not alter the long-term acyclic effect of the androgen.

It is technically impossible to do the obverse experiment and replace the hypothalamus or any of its nuclei: once they are cut, they are destroyed. It is necessary, therefore, to apply cutting as a technique to answer the question of whether a given hypothalamic nucleus does or does not contribute to the regulation of cycling of the gonadotropic hormones of the pituitary gland.

In addition to surgical cutting or ablation of neural fibers in order to localize and specify function in the hypothalamus, there is also the related technique of electrocoagulation, which is neater and permits greater precision. A microelectrode is implanted into the brain and an electrical current of sufficient intensity passed through it to "cook" and destroy the nearby cells. The exact location of the lesion is ascertained later, even years later, when the animal's brain is serially sectioned for microscopic study. It is then possible to correlate the functional effects of the lesion, measured while the animal was still living, with the nuclei or tracts in the brain that were intentionally put out of action.

In addition to its use for making a lesion, the implanted microelectrode may be used to measure the electrical activity of the fibers of the brain surrounding its tip. In the most delicate of such experiments, it has proved possible to measure the electrical activity of a single, isolated neuron. Instead of picking up electrical impulses to measure them, the implanted electrode may also release an electrical impulse strong enough to stimulate, without harming, neurons in the brain, in order to measure the effect that may be produced—the effect from hypothalamic stimulation on the hormonal production of the pituitary, for example.

The same shaft that holds the hair-thin silver wire of a microelectrode may also be used as the passage way through which to pass a hair-thin glass tube through which mini-amounts of liquid hormones or other pharmacologic products may be applied directly to brain cells. The same substances may also be applied in solid form, in miniscule amounts. The sensitivity of the cells to the substance can then be measured in terms of the response elicited—again perhaps on the functioning of the pituitary (Harris, Michael, and Scott, 1958; Lisk, 1962; Harris and Michael, 1964; Palka and Sawyer, 1966a and b; Nadler, 1968, 1971).

In certain experiments, it is possible that the substance inserted into the brain will be radioactively labeled. The purpose is to see how far it spreads, and whether it is absorbed preferentially by some cells and nuclei, and not others. The uptake of labeled hormones or drugs can also be assessed if the substance reaches the brain after having been injected into the bloodstream. In either case, the technique of assessment is by means of autoradiography: the animal is eventually sacrificed and the brain sliced paper-thin. The slices are then, over a long period of time, developed in a photographic emulsion, to produce an image somewhat like an X-ray. The blackest granules represent the radioactive material. They may be evenly distributed or lumped together at sites where the living cells had absorbed the labeled substance more avidly. By means of autoradiography, it has been possible to trace labeled sex hormone to the nucleus of single cells (Glascock and Michael, 1962; Michael, 1962) as well as to groups of cells at preferred sites (see review by Lisk, 1967; Green, Luttge, and Whalen, 1969; Whalen and Maurer, 1969).

These various techniques for uncovering the brain's secrets are widespread in their application, and are not specific to problems of hypothalamic-pituitary cyclicity. Even with respect to the latter alone, there is a detailed and ever expanding technical literature. For present purposes, the main findings may be summarized as follows.

Synoptic Statement of Hypothalamic-Pituitary Cyclicity

(1) The neuroendocrine control system of the hypothalamus that regulates release of gonadotropin from the pituitary in laboratory rodents and the cat (the rabbit being different) is located in the preoptic and anterior region of the hypothalamus. (2) In the female, this system may actually be

two subsystems, one controlling ovulation, and the other the release of gonadotropins (Gorski, 1966). (3) The sexual dimorphism of this system can be attributed to the defeminizing presence of androgen (or substitute substances, see section on neonatal estrogen and progestin, below) at a critical or sensitive period in prenatal or neonatal life. Without androgen, the system differentiates as female, as can be shown by prenatally or neonatally castrating the male to deprive him of androgen. (4) Experimentally, androgen may reach the hypothalamus by way of the blood stream, after an injection, or be microimplanted directly into the hypothalamus in solid form (Nadler, 1968), with the same defeminizing effect. (5) There is a critical period effect. (6) The transferability of data between species can at best be only tentative and conjectural, as phyletic reproductive programing varies extensively even between closely related species. Empirical data need to be obtained for each species, separately.

Critical Period Effect

The degree to which the hypothalamic system in control of cycling becomes androgenized is partly a matter of timing (Gorski, 1968, 1971). There is a critical or sensitive developmental period (Goy, Phoenix, and Young, 1962) before which androgen has no effect on the hypothalamic system. Likewise, after the critical period is passed, androgen is without effect. In the rat, which is born extremely immature, the critical period does not begin prenatally. Therefore, it is possible to masculinize the external sex organs of the fetal female (by injecting the pregnant mother with androgen), so that the clitoris becomes a penis, without disturbing the normal female estrus-cycling mechanism of the hypothalamus (Swanson and van der Werff ten Bosch, 1964). Similarly, it is possible to affect the cycling mechanism but to leave intact the mechanism that permits subsequent feminine sexual behavior (Revesz, Kernaghan, and Bindra, 1963; Whalen, Peck, and LoPiccolo,[2] 1966; Napoli and Gerall, 1970). The critical period for androgenization of hypothalamic cyclicity peaks from birth until the

[2]In this experiment, the authors used Norlutin®, the synthetic progestin, and not testosterone. The biologic action of the synthetic progestins is puzzling and paradoxical. Some of them are known to masculinize or hermaphroditize the external genitalia of the female. Some are known to bring about a total inhibition of androgen secretion from the adult male testes, and so may be employed as an aid in the treatment of the male sex offender (Money, 1970c). It is quite possible, also, that they have a direct inhibiting effect on brain cells, since they are known to possess anesthetic properties. In the above experiment, Norlutin® may actually have had two effects: a masculinizing one on the genitalia, and a masculine-inhibiting one on the hypothalamus. This is an alternative explanation to the one given by the experimenters in terms of a critical period effect.

fifth day and tapers off by the tenth day of age. The onset of this critical period is earlier by a day or two than the one in which the hypothalamic regulator of behavioral dimorphism will be optimally sensitive to androgen (Clemens, Hiroi, and Gorski, 1969).

In animals like the guinea pig that are more mature than the rat at birth, the critical period begins and ends before birth (Goy, Bridson, and Young, 1964).

During the critical period, a quite brief exposure to androgen is all that is needed. Arai and Gorski (1968), by using an antiandrogen to cancel the effect of androgen, found a six-hour exposure to androgen to be sufficient to establish acyclic gonadotropin release.

The amount of androgen present during the critical period also affects the degree to which the hypothalamic cycling system will be androgenized. The optimal amount eliminates all estrous cycles throughout adult life. Lesser amounts may reduce the number of cycles that will be experienced, so that cycling begins on time, but ceases prematurely. Gerall suggested that this effect may be likened to interference with the setting of a biological clock (Napoli and Gerall, 1970).

The type of androgen (or other androgenizing substance) present during the critical period may also have a differential effect on the hypothalamus. Such an effect has been recently discovered to apply to androstenedione versus testosterone with respect to behavior (Goldfoot, Feder, and Goy, 1969; Stern, 1969; see also Chapter 5). Androstenedione will produce an androgen-sterilized female rat with no estrous cycles, but without inhibiting feminine mating behavior in response to the stud male (Luttge and Whalen, 1969b).

The critical period effect applies also to antiandrogenization of the male, as is well demonstrated for the hamster in the work of Swanson (1971), using cyproterone (see Chapter 5).

Neonatal Estrogen and Progestin Effects on Hypothalamic Cycling

Knowledge is seldom as orderly as one might like it to be, and this is precisely the case with respect to the role of androgen, prenatally or neonatally, as the substance responsible for defeminizing the neuroendocrine control system of the hypothalamus. In the rat, the fact is that the same effect can be obtained by replacing injected androgen with other pharmacologic substances, including closely related steroids. Heinrichs, Gellert, Bakke, and Lawrence (1971) administered DDT to neonatal rats and found that it produced persistent vaginal estrus later in life, following early onset of puberty and a brief period of normal estrous cycles.

The steroid most frequently used to mimic the prenatal androgenic effect is the estrogen, estradiol benzoate (Gorski, 1963; Levine and Mullins, 1964; Harris and Levine, 1965). The chemically unrelated estrogen substitute, stilbestrol (Gorski, 1971) has been used as well. At least one progestinic steroid also, the synthetic product, Norlutin® (Whalen, Peck, and LoPiccolo, 1966) can presumably be used as a substitute for androgen (see Note 2, p. 58). None of these alternatives is a naturally occurring hormone in the body,[3] but all have pharmacologic application—as estrogens and as a progestin, respectively.

Prenatal use of estradiol benzoate and other estrogens is not so feasible as its neonatal use, for estrogen injected into the pregnant mother induces failure of the pregnancy (see Chapter 3; Phoenix, Goy, and Young, 1967). For this reason, the rat and mouse, because they are born in an immature state prior to the critical period for differentiating hypothalamic noncyclicity, are better experimental animals on which to test the effect of early estrogen excess than are the hamster, the rhesus monkey, and other species born more mature.

Norlutin® (17α-19-nortestosterone), a synthetic pregnancy hormone (progestin or gestagen), is a representative of that class of gonadal steroids of which progesterone is the naturally occurring substance. As its chemical name suggests, Norlutin's action is capable of being androgenic even though its progestinic action is the one for which it is used in medical practice. It is one of the pregnancy-saving drugs that was found responsible for masculinizing an occasional female fetus into a female hermaphrodite (see Chapter 6). Such bipotentiality of action may be dose-dependent or time-dependent, and is not unique. The gonadal steroids are chemically related in such a way that progesterone, testosterone and estradiol form a natural sequence of production both in the body or in laboratory synthesis. It is not surprising, therefore, that some of the transitional and variant forms of each hormone are bipotential, ambiguous, or paradoxical in their biologic activity, dependent on timing, site of action, and dosage strength.

In the particular context of neonatal (or prenatal) hormonal effects, the antithesis of androgen is not estrogen, but nothing. If male rats are given estrogen injections neonatally, they do not develop a female cyclic pattern of gonadotropin release (though there may be an adverse effect on spermatogenesis after puberty). For a male rat to be able to function cyclically, the effective experimental treatment is withdrawal of gonadal

[3]One would like to know the prenatal effect of Premarin®, a combination of feminizing hormonal products extracted from pregnant mare's urine, and very effective as a replacement hormone for use with adult human beings.

steroids by either surgical or pharmacologic castration at or before birth. Castration ensures an absence of testicular androgen, and also of any other steroid the neonatal testis may happen to produce, and so prevents acyclic masculinization of the hypothalamic control mechanism of gonadotropin release (Grady and Phoenix, 1963).

Effect of Androgen Antagonists on Hypothalamic Cycling

Progesterone itself has not been tested as a neonatal androgenizing agent, partly because of the quantity that would be needed to make a powerful enough dose for a fair test. In lesser amounts, progesterone has been proved to have exactly the opposite effect, namely, antiandrogenizing. Kincl and Maqueo (1965) found that progesterone would counteract the masculinizing effect of the androgen, testosterone propionate, or of the estrogen, 17α-ethynyl estradiol 3-methyl ether, injected into newborn female rats. The progesterone had its protective effect if injected at the same time as either the androgen or estrogen. Stern and Eisenfeld (1971) found that progesterone diminished androgen uptake at the cellular level.

There are pharmacologic substances other than progesterone that have been used experimentally to counteract the masculinizing effect of neonatally injected androgen (Kobayashi and Gorski, 1970; Gorski, 1971). The substances so far tested fall roughly into three groups: antiandrogens; tranquilizers or hypnotics; and experimental antibiotics. The chief example of the first group is cyproterone acetate, a steroid which is chemically related to progesterone. In the second group, phenobarbital and pentobarbital seemed to be particularly active; and in the third group, actinomycin-D and puromycin. The mode of action of these androgen-inhibitors in the brain is largely unknown. Presumably they all inhibit the uptake of androgen by sex-regulatory neural cells in the brain. The antibiotics may effect inhibition by blocking specific molecular pathways whereby RNA controls protein synthesis in neural cells.

In experimental studies on the male, pharmacologic androgen inhibitors of the foregoing type may be used to induce pharmacologic castration. Timed to coincide with the critical period of hypothalamic differentiation, this type of functional castration will have the same effect as surgical castration in inhibiting masculine differentiation. The feminine or cyclic pattern of gonadotropin release is then permanently established in the male—at least in the laboratory animals that have been tested.

It is decidedly premature to attempt to apply these new findings on androgen inhibitors to human beings. They do, however, leave wide open the door of speculation as to a possible central nervous system effect of maternally ingested drugs or other substances on fetal demasculinization, affecting the unborn male. Perhaps there may be undiscovered parallels affecting the unborn female. One may speculate also on the possible central nervous system (and behavioral) effect of dysfunction or imbalance in the mother's own androgenic, estrogenic and progestinic steroidal chemistry on fetuses of either sex (see Chapter 11).

Primate Menstrual Cycling

There have as yet been no reports of attempts to antiandrogenize male fetuses in a primate species, so one as yet has nothing to relate, positive or negative, with respect to the effect of antiandrogen on a gonadotropic cycling or noncycling mechanism in the male primate brain.

On the opposite effect, namely, of early androgens on female cycling of primates, there is still only little to report. Some work has been initiated on the effect of fetal androgen injections on the menstrual cycling mechanism of the female rhesus monkey (Goy, 1970). The experimental animals are the hermaphroditic females already alluded to in Chapter 3. The long-term treatment of the pregnant mothers of these hermaphrodites with testosterone was sufficient to masculinize the daughters' external genitals completely. It did not, however, induce a condition of anovulatory sterility—the evidence is definite for at least five of nine adolescent hermaphrodites. The most conspicuous effect of prenatal androgen treatment has proved to be a delay in the onset of menstruation. The normal age of onset is approximately 29 months. In the hermaphrodites it was 37 months. The regularity or irregularity of cycles was about the same as in the control group. It is possible that a different prenatal testosterone-dosage strength, a different schedule of administration, or even a different variety of testosterone, may have had a different effect on menstrual cycling, but there is no answer to that question at the present time, in the rhesus monkey.

The question is of pertinence to human studies, because some few hermaphroditic girls with the adrenogenital syndrome (see Chapter 6) have manifested extreme delay in beginning menstruation, despite the fact that they were well regulated on cortisone from early infancy onward (Jones and Verkauf, 1971). The delay cannot at present be explained. In a past generation, before the discovery of cortisone therapy, women with this syndrome remained heavily androgenized by their own adrenal glands for years. Once begun on cortisone, they began to menstruate within a few weeks and continued to do so regularly, unless interrupted by pregnancy and lactation. So far, there has been no evidence of premature menopause.

Prolactin and Mammary Development

In the same way that FSH and LH relate indirectly to dimorphism of sexual behavior, so also does prolactin (alternatively known as LTH). A Hungarian research team (Kurcz, Kovács, Tiboldi, and Orosz, 1967), found that males and androgenized females differed from control females with respect to prolactin secretion from the pituitary. One infers that hypothalamic structures which regulate prolactin secretion are also influenced by the absence or presence of androgen at the critical time of neural differentiation of the fetal hypothalamus.

Fetal sex-hormone events may also influence the ability of breast tissue to respond, in later years, to the hormonal events of pregnancy or simulated pregnancy (pseudopregnancy). In adult rats, it is easy to induce a pseudopregnancy by means of experimental injection of progesterone and estradiol, to simulate the hormonal conditions of actual pregnancy. As in actual pregnancy, pseudopregnancy induces a considerable growth of mammary-gland tissue. Neumann and his colleagues (Neumann, Steinbeck, and Hahn, 1970) induced pseudopregnancy in rats of four experimental groups: males and females castrated in adulthood; ovariectomized females that had been masculinized in utero by androgen-injection of the pregnant mother; and castrated males that had been feminized in utero by antiandrogen injection of the pregnant mother. There were distinct differences in the growth of mammary glandular tissue in response to estradiol plus progesterone treatment. Male controls and virilized females showed much less breast development than female controls and feminized males.

Principle of the Differentiation of Cyclicity

The sexual differentiation of those parts of the hypothalamus that will be responsible for regulating the cyclic (female) or noncyclic (male) release of gonadotropic hormones from the pituitary gland is under the control of androgen (or an androgen substitute). There is a brief critical period in either fetal or immediate postnatal life when androgen has its effect, which is to abolish cyclicity. The effect is permanent and irreversible. There would appear to be an analogy with the effect of androgen on the masculinization of the external organs, for in both instances feminine differentiation requires only the absence of androgen. It does not require the presence of a feminizing substance. The homologous organs of the male and female external genitals differentiate from the same, not from parallel anlagen. The same principle of differentiation might well apply to the dimorphic organization of the hypothalamic neural control of pituitary cyclicity as masculine or feminine.

5

FETAL HORMONES AND THE BRAIN: EFFECT ON SEXUAL DIMORPHISM OF BEHAVIOR IN ANIMALS

Dimorphism of Mating Behavior

The reproductive anatomy is dimorphic. Therefore, it is foreordained, if a species is to reproduce, that sexual behavior must be sexually dimorphic enough to permit conception to take place. It would not much matter whether, instead of the copulatory act as we know it, the male should take his sperm to the female in a membranous bubble, or whether the female's egg, attached to an ovidepositor, should temporarily inhabit a sperm chamber in the male. The issue is whether the male and the female each carry out their complement of behavior appropriately. Assuming that they do, then the issue becomes one of the origin of the dimorphism or complementarity of their behavior.

Behavior that is sexually dimorphic is not necessarily sexually exclusive. It may be shared by both sexes—perhaps during an early developmental period, or seasonally, or episodically, or even through the entire life span except for interludes when complementarity is needed. Thus males may play at mounting males as well as females when they are young; and females may mount females and males as well. Then, at puberty, the balance may shift, so that males will ordinarily mount only females, and females will ordinarily only be mounted. One exception may be that a male will present his rump to another male, as an invitation to mount, as a sign of deference and subordination. The dominant male may or may not mount him. Only rarely does anal intromission occur, dependent, perhaps, on the mounting male's state of tension release and the length of time he has been segregated from females. A second exception may be that a female will present and be mounted by another female at a time when agitation and nervous excitability are running high.

Before it can be decided whether sexually dimorphic behavior is strictly exclusive and sex-specific, or to some degree shared by both sexes, it is essential to avoid the pitfall of global impressionism. To do so requires differentiating a gross pattern of behavior, like mating, into its component acts. In the mating of the rat, for example, experimentalists follow the convention of differentiating, in the male, mounts without intromission, mounts with intromission, and mounts with intromission plus ejaculation. In the female, they differentiate lordosis, ear wiggling, and darting or hopping. A female can mount. She cannot achieve intromission, but she may exhibit spasmodic movement corresponding to ejaculation. A male can assume the crouched, rump-up, tail-deflected posture of lordosis, and also do the copulatory hop-or-darting movement, and the ear wiggle.

Beach's analysis of dimorphic sexual behavior in the rat (Beach, Noble, and Orndoff, 1969) is pragmatic and empirically applicable. The analysis for the female is as follows:

Mount by stimulus male: The criteria here were very strict. It was required that the stimulus male mount directly from the rear, clasp the experimental animal firmly with the forelegs, palpate the subject's sides with the forelegs, and execute vigorous pelvic thrusts. Mounts which were oriented in any other fashion or which were not accompanied by palpation and thrusting were not included in the analysis of results.

Ear wiggle: The head is shaken rapidly in the lateral plane and the ears seem to vibrate.

Hop-and-dart: The rat runs or hops rapidly away from the stimulus male and then comes to an abrupt stop.

Crouch: The rat assumes a motionless pose with legs slightly flexed and back held parallel to the substrate.

Turn: The animal turns around when the stimulus male tries to mount.

Walk: When mounted, the subject walks away.

Flat: The mounted subject assumes a position in which the back is parallel to the floor but neither the head nor tail is elevated.

Arch I: The mounted rat raises both head and tail noticeably but not maximally.

Arch II: Like Arch I except that the head is raised with marked neck flexion and the tail is distinctly elevated or deviated laterally.

For the male, the analysis is:

Mount or intromission latency: Time from introduction of the female until the first mount or intromission.

Mount and thrust: The same response described earlier for the stimulus males during tests for feminine coital responses.

Intromission pattern: Identical to the mount and thrust response except that contact is terminated by a definite and vigorous backward lunge on the part of the mounting individual. In normal males this pattern almost always signals the occurrence of penile insertion and it is clearly distinguishable from a mount and thrust without intromission.

Ejaculation pattern: The mounted male executes several pelvic thrusts and on the final thrust achieves full insertion which is maintained for a considerably longer time than during simple intromission. The male then releases his clasp of the female, frequently elevating his forelegs slowly and dismounting in deliberate fashion without a backward lunge. Ejaculation invariably is followed by a pause of approximately 4 to 5 minutes before copulation is resumed.

It is necessary to differentiate the component elements of the mating pattern, species by species. In the rhesus monkey, for example, pelvic thrusts are differentiated from mounting and intromission. Other components include grooming and the sexual yawn. There is, as yet, no conventionally agreed upon differentiation of the components of human sexual performance. The lack no doubt reflects contemporary scientific reluctance to watch human beings copulate, as well as the relatively unstereotyped nature of human sexual activity, as compared with that of other primates.

The evidence of animal sexology to date (Beach, 1947; Whalen, 1968) is that sexually dimorphic behavior is not uniquely male or uniquely female, respectively. Rather, it is bisexual in potential, though predominantly male or predominantly female in manifestation. Each sex may, and does, on occasion, display mating behavior, or elements of mating behavior, that belongs primarily to the other sex. The circumstances, conditions, or individual history in consequence of which the reproductively less appropriate patterns may appear have not been catalogued. It is known, however, that excessive crowding may disrupt normal sexual behavior patterns in rats (Calhoun, 1962), as may infantile isolation in rhesus monkeys (Harlow and Harlow, 1965) and chimpanzees (Kollar, Beckwith, and Edgerton, 1968; Turner, Davenport, and Rogers, 1969).

In addition, it is also known that castration of adult rats, followed by treatment with the heterotypical (opposite-sex) hormone, may release heterotypical sexual behavior patterns (Beach, 1947). Swanson and Crossley (1971) report the same for the male hamster. Such observations are of cardinal importance with respect to the long-term effects of prenatal or neonatal hormonal treatment on behavior. The dimorphic type of sexual behavior observed will be a product not only of the early hormonal manipulation, but also of the animal's pubertal hormonal status at the time of testing. To illustrate: the postpubertal sexual behavior of a female rat, androgen-treated before ten days of age, will be different if she has been subsequently left with her own ovaries intact than if she has been castrated and left untreated, or castrated and later treated with injections of androgen.

The reason for singling out the rat for special mention, here and in what follows, is that this has been the favored laboratory animal in the majority of experiments. The hamster, guinea pig, rabbit, rhesus monkey, and beagle dog have also been used. They are identified when referred to in the remainder of this chapter.

Mating Behavior of Neonatally Androgenized Female Rats and Hamsters

A neonatally androgenized and surgically ovariectomized female rat, if given no subsequent treatment, will show no puberty and no pubertal sexual behavior. She will, in general, be sexually indifferent to males and females alike, and they will be without copulatory interest in her.

The animal that is neonatally androgenized but not ovariectomized will not necessarily be sexually indifferent, but she will manifest an inhibition of feminine sexual behavior. It may be either complete or partial inhibition, dependent on the dosage-strength and timing of neonatal androgen administration. On a dose as small as 10 μg administered on the fifth day of postnatal life, the animal might accept the male, but on a bizarre schedule, such as on nine consecutive days (Barraclough and Gorski, 1962). The normal female rat displays lordosis and the other behavioral components of feminine mating, ear wiggling and darting, cyclically on the day of estrus. The neonatally androgenized female rat manifests not cyclic estrus but persistent estrus, as a consequence of being gonadotropically acyclic. Persistent estrus is anovulatory, so that the animal is sometimes referred to by the acronym, TSR, testosterone sterilized rat. A large dose of neonatal testosterone, as large as 100 to 500 μg, does the same as a smaller dose in producing persistent estrus of the vaginal mucosa (the vagina is anatomically normal or only mildly deformed). Its inhibiting effect on mating behavior at estrus is more complete, however, for the animal actively rejects and repulses the advances of the male.

This same animal, in the presence of a normal estrous female, will display partial masculine mating behavior, namely mounting. Since all females do the same, the residual effect of neonatal testosterone, if in evidence, will be a matter of degree. Investigators have been neglectful in statistical reporting with respect to increased frequency of the uncastrated TSR's mounting of other females. This neglect perhaps reflects the habit of thought which biases most people toward juxtaposing male and female, and forgetting about the ambisexual potential of most mammals. Nonetheless, there is sufficient evidence from which to infer an increase in behavior that technically might be called homosexual. The chief effect of neonatal testosterone, however, is to inhibit normal female patterns from expressing themselves under circumstances, and in response to stimuli, sufficient to elicit them from normal control females.

The neonatally androgenized female who is not subsequently castrated has ovaries that secrete female hormone. If these ovaries are removed before puberty, and the animal is later given a replacement injection of estrogen plus progesterone, then her sexual behavior remains essentially the same as without castration. If, however, the replacement injection is with male sex hormone (testosterone propionate, most commonly), then the animal's behavior shows a change. It is the same kind of a change as observed when a normal female is prepubertally castrated and then injected with testosterone, namely an increase in the manifestation of components of male sexual behavior, particularly mounting. The neonatally androgenized female, however, shows a greater degree of this behavior, and perhaps a more complete form of it. Harris and Levine (1965) reported an increase in the number of mountings in which vigorous pelvic thrusts were followed by a backward fall, with subsequent licking of the genital area, in the manner of the male intromission pattern. Such behavior appears when the experimental animal is tested with a normal estrous female. When she is tested with a normal male, she avoids being mounted, but shows an increase in nosing and exploring the genital area of the male. Harris and Levine (1965) reported that two of their experimental females mounted the male with vigorous pelvic thrusts.

Swanson and Crossley (1971), obtained results from the neonatally androgenized female hamster that are in agreement with those from the rat. They added one new experiment, namely, testing their animals with an estrous female not only after priming with testosterone, but also after priming with estrogen plus progesterone. The female hormones induced the same masculine mounting behavior as did the male hormone. Exactly the same result was obtained from males that had been neonatally injected with testosterone propionate, castrated later in life, and then tested with estrogen plus progesterone. Males not testosterone-treated neonatally failed to show the response. Their only reaction to estrogen plus progesterone was to display feminine mating behavior (lordosis) in the presence of a stud male. In the hamster, it thus appears, neonatal testosterone injection induces an even stronger degree of masculinization of mating behavior than does androgen from the normal male's own testes. The neonatally androgenized females were, however, awkward in their mounting. They positioned themselves on the head or side as well as the rump, and tended to slip off.

The experimental females herein considered are, as a result of having been neonatally injected with androgen, and of having been given more of the same again in adulthood, following prepubertal castration, likely to manifest a slight virilization of the external genitalia (Beach, 1968; Swanson, 1971), especially enlargement of the clitoris—the normal clitoris in rodents such as the rat, hamster, and mouse carries the urethral tube to its tip (the clitorine urethra) in a manner not different from the male's penile urethra. Enlargement of the clitoris corresponding to that obtained by androgen was obtained by Levine and Mullins (1964) when they substituted estradiol benzoate, an estrogen which proved to be a neonatal masculinizer (see below). One must, therefore, ask the question as to whether neonatal androgen affected behavior only by changing sexual behavior centers in the brain, or by potentiating clitoral enlargement and changing neural sensory organization at the periphery. It is quite possible that both the centrum and the periphery are involved. If so, their respective roles have not yet been clearly distinguished.

The same issue arises in converse form with respect to deandrogenization of the male, when the effect is to diminish the penis in size or leave it incompletely formed (Whalen, 1968; Beach, Noble, and Orndoff, 1969; Nadler, 1969). Complete deandrogenization of the male early enough in fetal life results in completely feminine external genitalia, and the possibility of copulating as a female (see below, and Chapter 3). Though the peripheral organs have not been entirely overlooked, so much intellectual excitement has been generated by the idea of finding sex-regulatory centers in the brain that investigators tend to have been biased, in their hypotheses, in favor of the central functions of the brain.

Estradiol Simulating Neonatal Androgenic Effect on Mating Behavior of Female Rats

Estradiol benzoate, stilbestrol, and Norlutin® have been identified as simulating the neonatal androgenic effect on hypothalamic cyclicity. Undoubtedly, there are other substances that will eventually be added to the list. The first and only one to have been investigated for its effect on the behavior of genetic females is estradiol benzoate.

Levine and Mullins (1964) treated neonatal female rats with estradiol benzoate. They castrated them as adults and injected them with testosterone. A possible complicating factor was that after nine days on testosterone, they manifested greater enlargement of the clitoris than the neonatally untreated control animals. They also manifested an increased incidence of the components of masculine mating behavior as compared with control females. One experimental animal is said to have actually exhibited on two occasions a simulation of the male ejaculatory spasm.

Whalen and Edwards (1967) did a similar experiment except for the different timing of ovariectomy which was performed on the day of birth. The two groups thereupon treated with either testosterone propionate or estradiol benzoate were remarkably similar in response to further treatment with testosterone again in adulthood. They had high mounting scores, and low or negative lordosis scores. The reverse occurred in animals that had been either sham operated or only ovariectomized, neonatally, without neonatal hormone treatment of any kind.

These experiments issue a clear warning that one must not be so influenced by adjectives as to equate masculine behavior with masculine hormone, nor feminine behavior with feminine hormone. The correct inference is that, in the absence of gonadal steroids in the neonatal period, neural differentiation takes place that will subsequently favor the expression of the component patterns of feminine mating behavior. In the presence of gonadal steroids, administered by injection, feminine neural differentiation is likely to be disturbed. Such disturbance has been proved when the injected gonadal steroid is the androgen, testosterone, or the estrogen, estradiol benzoate. In both cases, the disturbance is in the direction of abolishing a feminine type of differentiation, either by disorganizing it, if the dosage had been small, or, if a larger dosage had been given, by potentiating a masculinizing trend.

Mating Behavior of Neonatally Estrogenized Male Rats

The same rule that applies to the dimorphic neonatal hormonal effect on gonadotropic cycling in the hypothalamus applies also to the effect on behavior: the antithesis of androgen is not estrogen, but no gonadal hormone at all—in fact, no substitute whatever. The evidence in support of this principle comes from experiments in which estrogen has been administered to neonatal males, and experiments in which newborn rats have been deprived of their own androgens by being castrated or treated with an antiandrogenic compound.

Levine and Mullins (1964) injected male rats neonatally with 100 μg of estradiol benzoate. In adulthood, these rats were mating-tested before and after castration, and again after seven days of replacement therapy. Their performance paralleled that of the oil-injected control males to some extent, rather than being like that of a female. The intromission and ejaculation rate was lowered, perhaps because of poor morphologic development of the accessory sex organs after castration and injection with estrogen. Mounting activity was adversely affected. It was, in fact, quite bizarre. The animals tried to mount from the head, the side, or high up on the back of the receptive female.

There is no report on the mating behavior of the normal male toward these animals while they were on substitution treatment with androgen. Nor is there a report on what might have occurred had the animals been given substitution therapy with estrogen and tested with both male and female partners.

Mating Behavior of Neonatally Deandrogenized (Castrated) Male Rats and Hamsters

Like his female counterpart, a male rat castrated at birth and given no hormone treatment whatsoever will, in adulthood, be sexually indifferent. The rat is one among many species in which the activation of sexual behavior requires an endogenous sex hormone as well as exogenous perceptual stimulation. Without the priming effect of the hormone, the perceptual stimuli of sexual arousal, chiefly visual, olfactory, and tactile, are devoid of arousal power. In other species, especially man, the central nervous system, as mediator of perceptual arousal, is somewhat less rigidly dependent on the sex hormones as prerequisite to sexual behavior.

If the neonatally castrated male rat is given sex hormone, either masculine or feminine, after reaching the age of puberty, then it will become apparent that the loss of the testes and the androgen they would have secreted during the critical neonatal period has left a permanent behavioral effect. This effect is not all or none, however, like the companion effect on the hypothalamic cycling mechanism. Loss of the masculinizing principle through neonatal castration does not induce simply a persistence of a primary feminine behavioral prototype. Rather, it lays bare that bipotentiality of sexually dimorphic behavior which persists beyond infancy more strongly in the normal female than in the normal male (Whalen and Edwards, 1966; Beach, Noble, and Orndoff, 1969). In the hormonally normal female, this bipotentiality may manifest itself spontaneously in her behavior from time to time, especially in mounting behavior in adulthood, interspersed with her far more frequent lordosis. If this normal, intact female's usual androgen level is exogenously augmented, however, then her latent masculine behavior pattern will be manifested with greater frequency, and augmented to include not only mounting, but also the movements that accompany intromission and ejaculation as well.

The neonatally castrated male rat resembles the normal female when he reaches adulthood, with respect to bipotentiality of sexual behavior, except that all behavior will be dormant unless exogenous hormone is administered. Then, as many different investigators have demonstrated (Grady, Phoenix, and Young, 1965), if he is primed with estrogen followed by progesterone,[1] he will manifest a fairly complete replica of normal female receptive behavior, when placed with a test male that tries to mount him. A normal intact male, similarly injected with estrogen and progesterone, would show far less receptivity, and would continue to show less, even if surgically castrated as well.

Instead of priming with estrogen and progesterone, the other alternative is to prime the neonatally castrated rat in adulthood with androgen. His behavior, when tested with a receptive female in estrus, then resembles more that of a control female injected with androgen than that of a control male. His behavior includes mounting, but intromission and ejaculatory behavior do not match that of a control male castrated in adulthood and treated with testosterone, in either frequency or perfection (Whalen, 1964). The neonatally castrated male is at a great disadvantage in having hypoplasia of the penis and seminal vesicles. This is a permanent and irreversible sequel of having been deprived of his own testicular androgens in the early days and weeks of life, which is obviously a period when the future growth program of the sex organs can be permanently affected by absence of the testes.

The caution against a too easy transfer of principles from one species to another needs again to be sounded in connection with the neonatally castrated hamster. Though the findings in this species closely follow those of the rat (Eaton, 1970; Swanson, 1970, 1971), they are not identical. Neonatally castrated male hamsters, later given an ovarian implant, replicated their female controls in cyclic display of feminine mating behavior in the presence of a stud male. By contrast, males castrated in adulthood and given an ovarian transplant displayed lordosis not in cycles but continuously in response to a mounting male. Their own hypothalamic-pituitary mechanism could not make the transplanted ovary function cyclically. When the transplant was removed from the animals of all subgroups, and the female hormones, estrogen plus progesterone, were given acyclically by injection, then all were continuosly, and not cyclically, receptive

[1]In the rat, among other species, the induction of estrus requires the presence first of estrogen, and then of progesterone about four hours later, on the day of proestrus. The exact time-relationship is relative to the stage of the estrus cycle. See Lisk (1969).

of stud males. This finding applied to neonatally castrated females as well as males.

Males castrated in adulthood resumed masculine mounting behavior if injected with testosterone propionate and tested with a receptive female; but this behavior could not be induced in the neonatally castrated males or females, nor in adult castrated females, injected with testosterone.

The resumption of masculine mounting behavior in males castrated in adulthood also occurred, paradoxically enough, if they were tested, as above, with receptive females, after receiving an ovarian transplant. Since the same effect could not be achieved by injecting female hormones, one may implicate ovarian androgens as the responsible hormones (Swanson, 1971).

All told, data from the hamster suggest that the primacy of feminine mating behavior is more pronounced in this species than in the rat. Even the normal male reveals a vigorous capacity for mating as a female, if he has been castrated, given female hormonal treatment, and paired with a stud male. In an uncastrated normal male, it is an absolute prerequisite to his masculine mating behavior that a small amount of androgen should have been present postnatally. The quantity is apparently very small: in the hamster, it is experimentally easy to suppress the feminine behavior potential in the female by neonatally androgenizing her. It is also experimentally easy to suppress such manifestations of feminine-type behavior as are displayed by the normal male by neonatally injected extra androgen. The suppression is then more complete than that usually induced by the normal neonatal testes.

To return to the rat—no one seems to have thought of testing the neonatally castrated male with a combination of estrogen, progesterone, and androgen, so as to imitate the experiment of injecting androgen into an intact adult female. Pfaff and Zigmond (1971) found that they could obtain the feminine pattern of response to a stud male if they injected the adult, experimental male (neonatally castrated) with estrogen and omitted the progesterone; or if they retained the progesterone and substituted the estrogen with androgen.

The story of neonatal (or prenatal) hormonal effects on behavior is like a story in which a juggler throws a ball into the air where it doubles and returns to him as two balls, each of which also doubles, so that there are four, each of which doubles until there are eight, and so on. The source of all this complexity is, of course, the very dimorphism of sex itself. Thus there are genetic male and female fetuses or neonates, each of which can be castrated and deprived of their natural male or female hormone, or exposed to more of either, or both. Hence, one has already, at the outset, 12 groups (Figure 5.1).

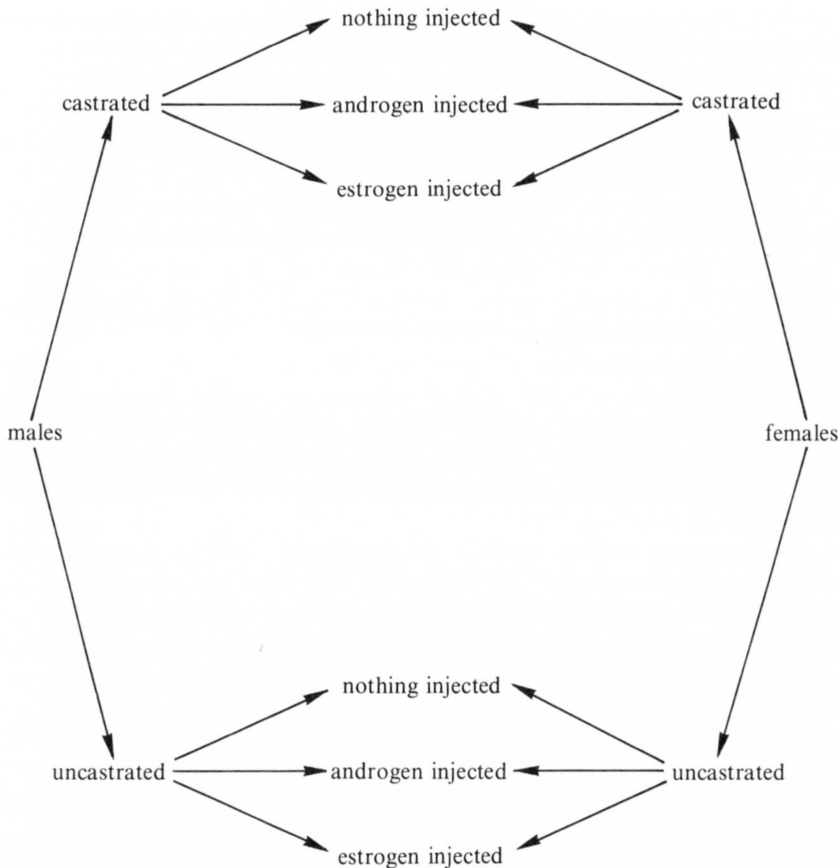

Figure 5.1. Diagrammatic representation of the exponential expansion of treatment groups in sex testing.

Each of these twelve groups may, at the age of puberty, be left untreated, or injected with androgen or with estrogen, making a total of 36 groups. Each of the thirty six groups may then be behaviorally tested with a partner of the same sex or opposite sex, making a total of 72 groups—to say nothing of testing with special partners themselves subject to experimental hormonal or other treatment. Add to all of this complexity a timing effect, necessitating that some experiments need to be repeated on perhaps as many as ten groups of differing age. Add also such other variables as the substitution of pharmacologic for surgical castration, the substitution of one form of androgen or estrogen for another, the substitution of different quantities of hormone administered, and the simultaneous use of a hormone and one of its pharmacologic antagonists. No wonder that investigators have had to limit themselves! They have focused their attention on selected programs of treatment and testing to the neglect of others, dependent on their chief theoretical interest and orientation in research. Understandable though it is, this selectivity has left some gaps in information which, hopefully, one day will be filled.

One of the gaps pertains to variation of the sex of the partner when testing behavior as a sequel to the various hormonal-priming conditions. The standard procedure has been followed of using a normal stud male as the partner when testing an experimental animal for feminine behavior, and a normal estrus female partner when testing the experimental animal for masculine behavior.

One exception is in the work of Swanson (1970), already quoted. Another is in the work of Dörner (1969), who has been theoretically interested in the relevance of animal studies to human homosexuality. He reasoned that the homosexual counterpart of man in rat experiments would be a neonatally castrated—and, therefore, deandrogenized—male rat, subsequently in adulthood maintained on replacement androgen (not estrogen plus progesterone) and mated not only with a normal receptive female in estrus, but, alternatively, with a normal stud male. The frequency of mounts on the estrous female could then be compared with the frequency of receptive, lordosis responses given to the stud male.

Making comparisons on the basis of five-minute testing sessions, Dörner found that neonatally castrated males which had been androgen-injected as adults showed a higher proportion of receptive, lordosis responses toward stud males than of mounting responses toward estrous females, despite the essentially masculine (albeit diminished) configuration of their own genitalia.

A control group of males, normal until adulthood when they were castrated and treated with androgen, showed no lordosis response at all toward stud male partners. A control group of females, normal until adulthood, when they were ovariectomized and treated with androgen, showed a lesser tendency than the experimental male animals to mount estrous female partners, and a greater tendency to be mounted by a stud male partner. Thus the neonatally castrated, deandrogenized males did not behave exactly like either males or females that had grown up uncastrated, insofar as their scores for dimorphic mating behavior were concerned. In this experiment, as in others involving neonatal castration, a peripheral neural effect from the hypoplastic genitalia cannot, by today's methods, be distinguished from a central, brain effect.

Dörner's data on the rat have not been fully replicated on the hamster, but there are some pertinent findings among those above-mentioned from the laboratory of Swanson (1971). Female hamsters castrated in adulthood and injected with testosterone propionate show no mating behavior with either a male or female partner. By contrast, normal males castrated in adulthood, and given estrogen plus progesterone, display feminine mating behavior with a male partner. Neonatally castrated males subsequently injected with testosterone propionate in adulthood show absolutely no sexual behavior with either a male or female partner—which is exactly the same as happens in neonatally castrated females injected with testosterone in adulthood.

Dörner (1968) has experimentally tested also a model of female homosexuality. Though the reason is not given, this model deviates slightly from its counterpart for male homosexuality in that female rats were neonatally androgenized and later ovariectomized and primed not with female hormones, but with androgen, at the age of puberty. They were then test-mated with estrous females versus stud males, so that lordosis versus mounting responses could be compared. In spite of their having a vagina and at most only a slightly enlarged clitoris, mounting of other females occurred significantly more often than lordosis responses to stud males. If androgens were administered not only neonatally but earlier still in the prenatal period as well, then the female rat was born masculinized with a penis and no vagina and, the remainder of the experimental treatment being the same as above, lordosis and other components of female coition were completely suppressed. In these animals, the frequency of mountings and ejaculatory-like patterns and the refractory periods that followed them did not differ significantly from those manifested by a genetic male control group, on the basis of 30-minute tests.

Swanson's data indicate that the female hamster, testosterone injected at birth, may be bisexual in mating behavior when tested with estrogen plus progesterone, later. She may crouch for the male, but will definitely try to mount the estrous female. A male, similarly treated, (see also Eaton, 1970) also will definitely mount an estrous female, whereas had he not been androgen-treated at birth, he would react only with feminine crouching (lordosis) when with a male as partner and do nothing when with a female as partner. The added testosterone at birth activates a bisexual potential in the female hamster, and inactivates or diminishes the routine, normal bisexual potential of the normal male.

As applied to the human condition, studies such as those of Dörner and Swanson cannot be explanatory in studies of human psychosexuality, but only suggestive of new hypotheses to be investigated.

Mating Behavior of Antiandrogenized, Hermaphroditic Male Rats and Hamsters

As already mentioned in Chapter 3, Neumann and his colleagues discovered the antiandrogenic properties of the steroid, cyproterone acetate (1,2α-methylene-6-chloro-$\Delta^{4,6}$-pregnadien-17α-ol-3,20-dione 17α-acetate), on behavior. They were engaged in testing a large range of newly synthesized steroids for biologic activity. When they injected this substance into newborn male rats, it induced a pharmacologic castrating effect not only on anatomical genital development, but also on subsequent sexual behavior. The behavioral effect closely parallels that of neonatal surgical castration (Neumann and Elger, 1966). When their own testes were left intact, the rats were capable postpubertally of a masculine type of response to an estrous female. If, however, they were castrated in adulthood and provided with implanted ovaries, they then displayed a marked feminine type of response when approached by a stud male.

This result was quite different from the observation on the control group of males, castrated later than the newborn period, who showed little or no female behavior, even when they were injected with up to fifty times as much estradiol as is sufficient to evoke the female response in males castrated at birth (Grady and Phoenix, 1963).

As in the case of bisexuality in the androgenized female (see above), the theoretical significance of the bisexual potential revealed by Neumann's investigations is considerable: one conjectures the possibility of a pharmacologic effect on the human male fetus, predisposing it to a potential for bisexual behavior after puberty (see Chapter 11). The dramatic and heuristic impact of this experiment is less, however, than the experiment in which Neumann and his colleagues began antiandrogenization of the genetic male offspring by injecting the pregnant mother rat with cyproterone acetate, during the critical prenatal period when the external sex organs of the fetus are being differentiated, and by injecting the newborn male for three weeks after birth.

The effect of this treatment is to produce a vagina that in anatomy closely approximates that of the normal female (Neumann and Elger, 1965; see also Figure 5.2). The treatment is not effective in feminizing the internal accessory reproductive organs, and it does not change the gonads from testes to ovaries. Thus, it is possible for the genetically male animal with an experimentally produced vagina to reach the age of puberty with two undescended testes which, being undescended, are subject to temperature-induced sterility, but secrete their normal quota of male sex hormone.

With their testes intact in adulthood, these animals behaved bisexually (Neumann and Elger, 1966). They were capable of a masculine type of response to an estrous female. They would pursue a female in estrus, sniff and lick her genitals, and mount her, though with less purposeful behavior than that shown by normal male controls. Their mounting attempts were reduced by 50 percent and only a small number of these mounts were normal performances. More than 80 percent of the attempted mounts were incomplete. The animals tried to mount from the side, over the head of the female, or even fled from the female altogether.

When the same animals were exposed to normal stud males, they were treated as females by their partners. The studs pursued them, and sniffed and licked the vagina and perineum, as they would normal females, and then attempted to mount them. The vaginalized males raised their tails, as a normal female would, but did not crouch in the normal lordosis position to effect copulation, as a normal estrus female would have done. Nonetheless, they sometimes allowed the stud male to mount. Alternatively, they exhibited the defense postures of a female not in estrus, or overtly repulsed the male (Figure 5.3).

In order to make comparisons, some of the vaginalized males were castrated at the age of three months and implanted with the ovaries of infantile female rats. As adults, many of these experimental animals then would undergo estrous cycles. They were then able to behave in the manner of normal females. They were responded to by stud males as if they were normal females. On the day of estrus, they frequently reacted to the mounting attempts of a stud male by going into the position of lordosis, with elevation of the tail, squeaking and manifesting other typical characteristics of the female response.

Because their sexual anatomy was changed, as well as their hormonal priming in adulthood, these animals raise a semantic issue about the definition of homosexuality. Did their behavior qualify as homosexual when they were mounted by the male? Or when they mounted the female without having a male penis with which to accomplish intromission? Common sense says that the anatomical, and not the genetic or hormonal sex is primary, in this context: the vaginalized genetic males were behaviorally homosexual when trying to mate with another rat that also had a vagina. Nonetheless, when they were mounted by a stud male, one might say that, though they did not qualify as anatomically or morphologically homosexual, genetically and gonadally they were homosexual. Whether or not they were also hormonally homosexual depended on their hormonal treatment status at the time.

What Neumann and his colleagues discovered in the rat, Swanson (1970) found to hold true also for the hamster feminized in utero and rendered partially hermaphroditic by cyproterone treatment of the mother during pregnancy. Swanson reported that, with their testes intact, the cyproterone treated males attempted to mount receptive females. They could not achieve intromission, however, presumably because of their genital maldevelopment, and frequently slid over the back of the female, or attempted aberrant mounts.

After castration, these animals resembled normal males that had been castrated in adulthood and that showed loss of mating behavior. They further resembled castrated normal males—already mentioned in the foregoing—in that testosterone, but not estrogen plus progesterone, would reinstate male mating behavior. The hormones released by ovarian implants, as contrasted with injected estrogen plus progesterone, were adequate to elicit male behavior toward receptive females. The same effect applied to the castrated normal males.

Female mating behavior in cyproterone-treated males could be elicited under the same conditions as in normal males, namely, when they were given estrogen plus progesterone, and tested with a stud male. Some, but not all, of the cyproterone-treated males manifested feminine mating cycles when given ovarian implants that could be cyclically programed by the cyclically functioning hypothalamic-pituitary mechanism.

The influence of prenatal cyproterone had a contradictory effect on nonmating dimorphic behavior in the open-field test. Cyproterone-treated males did not show the typical feminine response of uninhibited ambulation. In addition, female litter mates who also had been prenatally exposed to cyproterone became reticent instead of free roaming, and obtained low ambulation scores within the male range.

With respect to aggression, prenatal cyproterone did not make males either more or less aggressive than control males. Both were typically defeated by females, as is usual among hamsters, females being larger than males.

Effect of Homotypic Neonatal Hormone Injections on Subsequent Behavior

For the sake of completeness, one wants to know the effect of estrogen added to the neonatal female, and of androgen added to the neonatal male. It has been already noted that estrogen, specifically estradiol benzoate, simulates neonatally administered androgen in the female and has a masculinizing effect on behavior (Levine and Mullins, 1964; Whalen and Edwards, 1967).

The effect of androgen administered prenatally or neonatally to the male rat will depend on the type of androgen used. When the testosterone normally produced by the developing testis is augmented by injection of exogenous testosterone, then there is no observable effect on subsequent behavior (Whalen, 1968). If the neonatal rat is castrated prior to the injection of testosterone, then the injected hormone completely replaces the missing testicular secretion.

When the neonatal rat is castrated and given replacement treatment with androstendione instead of testosterone, the injected hormone is not identical in effect with the secretions of the testicles. In their subsequent behavior, male rats so treated will be able to display lordosis quite readily, when in the presence of a stud male, if given prior injections of estrogen plus progesterone. Conversely, if given prior injections of testosterone propionate, they will display mounting behavior, intromission, and ejaculation when paired with estrous females. This finding was independently established by Goldfoot, Feder, and Goy (1969) and Stern (1969).

The behavior produced experimentally in rats in the above experiments replicates that which can be elicited from male hamsters that have a normal untreated infancy. As already noted, if the intact male hamster is castrated in adulthood, and then injected with estrogen plus progesterone, he responds readily with lordosis when approached by a stud male. Injected with testosterone propionate, his behavior changes, so that he responds to the estrous female by mounting with intromission and ejaculation (Swanson, 1971).

When testosterone propionate, 300μg, is injected into the intact male hamster at birth, it is able to have an effect on the lordosis response above-reported—one which would have been entirely missed in the design of most experiments. Swanson (1971) was able to discover this effect, because she tested her experimental animals with both male and female partners after castrating and hormone-injecting them in adulthood. In this particular instance, to repeat what has been already noted in another context, the neonatally testosterone-injected males did not show the typical lordosis response when injected with estrogen plus progesterone and paired with a stud male. Instead, they manifested something entirely new: a mounting response in the presence of the estrous female, exactly the same as if they had been injected not with estrogen/progesterone, but with testosterone propionate instead.

The female hamster given parallel treatment responded similarly, that is with masculine mounting behavior in response to injected female hormones, when in the presence of an estrous female.

In the light of these experiments, one can speak of an ultramasculinizing effect of testosterone treatment of the intact neonatal male hamster. The criterion of ultramasculinism in the male is that he never shows lordosis behavior as the regular male may be induced to do. In his counterpart, the neonatally testosteronized female, the frequency of the lordosis response at the time of estrus, in the presence of a stud male, may be either reduced or unchanged.

These findings, suggesting as they do degrees of early masculinizing, may eventually prove to be of relevance with respect to the differentiation of gender identity in human beings. They may have special reference to the differentiation of gender identity as a homosexual (see Chapter 11).

The dramatic antimasculinizing effects of newborn castration on the male have no parallel in neonatal castration of the female (Whalen and Edwards, 1967).

Effect of Neonatal Hormones on Nonmating Behavior

Laboratory rats provided with a running wheel maintain extraordinarily regular daily running schedules (Richter, 1965). The intact female, as compared with the male, manifests cyclic fluctuations in running time, from day to day, in synchrony with her cyclic estrus. This sexual dimorphism of running schedules can be changed by neonatal hormone injections (see review by Gorski, 1971). Neonatally feminized males with an ovarian transplant secrete ovarian hormones cyclically as do females. They display corresponding cyclic fluctuations in running time. By contrast, rats with persistent estrus do not have cyclic running schedules, though the amount of running activity is not decreased to the male level, unless neonatal hormonal treatment happened to leave the animal, as an adult, in persistent diestrus.

Gorski (1971) reviews also various findings on saccharin preference, open-field behavior, and emergence behavior in rats. Unless the drinking water contains saccharin, water intake is the same for male and female rats. When the water contains saccharin, the females drink more. Neonatally androgenized females have a masculine saccharin-preference intake. The estrogen, estradiol benzoate, cannot be used neonatally to produce this effect, even though it will mimic some of the other neonatal effects of the androgen, testosterone propionate.

Placed in an open field, intact female rats move about more freely and drop fewer fecal pellets than do males. Neonatal testosterone propionate treatment changed this behavior in females, making them more reticent, like males. More of these animals then intact females were reticent also with respect to emerging from an enclosed box into an open arena. They thus resembled intact males. Neonatal castration did not, however, make males more venturesome in emerging from the box. These neonatally induced changes in open-field and emergence behavior in the female occur independently of the hormonal status of the animal being tested as an adult.

Open-field and emergence behavior were tested in the prenatally androgenized hamster by Swanson (1967). The findings were the same as above for the rat, namely, reduced ambulation and reduced emergence. The effect could be produced by estradiol benzoate as well as testosterone propionate, given neonatally. The change is not observed prior to puberty, but it persists postpubertally, even after gonadectomy and adrenalectomy (Swanson, 1969). There is, however, an interaction effect with experience, for hamsters that had been open-field tested in prepuberty failed to show the sexually dimorphic effect when tested in postpuberty.

Fighting for dominance is another pattern of nonmating behavior that may be influenced by the neonatal hormonal history, while not being exclusively dependent on it. Edwards (1969) found that male and female mice, given no treatment other than castration at 30 days of age, would when full-grown attack a juvenile mouse that intruded into the older animal's home cage. When it was experimentally arranged that the intruder would be of the same size, sex, and postneonatal history, then neonatal hormonal status was found to make a difference (Edwards, 1968, 1969). In particular, females that had been injected with testosterone propionate on the first day of life resembled control males in attacking an intruder—100 percent of control males attacked, 95.5 percent of androgenized females attacked, and only 20 percent of control females attacked. All three groups had been similarly injected, as adults, with testosterone propionate, prior to the fighting test.

In another experiment, Edwards (1970) found that even if ovariectomy was postponed until day 30, the masculine style of dominance attack could still be testosterone-induced later in 75 percent instead of the expected 25 percent of the fully grown females, if a large amount of testosterone had also been injected from day 30 through day 50. Thus it appears that early androgenization of the dominance-attack response has a long sensitive period and is subject to a dose-response effect.

Conner and Levine (1969) studied fighting in neonatally castrated male rats treated with testosterone in adulthood. These animals showed a female-like fighting frequency in a fighting test in which two same-sexed animals were placed into a wire-cage and given an electric shock. The neonatally castrated males differed significantly from normal males, and also from the other males castrated in adulthood and replaced with testosterone. They behaved like ovariectomized females treated with testosterone, that is, they fought less and needed a more intense shock before they displayed any fighting at all.

An essential part of the female role, after giving birth, is taking care of the young. Maternal behavior can also be influenced by early manipulation of gonadal hormones and their modification of neural differentiation. As yet, there are pitifully few reports. Neumann and his colleagues observed that antiandrogenized male rats that had been subsequently treated with female sex hormones to the point where they were capable of lactation cared for young rats and retrieved them into the nest. Caring for the young can be elicited from normal male rats only after they have been together with newborn pups for five to seven days. The care includes licking and retrieving the young to the nest, though not nest building or feeding the young (Rosenblatt, 1967). In Neumann's experiments, it was not possible to keep the newborns alive for more than a week in the care of antiandrogenized males, since induced lactation was not sufficient to nourish the litter (Neumann, Steinbeck, and Hahn, 1970).

The building of a nest is hormone-dependent but not sexually dimorphic behavior, according to the evidence of Lisk, Pretlow, and Friedman (1969) in a study of mice. They found that an estradiol injection would inhibit nest building, and that a progesterone injection would induce it. The optimal hormonal stimulus appeared to be high progesterone and very low estrogen. Similar reactions were obtained from males as females, though of some lesser degree in males. The difference between the sexes in manifesting nest-building behavior in ordinary life is, on the basis of this evidence, hormonally but not neurally determined; and it is not normally influenced by hormonal events at the time of neonatal sexual differentiation of the brain.

By contrast, in the rabbit, Anderson, Zarrow, and Denenberg (1970) discovered a delayed-action effect of fetal hormone injections on nest building in adulthood. They injected pregnant rabbits with testosterone and so produced daughters with masculinized genitalia. In adulthood, the same hormonal treatment that triggered maternal nest-building in 90 percent of the ovariectomized female controls induced maternal nest-building in only 11 percent of the fetally androgenized females and in none of the male control group. The typical maternal nest consists of straw and excelsior wood shavings, plus loose hair that the pregnant doe plucks from her fur to deposit into the nest as a lining and covering shortly before parturition. A castrated female, when treated with progesterone and estradiol, will begin to build such a nest, but a castrated male similarly treated will not (Ross, Sawin, Zarrow, and Denenberg, 1963; Zarrow, Farooq, Denenberg, Sawin and Ross, 1963).

Effect of Behavioral Experience

There is a tradition left over from the nineteenth-century biological materialism that makes some experimentalists of sexual behavior profoundly embarrased by the idea that life-experience might have any effect on the differentiation of behavioral dimorphism. The preference of such experimental traditionists is to assume that all sex differences in sexual behavior can be accounted for exclusively in terms of genetic and/or prenatal-hormonal or adult-hormonal engineering, so to speak, and to plan their experiments accordingly.

William C. Young (1961), a pioneer in hormones and behavior studies, was among the first to point out that individual differences among animals, including differences in social history, introduce variability into experimental results. Even so, today's investigators seldom systematically explore the interaction of hormones and past experience in producing a given pattern of sexual response. One exception is an experiment by Clemens, Hiroi, and Gorski (1969). These investigators injected 10μg of testosterone propionate into newborn female rats. As adults, they were spayed and injected with replacement hormone (estrogen plus progesterone). Then, tested with a stud male, they failed, as expected, to show the lordosis response. This failure was reversible, however, if the experimental animals were given a two-hour adaptation period in the test arena prior to the behavior test. Gorski (1971) conjectures that neonatal androgen may have rendered the females more sensitive to the copulatory environment, possibly to olfactory cues, in the manner that is usually typical of males. Once adapted to the environment, they became disinhibited. The behavior that was then released was not masculine in type, but the feminine response of lordosis.

In a different experiment, Clemens, Shryne, and Gorski (1970) found that the lordosis quotient of an adult group of neonatally androgen-treated female rats increased when the behavioral test was extended until the stud males had mounted them fifty times (under the conditions of the experiment, the females had been primed with estrogen alone, progesterone having been omitted). Here one sees an increase in lordosis in response to immediately prior experience.

Effect of Prenatal Siblings and Prenatal Stress

No one knows how many apparently normal genetic females not treated prenatally with hormones and born with normal-looking female genitalia might, in fact, have been subject to prenatal androgen excess insufficient to influence the external anatomy, though perhaps sufficient to influence the brain. A hitherto unsuspected example of such a possible prenatal influence was recently reported by Clemens (personal communication) from Michigan State University. He found that the larger the number of brothers in a litter of rats, the greater the likelihood that the sisters would display masculine mounting behavior when hormonally primed with androgen in adulthood. If the androgens of the brothers had influenced the brains of their sisters, then one has here an effect reminiscent of the freemartin phenomenon in cattle (Lillie, 1917).

The converse of the prenatally androgenized genetic female with normal genital anatomy would be the genetic male with normal genitalia but a prenatal history of androgen deficit. There is another recent discovery by Ingeborg Ward (1972) at Villanova University that points in the direction of an androgen-deficit effect on the brain of genitally normal males. She exposed pregnant female rats to the extreme stress of constraint under glaring light, in order to test the effect on the offspring of the mother's hormonal response to stress. The result was that the sons grew up to have lessened testicular weight and penis length. They were deficient in male mating behavior as adults when tested with receptive females. They also more readily displayed the lordosis response, typical of the female, if castrated and treated with estrogen/progesterone substitution therapy. These findings inevitably raise unanswered questions about the origins of masculine failure in some effeminate homosexual men (see Chapter 11).

Preliminary data from a new pilot study by Dr. Ward reveal that when prenatally-stressed males are castrated in adulthood, given replacement testosterone, and then mating-tested with stud males, some will show female behavior, an effect not seen in the control animals (personal communication).

Prenatally Androgenized Hermaphoditic Females: Mating and Nonmating Behavior, Guinea Pig, Rhesus Monkey, and Beagle Dog

The principles of anatomical differentiation as hermaphodite have already been delineated in Chapter 3. In essence, these principles are two: androgenization of the female and antiandrogenization of the male. The latter is exemplified in the rat experiments of Neumann and his colleagues, and the hamster experiments of Swanson and Crossley. Behaviorally, their findings were that prenatally antiandrogenized rats are capable of behaving bisexually in later life, dependent on the type of sex hormone then present in the bloodstream to activate sexual responsiveness, and the sex of the test partner.

The opposite experiment is prenatal androgenization of the female. The first experiment of this type, done for the purpose of examining subsequent behavior, was that of Phoenix, Goy, Gerall, and Young (1959) on the guinea pig. They reported that hermaphroditic female guinea pigs, completely masculinized prenatally and with a penis, were capable in adulthood of a lower feminine and higher masculine component in the bisexualism of mating-behavior as compared with the behavior of normal control females that had received the same adult hormonal injections. Their scores were also less feminine and more masculine than those of other females who received a lesser hormonal dosage prenatally and were, therefore, able to develop normal female external genitalia. These latter animals did, however, show on subsequent mating scores some defeminizing effect of the prenatal treatment.

These guinea-pig experiments are inconclusive with respect to the effect of the anatomy of the external sex organs on adult behavior, since none of the animals was subject to surgical feminization. They are further inconclusive insofar as all permutations and combinations of sex-hormone injection and sex of mate were not tested in adulthood. Nonetheless, they are experiments which occupy a very important place, historically, in opening up the whole question of a prenatal hormonal organizing effect on the central nervous system that will eventually mediate sexual behavior. They led directly to the first study of experimental hermaphroditism in a primate species. The same investigators produced hermaphroditic female monkeys with a penis by injecting the pregnant mother with large doses of testosterone (Figure 5.4).

The juvenile behavior of hermaphroditized females has shown some hermaphroditic changes, presumably as a sequel to prenatal androgenization, and prior to and independently of the priming influence of pubertal hormones (Phoenix, Goy, and Young, 1967; Goy, 1970). In the other species heretofore mentioned, changes in childhood behavior have been either not manifested or not looked for. The juvenile macaque female hermaphrodite behaves in a manner reminiscent of tomboyism in girls. More in the manner of her male than her normal female controls, she shows an increased amount of play initiation, rough-and-tumble play, chasing play, and playful threats. The frequency of mounting play is also increased in proportion to the frequency of hind-end presentation as a gesture of sexual invitation. Developmentally, the pattern of mounting also takes on a masculine stance. The juvenile hermaphroditic animal lifts its feet off the ground and clasps them around the shanks of the normal female's hind legs as she presents on all fours, and is mounted from behind (Figure 5.5). When a normal female mounts another, she keeps her own feet on the ground (Figure 5.6).

Developmental behavioral studies of the first generation of hermaphroditic female macaques continue at the Oregon Regional Primate Center. Retarded in the onset of menstruation by an average delay of nearly eight months, the nine oldest hermaphroditic females are now postpubertal (Goy, 1970). The full story of the adult sexual behavior of these animals remains to be investigated. The variables to be manipulated include the hormonal status of the hermaphrodite, replacing her own female hormones with androgen; the anatomy of the external genitalia, with surgical feminization and externalization of the vagina; and the sex of the partner.

Recently, another species in which female hermaphrodites have been experimentally produced and studied behaviorally is the beagle dog (Beach, 1970). Beach found that the size of the hermaphroditically masculinized external genitalia increased, and the degree of masculinization of subsequent mating behavior was more complete when the hermaphroditic female puppies continued their prenatal masculinization postnatally by having pellets of crystalline testosterone implanted beneath the skin on the day of birth. Then, when they grew up and were, under treatment with testosterone, experimentally tested for sexual response toward a bitch in heat, their social and copulatory scores were closer to those of control males than of control females or of hermaphroditic females not implanted with testosterone pellets at birth. Stud male dogs, when tested with these hermaphroditic females, reacted to them almost indistinguishably from normal control females. The hermaphroditic animals at the time of this test were receiving ovarian hormones (estrogen and progesterone) in amounts adequate to produce full feminine receptivity in non-hermaphroditic control females.

Another item of sexually dimorphic behavior manifested in the masculine way by the pellet-implanted, hermaphroditic female beagles is urination. They lift one hind leg, as does the normal control male and, like the normal male, urinate more frequently than does the normal, control female.

Fetal Hormones, Brain Dimorphism, and Behavior

The experimental task of identifying and tracing brain tracts, with all their tributaries and cross-connections, that mediate sexual behavior is difficult and delicate, regardless of sex (see Chapter 12). Tracing of the homologous tracts of sexual behavioral activation in the male and female brain is more than has been achieved at the present time. No wonder, then, that with today's state of knowledge, little can be said regarding the various structures of the brain and their various tracts and nuclei that are subject prenatally to dimorphism of hormonal organizing influence on subsequent behavior. No wonder, likewise, that little can be said with accuracy regarding the localization of brain changes when prenatal or neonatal male hormone injections change the subsequent balance of manifest sexual behavior in the genetic female—or, vice versa, when antiandrogenization or castration changes the balance of manifest sexual behavior in the genetic male.

The most direct evidence so far available comes from a rat experiment (Nadler, 1968) in which the behavioral changes of the anovulatory, persistent estrous, TSR syndrome could be induced by direct implantation of androgen into the hypothalamus of the newborn.

Another method of tracing brain changes related to sexual behavior is by tracing the focalized uptake, in the brain, of radioactively labelled hormone (see review by Gorski, 1971), the animals first having been hormone treated in infancy or fetal life. So far, this method has yielded no definitive information concerning brain loci that regulate sexually dimorphic behavior.

A large part of today's knowledge of where early hormonal treatments might exert their action on the brain is derived, by inference, from brain lesion studies in normal males and females that are subsequently treated and tested with extra sex hormone. Lisk (1967) summed up the prevailing point of view with respect to the hypothalamus: in addition to the regulator of the pituitary-gonadal axis (see Chapter 4), in the region of the median eminence, there is another hormone-sensitive system essential for feminine lordosis behavior in several species. It is situated in the preoptic region of the anterior hypothalamus. This same area, especially its midline structures, must be intact for expression of the sexual behavior patterns of the male.

As for hormone-sensitive centers in other brain structures, the full story yet awaits to be unraveled. The same is true with respect to prenatal and neonatal influences of sex hormones on neural cells at the periphery.

Principle of Dimorphic Behavioral Differentiation

There are two paradigms of differentiation of the sexual anatomy. One applies initially to the gonads, which differentiate first, and then also to the internal reproductive tracts. In both instances, Nature initially lays down the anlagen for both the male and the female organs; and then allows one set to regress and wither away permanently. The other set proliferates and develops into the adult organs of generation. The chemistry that regulates gonadal differentiation is not known. The differentiation of the internal organs is chemically supervised by hormones released by the embryonic gonads. No gonads, no male. Female differentiation takes place if no male hormone interferes. Moreover, female differentiation requires neither female hormone nor any kind of gonadal hormone at all. Male differentiation takes place only if the embryonic testis releases its chemical messengers.

The same principle of male hormone for male differentiation, and no male hormone for female differentiation applies to the external genitalia. Here the second paradigm applies: from the same anlagen, homologous female and male structures differentiate. The end result is fixed and irreversible.

With respect to differentiation of the brain, the evidence of Chapter 4 suggests that the nuclei of the hypothalamus in charge of pituitary-gonadal cycling follow the same paradigm as the external genitalia: without androgen they differentiate a permanently cyclic, feminine function; with androgen (or a substitute), feminine cycling is irreversibly abolished.

The evidence that emerges from this chapter suggests that, insofar as brain and behavior are prenatally or neonatally hormone-influenced, differentiation of certain patterns of mating behavior, and by inference of the brain that programs them, follow the paradigm of internal-organ differentiation. The rule would appear to be: male-female bipotentiality applies initially, prior to any hormonal influence. In other words, the original disposition of the organism is to be bisexually competent in mating behavior. The bipotentiality persists, in the presence of no hormonal influence during the early, critical period of differentiation. Bipotentiality also continues in existence if the early hormonal environment is feminine, so that either component of mating behavior can be elicited in adulthood, dependent, among other things, on whether the eliciting hormone is androgen or estrogen (or estrogen plus progesterone).

Bipotentiality is resolved in favor of unipolar masculinity of mating behavior if the early hormonal influence at the critical differentiating period is androgenic. The feminine component is inhibited.

Once this is accomplished, the feminine component will, in many though perhaps not all species, manifest itself only in response to special conditions (for example, direct brain stimulation), or will remain latent. The initial completeness of inhibition of feminine behavioral potential, in the course of normal differentiation, varies across species. For example, it is more complete in the rat than the hamster. In man, as will become evident in the next four chapters, it is probably not very complete, and is perhaps individually variable as well.

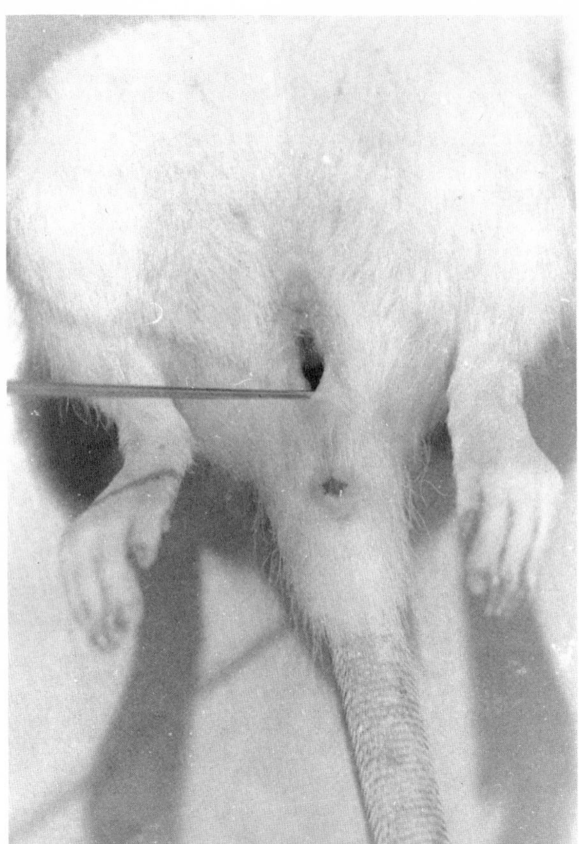

Figure 5.2. Feminized external sexual organs of a genetic male rat with two undescended testes. Feminization was induced by injecting the pregnant mother with the antiandrogen cyproterone acetate (photo courtesy of Friedmund Neumann).

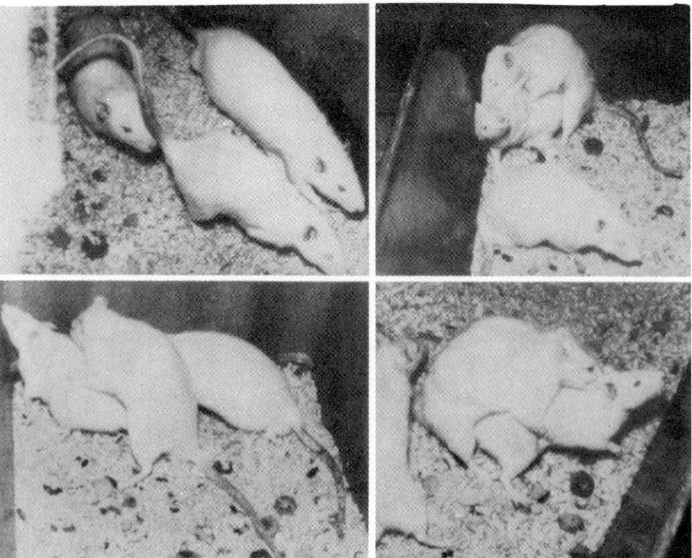

Figure 5.3. Feminized mating responses to stud males in prenatally antiandrogenized rats, subsequently castrated and treated with ovarian grafts (photo courtesy of Friedmund Neumann).

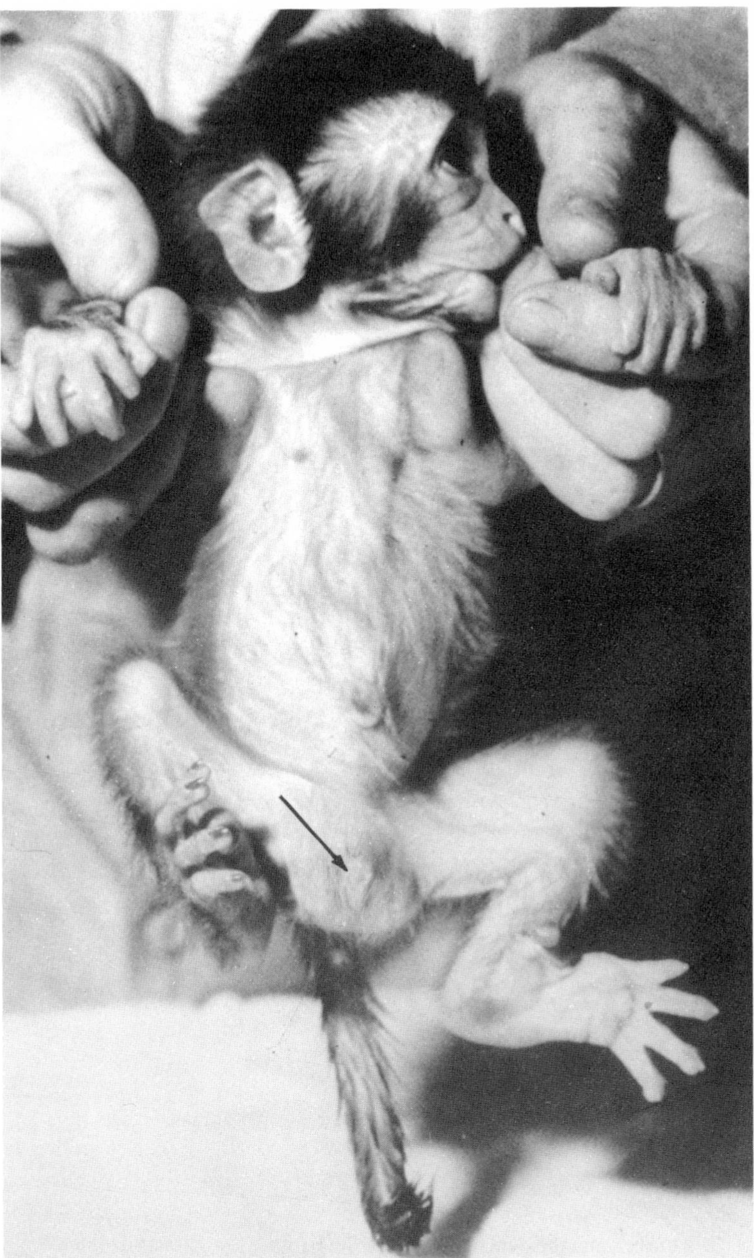

Figure 5.4. Masculinized external sexual organs of a genetic female rhesus monkey with two ovaries, uterus and Fallopian tubes. Masculinization was induced by injecting the pregnant mother with the androgen, testosterone propionate (photo courtesy of Robert Goy and Charles Phoenix).

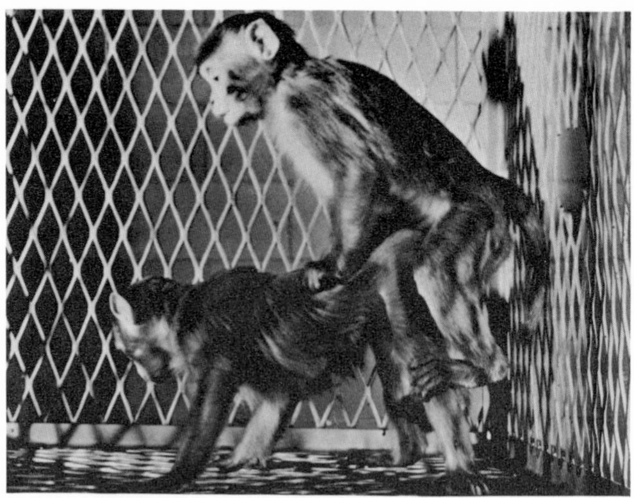

Figure 5.5. Adult mounting position rehearsed in the juvenile play of a prepubertal genetic male rhesus monkey. Though not typical of the childhood or adult behavior of normal genetic females, this position is manifested by hermaphroditic females masculinized in utero (photo courtesy of Robert Goy and Charles Phoenix).

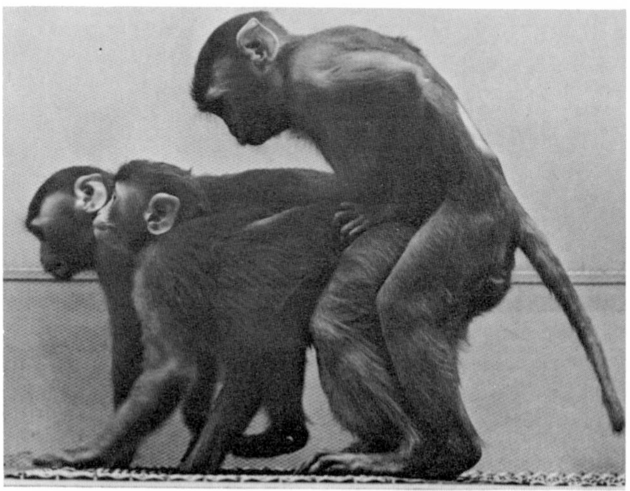

Figure 5.6. Mounting position seen in the early infantile play of rhesus monkeys of either sex, prior to maturation in the male and hermaphroditic female, but not the normal female, of the position seen in Figure 5.5 (photo courtesy of Robert Goy and Charles Phoenix).

6

FETAL HORMONES AND THE BRAIN: HUMAN CLINICAL SYNDROMES

Fetally Androgenized Genetic Females: The Syndrome of Progestin-Induced Hermaphroditism

The closest approximation in human beings to the planned experimental masculinization of genetic female animals before birth is the syndrome of progestin-induced hermaphroditism. This condition of prenatal masculinization was, two to three decades ago, inadvertently induced in a few genetic female fetuses by pregnancy-saving hormones given to the mother to prevent a miscarriage. These hormones belong to a recently synthesized group of steroids which, though related in chemical structure to androgens, are, in biological action, substitutes for pregnancy hormone (progesterone) and hence are named progestins. When they were first synthesized, it was not known that certain of them would exert, in rare instances, a masculinizing influence on a daughter fetus. Thus, before this effect was discovered and before the use of the hormones was discontinued, there were in the 1950's a few mothers who gave birth to daughters with masculinization of the clitoris. Usually the masculinization was restricted to enlargement of the clitoris plus or minus a certain amount of labial fusion (Figure 6.1) but, in rare instances, masculinization became complete, producing a penis and empty scrotum (see Figure 3.7 for corresponding examples).

The more complete the degree of masculinization, the deeper within, and closer to the neck of the bladder, would be the opening of the vagina.

But the internal organs of the female would always be present. The internal organs of the male would not be differentiated, apparently because of a timing effect. The masculinizing effect of the progestinic medication has proved to be confined to the fetal period of external sexual differentiation.

Because the influence of synthetic progestin pills taken by the mother ceases at birth, and because there are no other tell-tale signs or side effects to arouse diagnostic suspicion, the baby born with a penis would, naturally enough, be regarded as a boy with undescended testes, and brought up as a boy. The baby with only incomplete masculinization of the clitoris, however, would more likely be subject to diagnostic evaluation leading to the decision that, because the genetic, gonadal, and internal sex were female, the sex of assignment should be as a girl. Upon completion of surgical feminization of the external genitalia, no further surgical or hormonal treatment would be required. At the age of puberty, the girl's own ovaries function normally, totally feminizing the body and inducing menstruation, though possibly a little late.

Fetally Androgenized Genetic Females: The Female Adrenogenital Syndrome

The hermaphroditism and development of genetic females with the progestin-induced condition has a parallel in genetic females with the adrenogenital syndrome. The parallel exists only if the adrenogenital child is hormonally regulated from birth onward by treatment with cortisone to prevent postnatal continuance of developmental masculinization.

The adrenogenital syndrome is so named because, in this condition, the adrenal glands have a defect of function, beginning in fetal life, which in turn causes a defect of the genital anatomy, if the fetus is female. The primary defect is a genetic one, transmitted as a genetic recessive, which prevents the adrenal cortices from synthesizing their proper hormone, cortisol. Instead, they release a precursor product which is, in biological action, a male sex hormone—an androgen. This androgen enters into the blood stream of the fetus too late to induce extensive masculinization of the internal reproductive ducts (the wolffian ducts), but in time to masculinize the external genital anlagen. As in the progestin-induced syndrome, the result may be complete masculinization to form a penis and empty scrotum, or less complete, to form a grossly enlarged clitoris that resembles a hypospadiac penis, with partial fusion of the labia majora (Figure 6.2). In either case, the internal female reproductive organs will have differentiated. The vaginal orifice will be near its expected location if masculinization has been minimal. Otherwise, its opening will be into the wall of the urethra, internally, and will need to be brought surgically to its normal external location.

Such is the nature of adrenal malfunction in the adrenogenital syndrome that some babies born with this condition are also lacking in correct salt and fluid balance in the body, and some lack in blood-pressure regulation. In consequence, they may become desperately sick and rapidly die unless the condition is recognized and cortisone regulation promptly established. Especially because of the tell-tale symptoms associated with salt loss, even the baby masculinized to the extent of having a full penis is likely to be diagnostically recognized soon after birth as a genetic female with two ovaries and a uterus internally. There are some who, lacking serious symptoms, escape recognition and grow up successfully as boys; and in times past, there have even been a few born with an incomplete penis who, because of an incomplete diagnostic work-up, were surgically corrected as boys, and also grew up to have a masculine gender identity.

The adrenogenital female hermaphrodites of special interest in this chapter, however, are those whose diagnosis is promptly established neonatally so that they are assigned to grow up as girls. They are given at least the first stage of surgical feminizing repair of the genitalia within the first weeks or months of life. Sometimes additional, minor vaginal surgery may be needed in teenage. Their early surgery taken care of, the girls grow up to see themselves as girls, as well as to be seen as girls by the people who take care of them or otherwise see their genitalia.

Because the abnormality of adrenocortical function does not correct itself postnatally, it is necessary for children with this condition to be regulated on cortisone therapy throughout the growing period and, indeed, in adulthood also. This regulation is imperative to prevent growth and maturation in childhood which is too rapid, too early, and too masculine. Otherwise, the physique would simulate that of normal male puberty, but eight to ten years ahead of the normal time of male puberty. Of course, masculine puberty in a child living as a girl is unsightly and wrong. In later years, a girl also does not desire to be hairy, deep-voiced and masculine in appearance, for which purpose hormonal regulation on cortisone must be maintained. Properly treated, she will develop a feminine physique at the expected time of puberty. Her menses may be about a year late in appearing. In a few instances, they may be excessively delayed (Jones and Verkauf, 1971). Otherwise she can expect to be able to conceive, though perhaps not as expeditiously as she might desire. She can expect to give birth to a normal child, but proper cortisone regulation is imperative to prevent miscarriage. Lactation is also possible.

Cortisone therapy for the adrenogenital syndrome was discovered in 1950. It was just prior to this time that the first babies with progestin-induced hermaphroditism were born. Thus, the oldest adrenogenital girls treated with cortisone since babyhood, and the oldest of the progestin-induced group are now young adults. In the years 1965–67, when our special follow-up study of their behavioral development and psychosexual identity was undertaken, the oldest was sixteen.

Behavioral Sequelae: Fetally Androgenized Genetic Females, Not Additionally Androgenized Postnatally

The purpose of this follow-up study was to compare some aspects of sexually dimorphic behavior in fetally-androgenized, genetic females of the human species in childhood and adolescence with that of matched controls, in order to see if prenatal androgens may have left a presumptive effect on the brain, and hence on subsequent behavior. The sample comprised a census of all ten available genetic females with progestin-induced hermaphroditism, all given early corrective surgery, if needed, and all reared as girls; and an unbiased selection of fifteen early-treated genetic female adrenogenital hermaphrodites of suitable age, hormonal history, surgical history, and geographic proximity. They ranged in age from four to sixteen years, the majority being in middle childhood.

For each one of these twenty-five fetally androgenized girls, a normal girl as a matched control was found through the courtesy of local school authorities. Matching was on the basis of age, IQ, socioeconomic background, and race. All fifty girls and their mothers were interviewed with a standard schedule of topics, and were tested with sex-role preference procedures. Further details of methodology are in Ehrhardt and Money (1967), Ehrhardt, Epstein, and Money (1968), and Ehrhardt (1969).

Since the findings on the two diagnostic groups closely paralleled one another, they are presented together. Tables 6.1 to 6.3 are on pp. 106–8.

TOMBOYISM

Table 6.1 shows that fetally androgenized girls differed from their matched controls in regarding themselves as tomboys, a status of which they were proud. There were actually 9 of the 10 girls with the progestin-induced syndrome and 11 of the 15 with the adrenogenital syndrome who claimed they were tomboys. This status was confirmed by the mother, and was recognized and accepted by playmates and others. A statistically unimportant number of girls in the matched control sample identified themselves as tomboyish, and in most cases for only a limited episode, whereas for the patient groups tomboyism was a long-term way of life.

Tomboyism did not necessarily include explicit dissatisfaction with being a girl, although the difference between patients and controls on this criterion reached the 5 percent level of significance in the case of the adrenogenital syndrome. Some girls in the patient groups said they would rather have been born a boy, had there been a choice. Others were ambivalent in the sense that they could not make up their minds whether it would be better to be a boy than a girl. None of the girls actually wanted to change her sex, as some hermaphroditic children do (see Chapter 8), and none had entertained a conception of sex reassignment.

ENERGY EXPENDITURE IN RECREATION AND AGGRESSION

The common denominator of many tomboyish activities in girls is a high level of physical energy expenditure, especially in the vigorous outdoor play, games, and sports commonly considered the prerogative of boys. Such activities correspond, it would appear, to the rough-and-tumble play of prenatally masculinized female rhesus monkeys. Table 6.1 shows that the girls of both diagnostic groups tended to outstrip their matched controls in preference for athletic energy expenditure, and definitely to have more interest in joining with boys in their energetic play. Team games with a ball, especially neighborhood football and baseball games, received frequent mention. Some of the girls in the diagnostic groups liked to play with girls as well as boys, though some preferred boys as playmates. Most of the control girls preferred to play with other girls rather than boys, if they had a choice.

In the Oregon studies, experimentally masculinized female monkeys showed not only an elevated incidence of rough-and-tumble play, but also of threat in play (Goy, 1970). One might speculate, therefore, that fetally androgenized girls might have evidenced more aggression against their playmates than did their matched controls. In point of fact, this did not prove to be true. The fetally androgenized girls were well able to take up for themselves if attacked, but they were not rated by themselves or their mothers as aggressive children who liked to pick fights. In this respect they did not differ from their matched controls (Table 6.1).

This lack of predisposition to aggressive attack suggests that aggressiveness, per se, is the wrong variable on which to expect gender-dimorphic behavior, despite popular stereotypes to the contrary. It is more likely that the correct variable is dominance assertion, and striving for position in the dominance hierarchy of childhood. Though this variable was not identified in advance, so that specific data pertaining to it were not collected, in retrospect it appears that the girls of the two diagnostic groups did not strive for dominance in competition with boys, and they were not interested in the rivalries of other girls. Quite possibly, they may have exempted themselves from competitive rivalry with boys, sensing that, because they were socially identified as girls regardless of their skills and accomplishments, they were obliged not to trespass on the culturally defined right of male superiority. Such trespassing might have resulted in their being evicted by the boys from their recreational groups. Under the circumstances, they were better off to avoid dominance rivalry than to be rejected.

CLOTHING AND ADORNMENT

In keeping with their energetic outdoor recreations shared with boys, girls of the two diagnostic groups preferred the utilitarian and functional in clothing, rather than the chic, pretty, or fashionably feminine. Usually they chose to wear slacks or shorts and skirts rather than dresses. They were not, however, compulsively averse to dressing up on special occasions as a genuinely transvestic or transexual child might be. They simply preferred more practical clothes, and in this respect were significantly different from their matched controls. The same trend carried over to accessories, namely jewelry, perfume, and hair-styling, though there was a sufficient frequency of moderate interest in these personal adornments to make the contrast with frequency of interest in the matched control group not statistically significant.

CHILDHOOD SEXUALITY

Sexual play among the primates in childhood serves a rehearsal function in preparation for the reproductive behavior of adulthood. It is normally observed in human juveniles, provided it is not socially tabooed and inhibited. In rhesus monkeys, there is no absolute difference between the sexual play patterns of males and females, but there is a relative difference: males mount more than females do, the females being more often mounted. Moreover, males progress from keeping both feet on the ground while they mount to using their feet to climb onto and grasp the shanks of the female. Normal female monkeys do not practice this skill in their play, but fetally androgenized females do (Chapter 5).

Among the fetally androgenized human subjects and their matched controls, reports of manifest childhood sexual activity did not differ statistically (Table 6.2). There were only a few girls for whom manifest sexual behavior was reported. Presumably all of them, subjects and controls, had established obedience to the cultural norms and either avoided sexual play or kept it private. The important point is that a history of fetal masculinization did not, per se, bring about an observable change in the sexual play of childhood. Nor did it bring about a greater degree of verbal curiosity or interest. The amount of sex education received was more complete for the diagnostic than for the control groups, because what they learned at home was augmented in discussions at the hospital.

MATERNALISM

From the point of view of gender dimorphism of behavior, there is a certain unity to energetic recreation, dominance assertion, relative indifference to personal adornment and, possibly, masculine positioning in sexual play, all of which belong to the stereotype of boyishness. Conversely, there is a unity that belongs to the stereotype of girlishness. It pertains to rehearsals in childhood play and fantasy of maternalism, marriage, and boyfriend romance. Developmentally, maternalism appears first, in connection with its rehearsal in doll play.

Table 6.3 shows that fetally androgenized girls differed from their matched controls in the preferred toys of childhood. They were indifferent to dolls, or openly neglectful of them. They turned instead to cars, trucks, and guns, and other toys that traditionally belong to boys.

Lack of interest in dolls later became a lack of interest in infants, that is, in doing things for their care, or in expecting to do such things, even as a paid baby sitter, in the future. The discrepancy between the diagnostic groups and their controls reached statistical significance on the criterion of baby care in the adrenogenital syndrome only. Some girls in this group distinctly disliked handling little babies and believed they would be awkward and clumsy. By contrast, many of the control girls rated high in enthusiasm for little children; they adored them and took every opportunity to get in close contact with them.

All control girls were sure that they wanted to have pregnancies and be the mothers of little babies when they grew up, whereas one third of the fetally androgenized girls with the adrenogenital syndrome said they would prefer not to have children. The remainder, as well as the ten girls with a history of fetal progestin, did not reject the idea of having children, but they were rather perfunctory and matter-of-fact in their anticipation of motherhood, and lacking the enthusiasm of the control girls.

CAREER VERSUS MARRIAGE

When queried about the priority of a nondomestic career versus marriage and being a housewife in the future (Table 6.3), the majority of fetally androgenized girls subordinated marriage to career, or else wanted an occupational career other than housewife concurrent with being married, and regarded occupational and marital status as equally important. Among the control girls, the emphasis was in favor of marriage over nonmarital career. For the majority of these girls, marriage was the most important goal of their future.

At first glance, it might appear that preference for career versus housewife in the fetally androgenized girls was related to their generally high IQ level (Money and Lewis, 1966; Ehrhardt and Money, 1967; Ehrhardt, Epstein and Money, 1968; Lewis, Money and Epstein, 1968; Money, 1971). This finding of a trend toward IQ elevation in children exposed to an excess of fetal androgen (it occurs also in genetic males similarly exposed) was a serendipitous one, and one concordant with a high level of attainment academically. It raises questions, as yet unanswered, regarding the relationship of gonadal steroids to development of the cerebral cortex in the fetus, as well as questions regarding the relationship of high IQ to tomboyism, or vice versa in genitally normal females (Maccoby, 1963, p. 33). Obviously high IQ per se is not the determinant of tomboyism, for the fetally androgenized girls of the present sample were matched with the controls on the criterion of IQ; and the controls were not persistent tomboys.

ROMANTICISM, BOYFRIENDS, HOMOSEXUALITY

Paralleling their preference for a career over and beyond marriage, the fetally androgenized girls did not carry forward the precursor interest in romance and boyfriends from their play and daydreams into adolescent dating, as did the control girls in their play and daydreams. Those few who were already adolescent lagged behind their agemates in beginning their dating life and venturing into the beginnings of love play. Though the sample of adolescents was too small for any definitive conclusion, subsequent observations on additional teenaged patients bear out the impression that they are late in reaching the boyfriend stage of development and in getting married.

In view of all the foregoing signs of tomboyism, it is of considerable importance that there were no indications of lesbianism in the erotic interest of the fetally androgenized girls, nor in their controls (Table 6.3). Thus, it appears that in the fetally androgenized girls it may have been that the biological clock for falling in love was in arrears, but not that it was set to respond to a member of the same sex. It may, indeed, be easier for a fetally androgenized girl than for her control to grow up with a lesbian's biography, but so far this has not been observed, either in the girls of the study sample or in other adolescent patients who have since augmented it. The only exceptions are those patients who, having been assigned as males, and surgically corrected and hormonally regulated as males, grow up to have a psychosexual status that might be defined as iatrogenic homosexuality (see Chapters 8 and 11). Since they have a penis and a masculine body build, however, they can be regarded as homosexual only on the basis of genetic sex and gonadal sex, not of morphologic sex.

COMMENT

The most likely hypothesis to explain the various features of tomboyism in fetally masculinized genetic females is that their tomboyism is a sequel to a masculinizing effect on the fetal brain. This masculinization may apply specifically to pathways, most probably in the limbic system or paleocortex, that mediate dominance assertion (possibly in association with assertion of exploratory and territorial rights) and, therefore, manifests itself in competitive energy expenditure. Fighting and aggression are not primarily implicated.

Masculinization of the fetal brain may apply also to the inhibition of pathways that should eventually subserve maternal behavior. More correctly, one might say partial inhibition of these pathways, for normal males are capable of paternalism, much of which is identical with maternalism, both being manifestations of parentalism or caretaking.

The noteworthy lack of masculinization in fetal androgenization pertains to those pathways of the brain that subsequently will mediate love and eroticism in response to a mating partner. Evidently, the deciding factor as to the characteristics of the sexual mate as male or female operates postnatally and not prenatally. It remains to be explained why the timing of dating, romance, and the first love affair appeared to be delayed in fetally androgenized girls, until later than their occurrence in their agemates of either sex.

In the lower species, fetal androgenization may automatically reverse gender dimorphic behavior by prenatal hormonal decree, so to speak. In human beings there is no such automatic decree. So much of gender-identity differentiation remains to take place postnatally, that prenatally determined traits or dispositions can be incorporated into the postnatally differentiated schema, whether it be masculine or feminine.

Behavioral Sequelae: Fetally Androgenized Genetic Females, Additionally Androgenized Postnatally

Prior to 1950, when cortisone therapy was discovered, all genetic females with the adrenogenital syndrome had no choice except to grow up severely virilized by chronically high levels of adrenocortical androgen. They were not only prenatally masculinized, but postnatally also. In teenage and adulthood, they were in a position to report on erotic and sexual arousal before their excessively high androgen levels were brought down to normal under the influence of cortisone therapy, after 1950.

The study of 23 of these older adolescents and adults living as virilized women (Ehrhardt, Evers, and Money, 1968) corroborated, in general, the findings on the early-treated group reported in the foregoing. The majority of the 23 reported that they had been tomboys throughout childhood, and in adulthood their first preference was for a career other than full-time housewife.

Among the 23 there was a relatively high incidence (in 10 individuals) of homosexual as well as heterosexual imagery in dreams and fantasies. Three of these ten, plus one other, reported bisexual experience also. No woman, however, considered herself to have been erroneously assigned as a female, and none had entertained the idea of a sex reassignment.

A complicating factor in the bisexuality of imagery and experience in these women is that several of them still had a hypertrophied clitoris or clitoral stump capable of erecting under the influence of excess androgen, but not after the excess had been cortisone-controlled. Their sexual behavior may have been indirectly influenced also by their image of their bodies under the influence of postnatal virilization, even if the virilization had been partially corrected.

Among the 23 women, 13 are now known to have married, all but two of them after being feminized on cortisone. Five are known to have had at least one pregnancy and delivery. One had three. The babies are nonhermaphroditic and usually healthy. In some instances, the mothers worried about the wisdom of their becoming pregnant, for they felt insecure and feared they would be clumsy with small infants and would fail in mothering them. Actual practice with the baby enabled them to overcome their misgivings. At least one mother was able to breast feed her infants, of whom she had three (Money and Raiti, 1967).

Among the 23 women, there were 11 (52 percent of the 21 for whom sufficient data were available) who stated that having a child usually would not enter their thoughts, fantasies, or dreams. In the files of 12 patients, there was also information about how they expected they might feel, prior to actual experience, if having to hug and cuddle a tiny infant. Only two of them (17 percent) expressed a positive and genuine desire to be affectionate with small children. The other ten were noncommittal and preferred children who were at least at the toddler age.

There were some late-treated women with the adrenogenital syndrome who, even prior to cortisone treatment, manifested relatively little behavior that might be classified as more typically masculine than feminine. These women show that postnatally elevated androgen levels, persisting into adulthood, do not in and of themselves dictate a masculine gender role or gender identity. They also show that, if there is a permanent prenatal hormonal effect on a part of the central nervous system that mediates sexually dimorphic behavior, then it obviously is in some manner selective. The selectivity may pertain to the timing and/or amount of fetal androgen exposure. An alternative explanation may be that postnatal gender-identity differentiation may be capable of overriding prenatal precursors, or at least of modifying them to an extensive degree (see Chapter 8).

Fetal Absence of Gonadal Hormones: Turner's Syndrome

The antithesis of a genetic female masculinized in utero is not a genetic male feminized but, more accurately, a genetic male nonmasculinized (see Chapter 3). In the absence of androgen, the genetic male differentiates genitally as a female. In the absence of estrogen, the genetic female differentiates as a female. In the absence of gonads and their hormones in entirety, the fetus develops as a female, regardless of genetic sex.

The fetus with Turner's syndrome is one that has no gonadal hormones whatsoever, for its gonads are primitive streaks of tissues instead of being fully formed and differentiated. The etiology of the gonadal defect is cytogenetic (see Chapter 2), for individuals with the condition most commonly have only one sex chromosome, an X, the other one having been lost either prior to, or immediately after, fertilization. In the cytogenetic variants of the syndrome, for example in a 45,X/46,XX mosaic, it is presumed that the second X chromosome was by reason of its infrequency or location unable to exert its expected influence, for the gonads may be the same primitive streaks as in the simple 45,X chromosomal version of the condition.

The baby born with Turner's syndrome will look like a girl genitally, and so will be assigned and reared as one. Lack of gonadal hormones will be without known effect during the years of childhood, until the time arrives for the beginning of puberty. Then it will be necessary to give estrogen by pills, or possibly by injection. Without this substitution therapy in teenage, it will be extremely difficult for the girl to establish the same degree of psychosocial maturity as her agemates, or to be treated by them as their psychosocial equals, all the more so because of her typically short stature.

The biography of a girl with Turner's syndrome is of special interest with respect to gender-identity differentiation, insofar as it can be expected to show whatever effect, if any, may appear on account of prenatal absence of gonadal hormones. For this reason, and in connection with the study on fetally androgenized girls already presented in the foregoing sections, we undertook a comparison of 15 girls with Turner's syndrome and their matched controls, on the basis of the same criteria as those used to compare the fetally androgenized girls and their matched controls (Ehrhardt, Greenberg and Money, 1970). The girls ranged in age from eight to 16½ years, with a mean and a median of 12½ years. Only the oldest Turner girl was menstruating on cyclic estrogen substitution therapy when last seen at the time of the study. The patient sample was selected from a larger group seen in the pediatric endocrine clinic and the psychohormonal research unit without known sampling bias.

Table 6.1 Tomboyish, Energy Expenditure, and Clothing Adornment Preference in Fetally Androgenized Girls versus their Matched Controls, plus Girls with Turner's Syndrome versus their Matched Controls

BEHAVIORAL SIGNS	*PI vs C*	*AGS vs C*	*C vs TS*
EVIDENCE OF TOMBOYISM			
1. Known to self and mother as tomboy	$p \leq .05$	$p \leq .01$	o
2. Lack of satisfaction with female sex role	o	$p \leq .05$	o
EXPENDITURE OF ENERGY IN RECREATION AND AGGRESSION			
3. Athletic interests and skills	$p \leq .05$	$p \leq .10$	$p \leq .05$
4. Preference of male versus female playmates	$p \leq .05$	$p \leq .01$	o
5. Behavior in childhood fights	o	o	$p \leq .05$
PREFERRED CLOTHING AND ADORNMENT			
6. Clothing preference, slacks versus dresses	$p \leq .05$	$p \leq .05$	o
7. Lacking interest in jewelry, perfume and hair styling	o	o	$p \leq .05$

Legend:

PI = Progestin-induced hermaphroditism (N=10)
AGS = Adrenogenital syndrome (N=15)
TS = Turner's syndrome (N=15)
C = Matched controls
o = No significant difference

In Table 6.1, it can be seen that girls with Turner's syndrome did not differ from their matched controls on four counts, being equally feminine as the normal girls in these respects. On the three other counts they were even more extremely feminine than their controls: as a group they manifested a lesser incidence of athletic interest and skill, a lesser incidence of childhood fighting, and a greater interest in personal adornment.

Table 6.2 Sexual Play of Childhood in Fetally Androgenized Girls versus their Matched Controls, plus Girls with Turner's Syndrome versus their Matched Controls

EVIDENCE OF CHILDHOOD SEXUALITY	*PI vs C*	*AGS vs C*	*C vs TS*
1. Attention to genital morphology	o	o	o
2. Masturbation	o	o	o
3. Shared genital inspection and play	o	o	o
4. Shared copulation play	o	o	o

Legend:
PI = Progestin-induced hermaphroditism (N=10)
AGS = Adrenogenital syndrome (N=15)
TS = Turner's syndrome (N=15)
C = Matched controls
o = No significant difference

Table 6.2 shows that girls with Turner's syndrome were similar to their matched controls in their limited manifestation of childhood sexuality. Table 6.3 shows that they also resembled their matched controls in childhood manifestations and anticipations of maternalism, marriage, and romance. Despite the handicap of their stature and infertility which all the older Turner girls knew about, all but one explicitly hoped to get married one day. They all reported daydreams and fantasies of being pregnant and wanting to have a baby to care for one day. All but one had played with dolls exclusively, and the one preferred dolls even though she played with boys' toys occasionally. Twelve of them had a strong interest in taking care of babies, tending to their younger siblings, or babysitting for other parents; two had a moderate interest in such maternalistic activities; for the one remaining girl, information was missing.

Taken as a whole, these findings indicated that girls with Turner's syndrome differentiate an unequivocally feminine gender identity. Thus one may infer that, in order to differentiate postnatally as feminine, gender identity is not dependent on prenatal gonadal hormones (estrogen and/or

Table 6.3 Anticipation and Imagery of Maternalism, Marriage and Romance in Fetally Androgenized Girls versus their Matched Controls, plus Girls with Turner's Syndrome versus their Matched Controls

ANTICIPATION AND IMAGERY	*PI vs C*	*AGS vs C*	*C vs TS*
MATERNALISM			
1. Toy cars, guns, etc. preferred to dolls	$p \leq .05$	$p \leq .05$	o
2. Juvenile interest in infant care-taking	o	$p \leq .001$	o
3. No daydreams or fantasies of pregnancy and motherhood	o	$p \leq .05$	o
MARRIAGE			
4. Wedding and marriage not anticipated in play and daydreams	o	$p \leq .05$	o
5. Priority of career versus Marriage	$p \leq .05$	$p \leq .05$	o
ROMANCE			
6. Lack of heterosexual romanticism in juvenile play and daydreams	o	o	o
7. Lack of adolescent (age 13-16) daydreams of boyfriend and lack of dating relationships	o	o	o
8. Lack of homosexual fantasies reported	o	o	o

Legend:
PI = Progestin-induced hermaphroditism (N=10)
AGS = Adrenogenital syndrome (N=15)
TS = Turner's syndrome (N=15)
C = Matched controls
o = No significant difference

androgen) acting presumptively on the brain. Nor is a feminine gender identity dependent on the presence of a second X chromosome. A feminine gender identity can differentiate very effectively without any help from prenatal gonadal hormones that might influence the brain and perhaps, in fact, all the more effectively in their absence.

Fetally Nonandrogenized Genetic Males: Androgen-Insensitivity Syndrome

The individual with Turner's syndrome is not a genetic male who feminized in utero. She is not, therefore, the genetic male counterpart of the genetic female who masculinized in utero. The human clinical syndrome that most closely approximates the antithesis of fetal androgenization of the genetic female is the syndrome of androgen insensitivity (testicular feminization) in the genetic male (see Chapter 3). That the antithesis is not total is due to the fact that the syndrome represents not fetal estrogenization of a genetic male, but failure of androgenization of the genetic male. Without androgen, the genetic male fetus, like the 45,X fetus of Turner's syndrome, differentiates morphologically as a female. The same feminization occurs if the fetus is supplied with androgen but is unable to use it, which is precisely what happens in the androgen-insensitivity syndrome.

The defect in adrogen utilization in the testicular feminizing syndrome is known to be a genetically transmitted trait that travels down the generations among some of the fertile females of an affected pedigree. Three modes of genetic transmission have been postulated, an X-linked recessive, a male-limited autosomal dominant, or possibly a male-limited X-linked dominant, and it cannot yet be decided which applies. Whether a genetic male offspring will be affected or not will depend on which one of the pair of maternal chromosomes, the carrier or the non-carrier, happens to get into the egg when the pairs of chromosomes separate so that the egg receives only one-half of the total number of the mother's 46 chromosomes. If the egg does carry the affected chromosome, then the resultant baby will manifest the clinical defect only if it is fertilized by a Y bearing sperm from the father. If the sperm bears a second X chromosome, then the baby will be a fertile female, and a covert carrier of the genetic defect, capable of transmitting it in the succeeding generation.

The nature of the biochemical defect responsible for inability to utilize androgen in the testicular feminizing syndrome has not yet been identified. It is probably enzymatic. The site of action is presumed to be within the cell and to affect virtually every cell in the body that should be responsive to androgen. The exception may be the cells of pubic and axillary hair follicles which, in the normal female, are believed to be stimulated by adrenocortical androgens. Even these cells may be unresponsive in the individual with the androgen-insensitivity syndrome, for there are some patients who have no pubic or axillary hair in adulthood. Head hair is not affected, but hair on the face and body does not appear.

The testes in the androgen-insensitivity syndrome secrete androgen into the blood stream in amounts normal for a male. They also are the source of the much lesser amount of estrogen normal for a male. This estrogen proves sufficient at the age of puberty to bring about complete feminization of the bony structure and outer contours of the body, including normal feminine growth of breasts.

The effect of androgen insensitivity in fetal life is suppression of masculine differentiation of the wolffian ducts and of the anlagen of the external genital organs (see Chapter 3). The suppression is so complete that many affected babies are born indistinguishable in genital appearance from normal females. Since it is not usual to do a detailed pelvic examination on a newborn girl, it is not discovered that the vagina may be represented only by a dimple, or by a shallow cavity which ends blindly and which will need surgical lengthening in (or later than) mid-teenage. Such a vagina has no connection with a cervix or uterus. The uterus itself is not properly formed, but is a cordlike structure without an interior cavity. The embryological explanation for this defect of the uterus is that, in the early stages of sexual differentiation, the testes released not only their androgenic substance which the body failed to use, but also their mullerian inhibiting substance which the body did not fail to use. Thus the mullerian ducts began the process of becoming vestigial, as expected in a male, instead of enlarging and growing into the uterus and fallopian tubes of the female. This circumstance of prenatal development accounts for the fact that, at adolescence, even though feminization is otherwise complete (Figures 6.3 and 6.4), there is no menstruation.

Though there are some babies with the androgen insensitivity syndrome whose anomaly easily passes completely undetected in infancy and childhood, there are some who present the tell-tale sign of lumps in the groin or in the labia majora, which are actually the feminizing testes trying to descend from their original abdominal position. If they are then surgically removed, the child will need replacement therapy with estrogen at the age of puberty.

Another tell-tale sign, present at birth, may be a slight enlargement of the clitoris, insignificant in itself, but enough to lead the alert physician to make further diagnostic investigations. In a very small number of recorded cases, the clitoral organ may be large enough that, in combination with the fact that the testes can be palpated in the groins, the physician may decide the baby should be declared a boy, and surgically corrected as much as possible as a boy. From puberty on, these boys are imprisoned in a body that develops like that of a female and absolutely refuses to masculinize despite all therapeutic efforts, however heroic. The breasts can be removed surgically, of course, but it is impossible to induce deepening of the voice and masculine hair distribution. A particularly disheartening feature of failure to masculinize is that it also creates the impression of failure to age in appearance and look mature enough for one's age. As a husband, if a man with this condition surmounts the obstacles of his physique and sexual anatomy and gets married, he may scarcely be able to cope with the indignity of being mistaken for his wife's son.

It is fortunate for most babies with the androgen insensitivity syndrome that they are so completely feminized in genital appearance that, even if their testes are palpated neonatally, they are assigned to be reared as girls. As these patients grow up, their biographies are of special value as test cases of whether sexually dimorphic behavior will have been influenced by either the genetic or the gonadal status of the fetus as a male, in the absence of fetal hormonal masculinization.

Behavioral Sequelae: Androgen-Insensitivity Syndrome

Though it is exceptionally rare, and also exceptionally difficult to explain embryologically, it may happen that a genetic male is born with the external genitals differentiated as a female, and with two undescended testes that will not feminize but masculinize the body at the time of puberty. For this reason, it is preferable that psychologic studies of androgen-insensitivity pertain to individuals who, even though they have been followed through childhood, are old enough to have shown the signs of testicular feminization at puberty. There were ten patients in this older age range, at the time we undertook a survey of our clinical data (Money, Ehrhardt, and Masica, 1968; Masica, Money, Ehrhardt, and Lewis, 1969; Masica, Money, and Ehrhardt, 1971), who had been born with normal-appearing female sex organs. Since then, there have been four more patients, on whom the findings confirm those of the other ten. The psychohormonal files on these ten patients were abstracted and tabulated according to the same categories as those used for the fetally androgenized and the Turner-syndrome girls.

With respect to marriage and maternalism, the girls and women with the androgen-insensitivity syndrome showed a high incidence of preference for being a wife with no outside job (80 percent); of enjoying homecraft (70 percent); of being resigned to their permanent incapacity for pregnancy (70 percent); of having dreams and fantasies of raising a family (100 percent); of having played primarily with dolls and other girls' toys (80 percent); of having a positive and genuine interest in infant care, even though they had to forfeit the care of the newborn (60 percent); and of high or average affectionateness, self-rated (80 percent). Two of the married women each had adopted two children, and they proved to be good mothers with a good sense of motherhood.

On the criteria of sex and eroticism, when the findings on the 10 androgen-insensitive patients were compared with those of the 23 late-treated adrenogenital women (see above) by way of contrast, the androgen-insensitive stood out as strongly feminine. The findings can be summed up by saying that nine of the androgen-insensitive women pretty much conformed to the idealized stereotype of what constitutes femininity in our culture. The tenth, a teenaged girl with an exceptionally troubled home background and adverse surgical and medical history, was going through a troubled period of adolescent development in which she rejected herself, her sex, her family, and her religion.

The group incidence of exclusive heterosexual relations among the 10 androgen-insensitive patients was 80 percent, and the incidence of adult homosexual experience was nil, with only one case of homosexual activity and bisexual imagery in adolescent fantasy (not admitted until several years later); the remaining girl was sexually unexperienced. Six of the women rated themselves as having an average level of libido, having orgasm most of the time, and being reserved and passive in coitus; two rated themselves as above average in libido, always having orgasm, and predominantly initiating sex. The remaining two had not begun their sex lives. Seven considered themselves conservative with respect to coital positions, using one or two positions only. The breasts and clitoris were regarded as erotic zones by 80 percent, the vagina by 80 percent, with no information from the one inexperienced girl. Sensory erotic arousal was predominantly through the sense of touch (80 percent).

The majority (90 percent) of androgen-insensitive women rated themselves as fully content with the female role, with only one being ambivalent. By contrast, only 47 percent of adrenogenital girls (the 15 early-treated ones are here used for comparison) so rated themselves, with 33 percent ambivalent and 20 percent preferring to have been born a male. Only one (10 percent) androgen insensitive patient, the disturbed adolescent girl, disliked feminine clothing style, with 90 percent favoring it. The corresponding percentages in the adrenogenital girls were 60 percent and 40 percent, respectively. A strong interest in personal adornment was declared by 80 percent of the androgen-insensitive group as compared with 13 percent of the adrenogenital group.

These various percentages clearly tell a story of women whose genetic status as males was utterly irrelevent to their psychosexual status as women, as also was the histology of their gonads. Their behavior and outlook were feminine, concordantly with the feminine hormonalization of their bodies at puberty and thereafter. Insofar as there had been any prenatal hormonal influence on pathways in the brain that would subsequently mediate gender dimorphic behavior, including sexual behavior, one must infer that it had been a nonmasculinizing influence. In these cases the presumptive prenatal influence was thus nicely congruent with the postnatal influences of feminine rearing and feminine gender-identity differentiation. This congruence stands in contrast with what is the presumed incongruous prenatal androgenization effect when genetic females with either of the prenatal androgenization syndromes are reared as girls and differentiate a tomboyish version of a feminine gender identity.

Incongruence of a different type is manifested when a baby with the androgen-insensitivity syndrome is declared a boy because of palpable testes and a slight enlargement of what could otherwise be considered a clitoris. In this case, the boy differentiates a male gender identity in spite of the limits set by the obstacle of an absence of presumed fetal masculinizing effects on the brain, and absence of postpubertal androgen effects. The impairment of his masculinity is particularly noticeable when he talks about his erotic arousal, sensations and feelings, as well as about the sexual functioning of his genitalia (Money, unpublished data). Just as a colorblind person cannot talk from the vantage point of color-seeing, so also such a man cannot talk from the sexual vantage point of the ordinary male.

For the systematic accumulation of knowledge, it would be ideal if there existed a clinical syndrome in which lack of, or insensitivity to androgen in fetal life could be fully corrected at birth. Such a syndrome would correspond to the two syndromes of fetal androgenization both of which can be corrected at birth by surgical feminization of the external genitalia, with hormonal correction by means of cortisone added in cases of adrenogenital syndrome. There is no such nonandrogenization syndrome which is fully correctable, for the problems of plastic surgery in attempting to construct a simulated penis from the patient's own skin grafts are virtually insurmountable, and promise to remain so at least until the technical problems of a genital-organ transplant have been solved. In addition to the surgical challenge, the hormonal challenge still remains unmet in the androgen-insensitivity syndrome. There is no known way of correcting the basic cellular resistance to androgen, either at birth or subsequently. The hormonal challenge can be met in the other known syndrome of fetal nonandrogenization, namely that very rare form of hermaphroditism characterized by a 17α-hydroxylase deficiency in a genetic male. This enzyme deficiency prohibits the synthesis of androgen by the adrenal cortex and by the testes. If the baby survives, and if the rearing is mistakenly as a boy in contradiction of the female external organs, but in agreement with the chromosomal and gonadal sex, then at puberty it is possible to induce pubertal masculinization of the body by means of replacement androgen therapy (New and Suvannakul, 1970). No amount of androgen replacement, however, will change the phallus from its clitoral structure to a penis.

Lacking all the evidence that might be desirable, one must be satisfied with such evidence as is available. The human clinical syndromes reviewed in this chapter suggest that there is in human beings a counterpart of experimental animal data on the influence of prenatal hormones on gender behavior. Nonetheless, as compared with the lower species, much that pertains to human gender-identity differentiation remains to be accomplished after birth, not in a developmental vacuum, so to speak, but, like language, in interaction with the social environment. The prenatal determinants of gender identity can be perhaps not entirely overridden, but they can be and are incorporated into the postnatal program of differentiation—of which more in the next chapter.

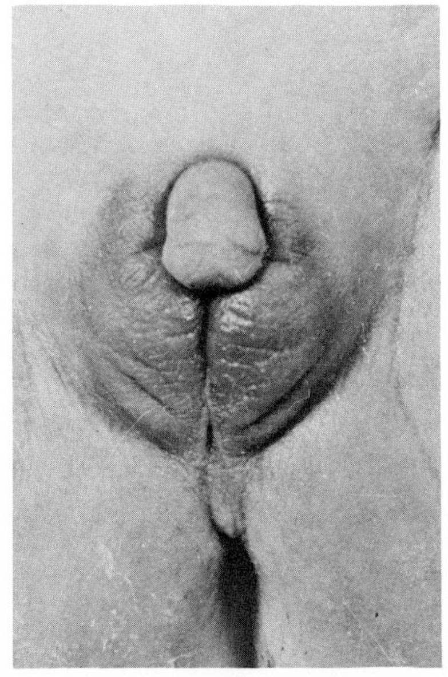

Figure 6.1. Incomplete masculinization of the external genitalia in a genetic female whose hermaphroditism was induced by synthetic progestinic hormone given to the pregnant mother to prevent miscarriage.

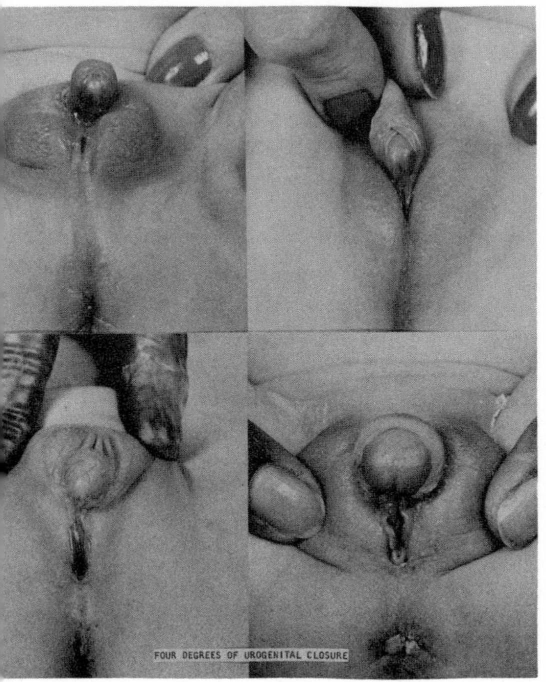

Figure 6.2. Four degrees of clitoral enlargement and partial urogenital closure, producing hermaphroditic ambiguity of appearance of the sex organs, in four cases of the masculinizing adrenogenital syndrome in genetic females. Exactly the same degrees of genital ambiguity may occur also in genetic males with incomplete masculinization.

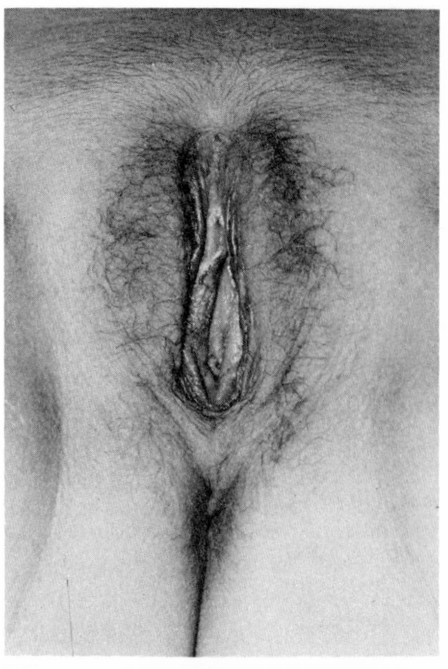

Figure 6.3. Female appearance of the external genitalia in an adult with the androgen-insensitivity, testicular feminizing syndrome. The sexual life is that of a female, in conformity with assigned sex, hormonal sex and gender identity.

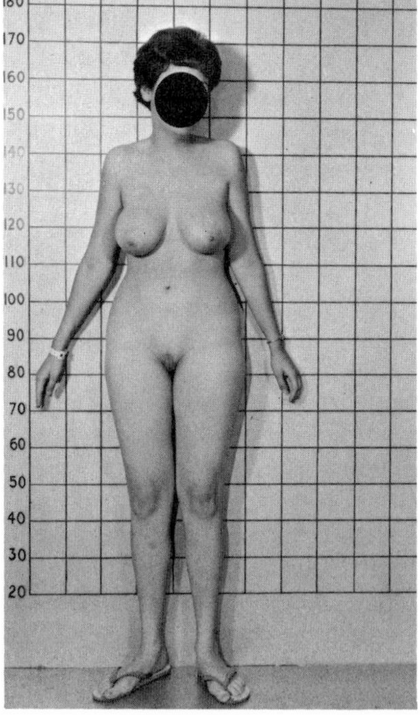

Figure 6.4. Body morphology in an adult with the androgen-insensitivity, testicular feminizing syndrome. Feminizing puberty occurs with no hormal treatment needed, under the influence of estrogens normally secreted by the testes in males, since the body is unresponsive to the competitive effect of testicular androgen.

7

GENDER DIMORPHISM IN ASSIGNMENT AND REARING

Dimorphism of Behavior, Parental and Cultural

It is easy to get trapped in circular argument as to whether boys and girls develop different patterns of preferred behavior because they are treated differently, or whether they are treated differently because they demonstrate different behavioral patterns right from the beginning. The evidence of Chapter 6 shows rather conclusively that there are in human beings some gender-dimorphic behavior differences based on antenatal hormonal history, but that these differences do not automatically dictate or totally preordain the course of postnatal dimorphism of behavioral differentiation. Chapter 8 produces further evidence of the weighty importance of postnatal events in determining how the prenatal determinants or dispositions will be incorporated into the final gender-dimorphic behavioral product.

The purpose of the present chapter is to assemble some evidence that demonstrates the proposition that cultural tradition does indeed prescribe what no one seriously doubts, namely, that parents behave differently toward and have different expectations of their infant sons and daughters; and also that these gender-dimorphic expectancies may be very differently defined in the traditions of different societies. The evidence is drawn from two quite different sources.

First, there is the testimony of two different pairs of parents who actually went through the experience of treating a baby as a son for the first seventeen months of life, and, thereafter, following an obligatory sex reassignment, as a daughter.

The second line of evidence comes from cultural anthropological studies, two of them original, each of which shows that gender-dimorphic expectancies and traditions of behavior can vary to an extraordinary degree and yet still remain dimorphic. This variability may be so great as to appear contradictory on such a fundamental issue of gender dimorphism of behavior as that concerning the sex of one's sexual partner. Three of the cultural examples are drawn from the great geographical arc that stretches from Sumatra in the west, through southern New Guinea, to the eastern Melanesian Pacific islands, in which one finds ethnic groups that prescribe homosexuality for males in the period between puberty and parenthood, and proscribe heterosexuality apart from marriage and parenthood. The other two societies, one in Australia, and the other, Argentina, institutionalize heterosexuality in the rehearsals of childhood play, and have no prescribed place for homosexuality or bisexuality in the cultural institutions of adolescence or adulthood.

Rearing of a Sex-Reassigned Normal Male Infant After Traumatic Loss of the Penis

The extreme unusualness of this case of sex reassignment in infancy lies in the fact that the child was born a normal male and an identical twin, without genital malformation or sexual ambiguity. The idea of sex-reassignment would never have been entertained were it not for a surgical mishap at the age of seven months in which the penis was ablated flush with the abdominal wall. The mishap occurred when a circumcision was being performed by means of electrocautery. The electrical current was too powerful and burned the entire tissue of the penis which necrosed and sloughed off.

The parents were young people of rural background and grade-school education. They were understandably desperate to know what could be done and suffered through a rather long saga of finding no answer. Then a consultant plastic surgeon, familiar with the principles of sex reassignment, recommended reassignment as a girl. The parents agonized their way to a decision, implementing it with a change of name, clothing and hair style when the baby was seventeen months old. Four months later, the surgical first step of genital reconstruction as a female was undertaken, the second step, vaginoplasty, being delayed until the body is full grown. Pubertal growth and feminization will be regulated by means of hormonal replacement therapy with estrogen.

At the time of surgery, when we saw the parents in person for the first time in the psychohormonal research unit at Johns Hopkins, we gave them advice and counseling on the future prognosis and management of their new daughter, based on experience with similar reassignments in hermaphroditic babies. In particular, they were given confidence that their child can be expected to differentiate a female gender identity, in agreement with her sex of rearing. They were broadly informed about the future medical program for their child and how to integrate it with her sex education as she grows older. They were guided in how to give the child information about herself to the extent that the need arises in the future; and they were helped with what to explain to friends and relatives, including their other child. Eventually, they would inform their daughter that she would become a mother by adoption, one day, when she married and wanted to have a family.

During the follow-up time of nearly six years since surgery, the parents have kept in close contact with us, making visits on an annual basis to get psychological support and guidance. The mother's observations and reports have provided us with an insight into changes in her rearing practices towards the sex-reassigned child, and into the different way that she rears this child as compared with the twin brother.

The first items of change were clothes and hairdo. The mother reported: "I started dressing her not in dresses but, you know, in little pink slacks and frilly blouses . . . and letting her hair grow." A year and six months later, the mother wrote that she had made a special effort at keeping her girl in dresses, almost exclusively, changing any item of clothes into something that was clearly feminine. "I even made all her nightwear into granny gowns and she wears bracelets and hair ribbons." The effects of emphasizing feminine clothing became clearly noticeable in the girl's attitude towards clothes and hairdo another year later, when she was observed to have a clear preference for dresses over slacks and to take pride in her long hair.

Related to being dressed nicely is the sense of neatness. The mother stated that her daughter by four and a half years of age was much neater than her brother, and in contrast with him, disliked to be dirty: "She likes for me to wipe her face. She doesn't like to be dirty, and yet my son is quite different. I can't wash his face for anything. . . . She seems to be daintier. Maybe it's because I encourage it." Elsewhere in this same recorded interview, the mother said: "One thing that really amazes me is that she is so feminine. I've never seen a little girl so neat and tidy as she can be when she wants to be. . . . She is very proud of herself, when she puts on a new dress, or I set her hair. She just loves to have her hair set; she could sit under the drier all day long to have her hair set. She just loves it."

There is a whole pattern of dimorphism of rearing girls and boys with respect to genitalia, sex and reproduction. Boys and girls learn differently how to urinate—boys to stand up and girls to sit down. This child had not, of course, been able to stand when the penis was ablated at age seven months. When, at the age of two, she tried standing up, as many girls do, her mother made a special point of teaching her how little girls go to the bathroom. In this case it needed perhaps more training than usual, because after surgery the girl's urethral opening was so positioned that the urine sometimes would overshoot the seat of the toilet. At the last follow-up, when the girl was five years and nine months old, her mother reported that she had learned to sit down and, with slight pressure from the fingers, direct the urinary stream downwards. Sometimes she still tried copying her brother, usually making "an awful mess," according to her mother.

The family was relatively open in regard to matters of sex and reproduction, so that one can study particularly well the differences in treating a girl and a boy regarding sex and their future adult reproductive role. When the twins were four and a half years old, the mother gave a good example of how parents react to boys' versus girls' genital play. Talking about the boy, the mother reported: ". . . in the summer time, one time I caught him—he went out and he took a leak in my flower garden in the front yard, you know. He was quite happy with himself. And I just didn't say anything. I just couldn't. I started laughing and I told daddy about it. . . ." The corresponding comment about the girl ran thus: "I've never had a problem with her. She did once when she was little, she took off her panties and threw them over the fence. And she didn't have no panties on. But I just, I gave her a little swat on the rear, and I told her that nice little girls didn't do that, and she should keep her pants on. . . . And she didn't take them off after that."

Once the children asked what their mother's breasts were for. She explained that whem mommies have babies, they give milk with their breasts, so that the baby is fed with the mother's milk. The boy answered that he wanted to be a mommy. His mother explained that he could only be a daddy—"and grow muscles so he could take care of mommy and baby, and go to work in car like daddy does. I finally convinced him he might have just as much fun as a mommy does. . . . I've explained to each what their function will be as a grown-up, where babies grow, and that a daddy has to have a wife to have a baby and vice versa."

When the girl once came across one of her mother's supply of sanitary pads, she was given an appropriate explanation about menstrual care and the fact that it is part of the female's role.

The mother of these two children was particularly good in pointing out the specifics of the female and male adult reproductive roles to her daughter and her son. When an incident happened that could be interpreted as penis envy in the girl and baby or pregnancy envy in the boy, she successfully offered explanations geared to the specific advantage of being a female on the one hand, and a male on the other. The incident happened some time when the children were five years of age. Both children were taking a bath together and the boy was bragging about his penis which was erect. The mother described the situation as follows: ". . . he managed to get a hard on, and he was standing there and saying, look what I got, look what I got, proud as a peacock and she (his sister) got so mad she slapped him—she didn't like it—right on his little penis. I think, she was a little jealous. So then I went and I told her you wait and see, women can have babies and boys can't." When the girl had been reassured about the advantage of being female and having babies, the boy was disappointed and jealous. His mother hastened to reassure him that "little boys could have babies, too," and she explained that the father was the one who had to provide the sperm or "seed" as she put it.

Of course, girls and boys are not only prepared differently for their future reproductive role as mother and father, but also for their other different roles, such as wife and husband or financial supporter of the family and caretaker of children and house. The mother of these two children gave a good example of how her children were copying aspects of the wife and husband role. The parents were quite open in showing affection to each other in the presence of their children. The mother observed how her son would copy some of his father's behavior: "Like he'll bend over and give her a kiss on the cheek or he'll give her a hug . . . and if he (my husband) gives me a swat on the fanny, he'll go and give her a swat on her fanny, too." The boy was clearly the initiator of affection, copying what he saw in his father's behavior. The girl copied some of her mother's responses—"If she's in an affectionate mood, she'll like it; but very often she'll say, don't do that. . . . If he's been playing some place and comes in the house to where she is helping me . . . then she'll give him a little hug like she's glad to see him."

Regarding domestic activities, such as work in the kitchen and house traditionally seen as part of the female's role, the mother reported that her daughter copies her in trying to help her tidying and cleaning up the kitchen, while the boy could not care less about it. She encourages her daughter when she helps her in the housework.

Rehearsal of future roles can also be seen in girls' and boys' toy preferences. The girl in this case wanted and received for Christmas dolls, a doll house, and a doll carriage, clearly related to the maternal aspect of the female adult role, while the boy wanted and obtained a garage with cars and gas pumps and tools, part of the rehearsal of the male role. His father, like many men, was very interested in cars and mechanical activities.

According to today's standards, not only boys, but also girls often pursue a career. Regarding school and future plans, the mother formulated her own hopes, when the children were a year and ten months old, by saying: "Oh well . . . . I am leaving it up to them, but I would like for both of them to go to college and university, and have some kind of career. That's what I would like for both of them. . . . As long as they get their high school, at least my daughter. My son, it's almost essential, since he will be earning a living for the rest of his life." This standpoint represents the opinion of many parents who encourage education and career plans to a stronger degree for boys than for girls. By the time the twins were five years and nine months of age, they expressed clearly different goals for the future. According to their mother's report:

> I found that my son, he chose very masculine things like a fireman or a policeman or something like that. He wanted to do what daddy does, work where daddy does, and carry a lunch kit, and drive a car. And she didn't want any of those things. I asked her, and she said she wanted to be a doctor or a teacher. And I asked her, well, did she have plans that maybe some day she'd get married, like mommy? She'll get married some day—she wasn't too worried about that. She didn't think about that too much, but she wants to be a doctor. But none of the things that she ever wanted to be were like a policeman or a fireman, and that sort of thing never appealed to her. So I felt that in a way that's a good sign. . . . I think, it's nice if your boy wants to be a policeman or a fireman or something and the girl wants to do girl things like a doctor, or teaching, or something like that, and I've tried to show them that it's very good. . . .

The girl had many tomboyish traits, such as abundant physical energy, a high level of activity, stubbornness, and being often the dominant one in a girls' group. Her mother had tried to modify her tomboyishness: ". . . of course, I've tried to teach her not to be rough . . . she doesn't seem to be as rough as him . . . of course, I discouraged that. I teach her more to be polite and quiet. I always wanted those virtues. I never did manage, but I'm going to try to manage them to—my daughter—to be more quiet and ladylike." From the beginning the girl had been the dominant twin. By the age of three, her dominance over her brother was, as her mother described it, that of a mother hen. The boy in turn took up for his sister, if anyone threatened her.

The examples of different rearing practices towards girls and boys here presented, are by no means a complete sample of the cues and reinforcements parents offer to their children. Most parents give them without conscious effort, routinely. It is unusual to have a mother to be as observant, and as good a reporter as this woman. Her husband, by contrast, was less alert in observing and reporting his own actions and behavior towards his daughter and his son, although he also was reinforcing different behavior in each one of his children. He is more typical than his wife in being relatively inarticulate regarding sex differences in rearing. He was more inclined to stress the idea of lack of favoritism in his responses to both children.

Rearing of a Genitally-Malformed, Sex-Reassigned Infant as a Girl

The diagnosis established for this baby born with ambiguous genitalia was that of genetic male (46,XY) with a hypospadiac microphallus. The phallus was 1 cm long, so small as to resemble a slightly enlarged clitoris, and like a clitoris, it did not carry a urinary canal. The urinary opening was at the base of this organ in approximately the female position. The scrotum was incompletely fused in the midline, but each half of it contained a palpable testis.

Though a female sex assignment was suggested to the parents at the time of birth, the suggestion was revoked after a few days. A specialist consultant, on the basis of the presence of testes, had decided that the child should live as a boy, despite the absence of a penis. Thenceforth, the parents lived through several months of indecision, while medical opinions differed as to the wisdom of assigning the baby as a boy. By the time the child was seventeen months old, following the necessary consultations, a decision was finalized to reassign the child as a girl. The first stage of surgical feminization of the genitalia was successfully completed. The second, vaginoplasty, would follow in teenage, after pubertal growth and feminization of the body shape by means of estrogen replacement therapy.

Both parents were in their late twenties when they had their second child, at which time the older brother was twenty-two months of age. The older boy had been born with a defect of the penis, a second degree hypospadias, which had been successfully repaired.

At the time of sex reassignment, the parents were given the same type of advice and counseling as indicated in the preceding case example, with particular attention to what to tell the older brother (Money, Potter, and Stoll, 1969). He needed to know that by no caprice of fate would a reassignment of sex be required of him.

The followup since sex reassignment has been nearly three years. Meantime the parents have been informative regarding their experience of making the change from rearing a son to rearing a daughter.

The first change was related to different clothes. The baby received a completely new set of female clothing and her hair was allowed to grow long. Another recent immediate change was a completely new set of girl's toys.

Shortly after the sex reassignment, the parents noted a marked change in the brother who was about 3½ years of age at that time. The parents had explained to the boy that his baby brother really was a baby sister and that the doctors had made a mistake. Subsequently, they showed him the surgically feminized genitalia and he had no difficulty in accepting the sex reassignment. The father reported: "My wife tells me, she has noticed a marked difference in his behavior towards his new sister . . . she sees a very evident degree of protectionism, now, on his part towards his sister, and a marked tendency to treat her much more gently. Whereas, before, he was just as likely to stick his foot out and trip her as he went by, he now wants to hold her hand to make sure she doesn't fall." The parents were not aware of making a special point that their son should treat his sister differently from the time she had been a boy. The only reason they could think of for the change in his behavior was that he copied other boys' behavior towards their sisters.

Two months after the sex reassignment, the mother reported that she and her husband thought the girl had really changed in her ways and had become much more feminine. They allowed that it may have something to do with their own perception, but that they thought it was a clear-cut, objective observation. The father described at that time his own feelings: "It's a great feeling of fun for me to have a little girl. I have completely different feelings towards this child as a girl than as a boy." He had noticed a change in his behavior towards his daughter compared to his son: "I treat my son quite differently—wrestling around, playing ball." He said that he had done the same with the second child before sex reassignment. Now he avoided such things with the girl. He attempted to distinguish between "things you associate with fun for boys, and things for girls."

During a follow-up visit when the child was two years and three months old, the mother reported that her daughter imitated many things from her such as doing dishes, cooking, kitchen work on her own kitchen sink and, in general, activities that are related to the woman's household role. At the same time, the child participated in boys' play activities and games together with boys, as do many tomboyish girls. Her mother was concerned whether she should discourage any tomboyish activity to a larger degree than she was doing. She was advised rather to let the child follow her own impulses in order not to evoke a rebellious counterreaction. Similar advice was offered to the mother three months later, when she became concerned that her daughter would say occasionally that she was a boy and not a girl. The mother was told that it would be better not to contradict the child, but to put the child's comment into a girl's perspective by saying that lots of girls wanted to become boys, sometimes.

At age three, the girl's behavior still seemed quite tomboyish to her mother who noticed that she tended to be louder and more aggressive than other little girls they came in contact with. She also still seemed to have more physical energy expenditure. The parents were quite aware that they were perhaps somewhat oversensitive about their daughter's behavior and that they kept comparing her too much with other little girls of her age. At age three, the girl also had clearly feminine wishes. For Christmas, she wanted glass slippers, so that she could go to the ball like Cinderella, and a doll. The parents were delighted. The girl continued to receive typically girlish toys from her parents. She continued more and more to show feminine interests, as in helping her mother.

The father gave an example, when the girl was three years old, of how girls and boys are differently treated with respect to rehearsal of their adult roles as a female or male romantic partner. The family had established the habit of dancing together to the record-player, after the father arrived home from work. The father usually picked his daughter up, or danced with her, holding her close to him, while the boy was doing rock and roll dancing of a more solo type, maybe including his mother as a partner. At first, the girl wanted to copy her brother, but then she began to enjoy the favoritism of dancing with her father.

Regarding toilet habits, the girl tried standing up to urinate (though, because of the genital deformity, the standing position had always been impossible) and had been told that little girls usually sit down on the toilet. At age three, this habit had faded, and the girl preferred to sit down on the toilet.

The two cases of sex reassignment illustrate that parents do indeed have different criteria of what to reinforce in the behavior and responses of boys and girls. These criteria apply to clothing, adornment and general appearance; to body movements and positions; to play and the rehearsal of future roles as romantic partner, and wife and mother, or husband and father; to genital play and sex education, and to academic and vocational choice. Some gender-conforming behavior is openly and explicitly reinforced by adults and other children, whereas in other instances the reinforcements are more subtle and covert.

Cultural Variability of Gender-Dimorphic Behavior in Sexual Partnerships

The members of any society, as participants in its cultural pattern, inevitably perceive some of the dictates of that cultural pattern as eternal verities, and perhaps even as expressions of immutable natural and moral law. The fact is that the canons by which human behavior is regulated are variable to an extraordinary degree, so that the most sacred rules of one society may be the heresies of another. This general principle applies to gender-dimorphism of behavior. For example, male homosexual relationships may be a negation of masculinity in a society like our own. By contrast, oral homosexual relations for the purpose of ingesting semen may be magically esteemed as essential to strength, virility, and growth into manhood, as is the custom among some Kukukuku people of the New Guinea highlands. According to this custom, homosexuality is prescribed for all preadolescent and adolescent boys and young men. Adolescent male homosexuality, along with headhunting, may also be a method of keeping the number of births in balance with the tribal economics of marriage and the bride price.

The point to be made about male homosexuality in the foregoing contradictory cultural extremes is that both the proscription and the prescription of the behavior represent masculine gender-dimorphic behavior. In the one case it is masculine for two males to avoid getting together genitally, and in the other it is equally masculine for them to ensure that they do get together. The key to this apparent paradox lies in the temporal criterion: the society that prescribes homosexuality does not prescribe it for all males all of the time. The society is, therefore, really prescribing bisexuality, for those who must follow the rule of homosexuality must also, at another phase of their lives follow the rule of breeding. The only other way that a society could both survive and prescribe male-male genital sexuality as a form of gender-dimorphic behavior would be by subdividing its males into breeders and nonbreeders. This is the kind of subdivision familiar in our own society with respect to prescribed celibacy in the religious and, in earlier era, with respect to prescribed castration of singers. Harem attendants, in other societies, constitute a similar group.

Another special point about homosexuality as a prescribed gender-dimorphic behavior is that cultural traditions as to what constitutes gender-dimorphic behavior are variable even with respect to the very partnerships upon which the renewal of the generations and the survival of a people depend. Whereas in the lower species the form and sequence of the sexual partnership in mating and reproduction is stereotypically programed, in the human species man's inventiveness edits and elaborates the program.

The variables around which behavioral dimorphism of the sexual partnership may be culturally and traditionally elaborated are as follows

—age: same or disparate

—physique: juvenile, adolescent, or adult

—sex: same or opposite

—kinship: related or not related by blood, clan, or race
—caste or class: same or different
—number: unity or plurality of partnerships
—overlap: sequential or contemporaneous partnerships, or one partnership only.
—span: transient or constant partnerships
—privacy: public or concealed
—accessories: plain or modified by material artifacts, e.g., personal ornament, wedding ring, contraceptive device, etc.

One may apply these ten categories to our own cultural traditions, and specifically in the context of what is happening by way of change in the present era of so-called sexual revolution. On the criterion of age, there has been no change of tradition with respect to a preference for pairing couples of similar age, while a continued tolerance of a few exceptions of age disparity is allowed within the adult years. There is still a rigid rule against juvenile sexual play, for both sexes, more strictly applied to girls than boys, though the age of academic sex education is subject to radical downward revision, amidst sometimes acrimonious social controversy. The taboo against pictures and writings of sex weakens, but the backlash is strong. There is no issue more heated than that of the rights of adolescents and young adults to have sexual partnerships and love affairs premaritally, with or without intention to marry and/or to have children. The trend is toward greater freedom.

Sanctions against homosexuality are being examined and eased, though ambivalently, in favor of consensual agreements between adults, to the neglect of the rights of younger people in this respect. Problems of kinship in mating continue to be singularly unimportant, so long as the incest taboo is respected. The issue of miscegenation is so explosive that it can scarcely be mentioned in public and political discussion, perhaps because it is a foregone conclusion that black-white intermarriage will become routine. Class and caste preferences and distinctions in sexual pairing remain otherwise about the same as ever.

The leading pressure point of change in our society's sexual traditions would seem to be toward a greater plurality of sexual relationships, for females as well as males, on a basis of mutual reciprocity. This change is registered in sequential more often than contemporaneous plurality of relationships, before or after marriage. Even multiple contemporaneous relationships tend to be constant, over a period of time, rather than transient. Despite the increasing option of plurality of partnerships, the preference is still for fidelity, or for episodic monogamy rather than for running more than one affair contemporaneously. However, a new institution, its future still uncertain, is the "swinging scene" of partner exchanging and group sex, coexistent and compatible with contractual marriage and long-term loyalty and emotional allegiance to one partner. Plural relationships are perhaps preferred more by men than women, but there may be an increase in the number of women who have more than one sexual partner, and in the number of partners they have, especially before settling down into the monogamy of marriage.

Coitus itself is still subject to the rule of privacy, though some group sex participants are indifferent to being observed or to engaging in activities with more than one partner simultaneously. Privacy amounting to at least a partial need for concealment applies widely to partnerships outside of marriage, though there is increasing freedom accorded to young adults of both sexes to be frank and open among their own age group about their nonmarital partnerships and living together.

Availability of contraception is undoubtedly the material artifact that underlies the cultural change toward plurality of sexual partnerships, especially for women. However, in the case of serial marriage and divorce, with children to be supported, the legal, economic and vocational emancipation of women is also a major factor.

The use of contraception is not a gender-dimorphic behavioral trait, but the type of device is gender specific. There is still a good deal of ambivalence between the sexes as to which partner should bear the aesthetic, moral, and physiologic responsibility of effecting conception control or timing.

Though there has been a highly visible amount of rejection of gender-dimorphism in the clothing and adornment of sexual partners in a small segment of the adolescent and young adult population, it is very rarely that males and females cannot be distinguished. Thus the change for men to wear their hair long, like women, is accompanied by the change from not baring the skin of the face, like women, but covering it fully with a beard or partially with sideburns or mustache as insignia of sex. Gender dimorphism of appearance cannot be successfully abolished after puberty except by people who assiduously cultivate the art of impersonation.

The ten criteria of dimorphism in sexual partnerships may be applied also to identify and better understand the differences between white or black middle class traditions versus the urban-ghetto and rural black traditions (Money, 1965b) in our own society. There is no difference on the criterion of age-matching, but some difference on the criterion of physique, insofar as pregnancy in black girls soon after the menarche is a stronger cultural tradition. This tradition represents a cultural lag from the days of slavery when females were obliged, even forced, to breed as soon as they reached maturity.

On the criterion of same- or opposite-sexed partnerships, the two traditions are little different, except for tolerance of casual male homosexual relationships in black youths, one of the partners being an obligatory effeminate male homosexual, and the other bisexual. By contrast, black lesbian relationships are perhaps less tolerated.

There is little difference between the two traditions to be noted with respect to kinship, caste or class, number, or overlap. There is a difference with regard to span, which is another example of a cultural lag from the time of slavery. Under slavery there was no marriage because slaves had no legal rights, and marriage is a legal right. Couples who wanted to stay together did so only at the master's will, and were subject to being separated and sold any time at his bidding. Couples owned by different masters might never be able to live in a permanent partnership on the plantation of one of them. Some young people were subject to forced breeding, in the manner of animal husbandry. The very condition of slavery thus favored temporary partnerships, or a series of them.

The system that decreed temporary partnerships was self-consistent with respect to childrearing, for that task was assigned to the grandparental generation, while the strong, young mothers and fathers left the yard to do heavy work.

The relationships of human beings who have personally and emotionally experienced no alternative examples of sexual partnerships to fall back on do not change by legal fiat. Thus, since the emancipation, the partnership system of slavery has lingered on. The master who provided subsistence has been replaced by the Department of Welfare. The old people responsible for childcare are now the young mother's own mother and her partner. The young mother goes out to work by day, probably for low pay that keeps her economically subservient to whites, as under the conditions of slavery. So does the children's father. He may live in the household with the children, or he may make regular visits and continue his sexual relationship with the mother of his child or children, or he may be away, established in another sexual partnership. Young parents may or may not be legally married. By tradition, they are more likely to settle down into a permanent partnership later in life, when they take on the old people's role and responsibility, staggered across the generations, of caring for the young ones. Without design or plan, they effectively maintain a system that, in legal technicality, might be called the system of illegitimate grandparenthood.

The criterion of copulatory privacy is not particularly different in black and white cultures, though the older black generation may be more able to turn a blind eye, so to speak, and provide privacy at night for young people, despite crowded living conditions. Accessories of partnerships also do not differ fundamentally, though there is some divergence regarding the basis of ambivalence concerning the use of birth control devices. This ambivalence has recently been given expression among some black groups in the political catch-cry of black genocide, while others prefer birth control and planned parenthood.

The black system of sexual dimorphism in sexual partnerships is a viable system, equal in status to that of the white middle class, if not in some ways superior and better adapted to modern urban conditions. But it is at odds with the majority system and so is branded as immoral and inferior, and is not bulwarked and supported by the economic institutions of our society. Therefore it cannot compete on equal terms to become the majority system—for the present, at least.

Gender-Dimorphic Traditions in Sexual Partnerships among the Batak People of Sumatra

As compared with our own changing traditions, the culturally defined gender-dimorphic behavior of sexual partnerships among the Batak people of Lake Toba, in northern Sumatra, is noteworthy for its relatively unchanging tradition, for its prescription of male homosexual relationships among boys and young men, and for its very strict requirement of unbreakable monogamy (Money, unpublished data).

The Batak cultural tradition permits an age difference in a sexual partnership spanning an age-spectrum in physique from puberty to young manhood, but only in partnerships that are homosexual, not heterosexual. In late childhood, it is not decent for children to stay sleeping in their parent's single-roomed house. A girl takes her sleeping mat to the home of a widow or an old woman who accomodates about half a dozen girls who range in age from puberty to late adolescence. If these girls make homosexual partnerships, the information is not disclosed to males, as talk about sexual activities, except between husband and wife, is taboo between the sexes. In the absence of a woman investigator, no certain information could be obtained with female informants.

At the same age as a girl begins to sleep away from the family home, a boy joins a group of a dozen to fifteen males, his own age and older, who sleep in a boys' house specially constructed for them. There he learns from adolescents and young unmarried men how to participate in paired homosexual play with them or with other boys beginning puberty: primarily mutual masturbation of penis held against penis, maybe anal coitus, but never fellatio. All members of the group may become one member's partner, in rotation. Relationships are not necessarily unobserved, but they are always in pairs, not in larger groups. Partnerships among group members do not involve falling in love, but they are constant up to the point where a young man opts to leave the group by marrying. No man is permitted to remain a bachelor.

When he is ready to marry, a young man asks his close friend to join him in a prescribed etiquette of approaching the chosen girl, in order to sound out her interest in him. The friend also approaches the prospective bridegroom's own family, to see if they have the wealth to pay the bride price proposed by the girl's family, and to put on a wedding festival.

The young man in search of a wife narrates the procedure of his courtship to his companions in the boys' house. Once married, he discloses details about sexual intercourse. In this way information is transmitted down the generations, and a young adolescent is prepared to anticipate his graduation from the era of homosexual experience to heterosexual falling-in-love and marriage.

The homosexual era in adolescence, by sequestering of the sexes, ensures that young women will be virgins until married. The sanctions against premarital sex are stringent, so that a girl who is discovered in transgression probably commits suicide. Once a marriage is effected, the husband discontinues homosexuality, though men away on working parties in the jungle may temporarily resume it.

By contrast with the allowable age disparities in homosexual partnerships, the heterosexual partnership is formed between people of like age in young adulthood, or else the girl may be younger, in her teens, than the man, in his twenties. The relationship between the pair may be as close as cousins, but there is no special kinship obligation in the choice of a partner. There is a preference for partnerships within the racial-linguistic group. Marriage is the first and only heterosexual partnership. Neither party is permitted additional heterosexual partnerships, except for remarriage after the early death of one of the spouses. A marriage cannot otherwise be broken. Being married is, of course, publicly announced. The coital relationship of marriage is, by convention, private and unobserved, except that young children may awaken when the parents are copulating. They then must not disclose their observation, but ignore it. According to the formalities of the culture, they learn about sex not at home, but from their adolescent and young adult friends.

These cultural traditions of a lakeside people in Sumatra have been able to survive intact for an unspecified number of generations, but now, under the impact of cultural contact through education and broadcasting, there are signs that they are about to yield to change.

Gender-Dimorphic Traditions in Sexual Partnerships among the Marind Anim people of New Guinea

Yet another culture with sex segregation and an institutionalized phase of homosexuality is that of the Marind Anim, a headhunting people of Southern New Guinea. Colonial influences have brought about changes in their way of life, as compared with what is reported here on the basis of the retrospective researches of van Baal (1966), but there are more isolated tribes in the mountains whose similar customs remain relatively unchanged (Gajdusek, unpublished field notes).

The Marind Anim live in small villages in different territorial groups according to a clan-system. The men are hunters, fishermen, and gardeners. Women and men live segregated, even after being married. Women sleep in women's houses located not too far distant from the men's houses, where their husbands sleep. Most of the domestic and social life between the sexes occurs outside, in the space between the houses. A husband enters the women's house only if he needs something from his wife and the same is true for a married women who wants to enter the men's house. Unmarried young people refrain from entering the house where members of the other sex sleep. Marital sexual relations are apparently always outside in the bush.

A married woman expecting a baby moves away from the women's house shortly before delivery, to live in a specially prepared maternity hut outside of the village. Her mother might join her, and her husband often moves into the vicinity until the child is born. When the baby is six to eight months old, husband and wife return to the village to have the child officially included in the community with a name-giving ceremony. Boys are more welcome and occasional infanticide of females has been reported.

Early childhood sex play is freely accepted, as is childhood nudity. Older people, when they play with young children, might touch their genitalia. Sex segregation starts some time between 4 to 5 and 7 to 8 years of age, with the boy joining his father in one of the men's houses. In middle childhood, boys and girls still run about together and play at their favorite playground on the beach. Sex segregation gradually progresses with girls preferring their mother's company in the house and garden, and boys spending more time with other male age-mates and their fathers.

Strict segregation of the sexes starts in early adolescence when the first signs of puberty occur. From then on, adolescent boys and girls are supposed to be completely apart during day and night. The adolescent boy leaves the village and the men's house early in the morning to spend his day in the *gotad*, the boy's house, which usually consists of a long platform under a roof, located in the bush. At night, the adolescent boy returns to the men's house, not to his father's side, however, but to that of his mentor, his *binahor-evai*, who might be his maternal uncle or another relative. It is the boy's duty to assist his binahor-evai in gardening and hunting, and to be instructed in the strategy and tactics of head hunting. The gotad is a favorite place also for married men, where they meet and discuss matters they do not want women to overhear. The gotad is also a place where boys may masturbate and have homosexual relations with their own age-mates or with older men. Homosexual relations are rumored to also take place sometimes at special ceremonies.

The adolescents' mentors are always a married couple, the binahor-evai and his wife, the *binahor-wah*, for the boy; and the *yarang-evai* and the *yarang-wah*, for the girl. The boy moves away from his father's side in the men's house when he is given binahor mentors or parents. He and his binahor-evai usually have a homosexual relationship including masturbation and anal intercourse.

The girl stays at her yarang-wah's home after she is given yarang parents. The yarang-wah watches over the adolescent girl's development, expects her assistance in gardening, and instructs the girl in hairdo and ornamentation. There is no evidence of a female homosexual relationship.

With marriage, kinship rules come into effect. Sister-exchange often occurs. The husband's family who get a new young female, namely the daughter-in-law, give in exchange a sister of their son to the daughter-in-law's family. The frequency of adoption was high in order to be able to provide an exchange partner for a son.

The young couple are approximately of the same age. Even young widowers usually are not allowed to marry again, because they are already above the age-limit. The young boys and girls themselves apparently have some say about whom they are going to marry: sex segregation of adolescents is not completely effective. Young girls promenade around near the gotad and boys and girls sometimes meet at night on the beach. A girl and a boy may have secret premarital sexual relations together in the bush, and also exchange some ornaments. However, the taboo against a child out of wedlock is rigid, so that any child born to an unmarried girl must not be allowed to live. An illegitimate baby is believed to be a child of the totem ancestors, a *dema* child and unfit to live.

Shortly before a young man marries, he returns from the gotad to the village and joins the group of adult men. Once married, he no longer must obey his binahor-evai. The same holds true for the girl and her yarang-wah. After the wedding ceremony, a few old women take the bride to an outside spot in the village, where sheets of eucalyptus bark are spread out and where sexual intercourse will take place. The bride must have sexual intercourse first with the male members of her husband's clan before the groom is allowed to copulate with his young wife. Sometimes this type of wedding night might extend over several nights. Supposedly it is not a particularly satisfying experience for the woman. This kind of sequential group sex with one woman and several men (the *otiv-bombari*) is repeated at various intervals, for instance, when the woman returns from her maternity seclusion after delivery of her baby, and on other ceremonial occasions.

Extramarital sexual relations are not confined to occasions of the otiv-bombari, but happen quite frequently, for example, if one of the husband's friends comes to visit, or in an exchange of favors between the husband and another man, who might have made a gift of tools or food.

Apart from this custom, most marriages are monogamous and break up rarely. The rule is apparently that affection and love exist between the spouses, and the husband may get violently jealous if his wife should have secret sexual relations with a man without prearrangements and the husband's consent.

Extramarital heterosexual relations are not supposed to become love affairs. They have the character of a ritual. The birth rate is low. Otiv-bombari are supposed to make women fertile. They are also used to collect semen, for semen is considered the essence of life, health and prosperity. Semen discharged from the vagina is ritually prized. After an otiv-bombari it is collected in a coconut bowl to be used in food or medicine, and for body creams. If a woman does not become pregnant, she is the preferred female for an otiv-bombari, to increase her fertility. Women may complain about the otiv-bombari sessions, but do not refuse them through fear of otherwise being infertile.

Along with the experience of the institutionalized phase of homosexuality and frequent extramarital sexual partnerships, marriage is desired by every young man. Those who remain bachelors are the exception and are pitied by the others. Being married means to participate in heterosexual relations with one's own wife as well as other men's wives. It gives prestige, socially. At the same time, homosexual relations remain available with boys and youths in the gotad or perhaps at occasional special ceremonies. Parallel homosexuality for the wives is not customary.

Analyzed according to the schematic categories of gender-dimorphic behavior in sexual partnerships, the Marind-Anim culture can be summarized thus: Sameness of age is a strict requirement for young people getting married. They are thus at a parallel stage of physical maturity, most usually adolescent. Marriage conforms to kinship rules, the husband and wife being from a different clan or subclan. Marriage is monogamous and a constant partnership, but both the husband and wife have extramarital, heterosexual partnerships also. These extramarital partnerships are not secret. They are sequential and transient. They occur on prescribed occasions, including a ceremonial one when many men have intercourse with one woman, or when the husband has a friend visiting. Marital coitus is typically kept private, and usually performed in the bush. Gender-dimorphic artifacts or accessories in the sexual partnership do not include contraceptive devices, population growth being limited by infanticide and head-hunting. Contemporaneously with marriage and heterosexual relations, men have also homosexual relations with young and adolescent boys while the younger ones are passing through an institutionalized phase of homosexuality. Here then one has a society in which the men but not the women are bisexual in experience, with some overlap from the homosexual to the heterosexual phase. Exclusive or obligatory homosexuality is lacking.

Gender-Dimorphic Traditions in Sexual Partnerships among a Melanesian People

There is a partial redundancy which is intentional in presenting this Melanesian culture that shares in common with the Batak and Marind-Anim cultures the tradition of prescribed male homosexuality prior to marriage and breeding. The three societies are spaced across approximately one sixth of the earth's circumference and have been autonomous and uninfluenced by one another presumably for thousands of years. Each of them obviously has a viable way of life. Their ways of life were recorded independently by observers who were not influenced by one another. Their traditions of sexual-dimorphism of behavior, which differ so greatly from those of our own culture, must be acknowledged by the scientists of our own culture—acknowledged not as fortuitous behavioral quirks, sins, or pathologies but as manifestations of potentially universal human behavior. This must be taken into account before any theory can be satisfactorily formulated to explain human sexuality and sex differences, whether from the point of view of genetics, prenatal hormones, postnatal hormones, the prenatally programed brain, or the postnatal brain programed by way of contingency learning.

Davenport (1965) and his wife, who studied this Melanesian people, chose to leave them anonymous by fictitiously naming their village East Bay, a large district on an unidentified Pacific Island. As Davenport tells of them, the people of East Bay are prosperously endowed with more agricultural resources than they need for themselves, so that they are able to export. Some individuals or their families are in the position of accumulating enough wealth to pay high bride prices for women brought from outlying islands. Men in East Bay outnumber women, with no known cause for this disparity, so that bringing women from another island helps to even the sex ratio.

As observed by Davenport and his wife, East Bay is a society in which children, wearing no clothes until the age of puberty, are allowed overt sex play in the early years of childhood. Toddlers of both sexes frequently finger and manipulate their genitalia, with little attempt on the part of the parents to discourage it, until they can talk and understand. From age four on, the parents' attitude changes and becomes somewhat different for boys and girls. Boys are made fun of for having an erect penis. They continue to play with it, nonetheless. At the same age, girls are severely scolded for touching their genitalia in public. Soon they cease to do so.

Girls are treated very differently from boys not only regarding sex play. From the time that children can walk, boys and girls begin to lead a different life. While boys are allowed to run freely all over the village, girls always stay with their mothers and older sisters who are engaged in household and garden work. Boys pursue outdoor, rough-and-tumble activities and form play gangs. While grabbing and pinching of their genitalia is part of their play among themselves, from age four on they do not touch the girls' genitalia any more, nor vice versa. From age five on, the taboo extends to not being allowed to touch a member of the opposite sex at all, finally resulting in the generalized sex-avoidance behavior of adults, with strict rules on who can meet and talk to whom in public.

Until early adolescence, both girls and boys are completely naked most of the time. In spite of their nudity, there is little evidence of heterosexual play, except sometimes between a sister and a brother, which, if it occurs, is immediately discouraged. The separation of the sexes and their involvement in completely different activities helps them to avoid breaking the rules of forbidden touch and sex play between girls and boys.

From middle childhood until early adolescence, boys rehearse and learn activities expected from them later as adult males, and girls become proficient in carrying out female duties. During this time, boys learn to shoot their bows, to fish, surf, and canoe. Girls learn to take care of the household and garden and to look after babies.

Sometime in early adolescence, between ages eleven and fifteen, a ceremony is performed for a boy and sometimes also for a girl. The meaning is quite different for both sexes. The boy has now the status of a young man, and will change his residence from his family's dwelling to the men's house. For the girl, the ceremony also signifies the threshold of young womanhood, but with no implication of change of residence.

Since heterosexual interactions are strictly forbidden, and even are considered harmful at this period of adolescence until young adulthood, premarital heterosexual relations usually do not occur. By contrast, masturbation in privacy is encouraged as a normal sexual outlet for both boys and girls at this stage. Boys typically go through a phase of homosexual relations. There are two kinds of male homosexual relations. One type applies to two adolescent youths of the same age and physical development who live in the men's house. No kinship or class rules come into effect in these adolescent homosexual partnerships. The partner can be a friend or a brother. The two engage in mutual masturbation and anal intercourse in privacy in the bush, and sometimes in the men's house at night.

The second type of homosexual relationship may exist between an older man and a younger boy, often too young to be living in the men's house yet. This relationship is age and physique disparate. It also is expressed sexually in privacy, usually in the bush. The only obligations of kinship to obey are related to the incest taboo. A father will not have a homosexual relationship with his son. However, the father's friend may.

Both types of homosexual relationships are completely acceptable and openly discussed. While mutual masturbation and anal intercourse are considered normal for these relationships, any type of oral-genital intercourse is unknown.

The data on female sexual activities indicate that girls and young women have no comparable phase of homosexuality. Their only substitute for heterosexual activities is self-masturbation.

Marriages are arranged by the boy's and girl's relatives and the future bridegroom's family has to provide an appropriate bride-price. The arrangements can be made at all ages of the children, from infancy on. However, the girl and boy have something to say about their future husband or wife at the time of marriageable age. Marital sexual enjoyment is considered a very important part of marriage, so that the girl's or boy's doubt that the selected partner is sexually attractive to her, or him, is a valid reason for the parents to call all negotiations off.

Usually people who get married are of the same age group. The girl is typically 18 or 19 years old, and the boy about 20. Because men outnumber women, it sometimes happens that there are not enough girls, so that marriages are also arranged between an older widow and a younger man. If the family of the young man can afford it, a bride from another island may be sought, but never do girls become brides of men from other islands. Sometimes it also happens that older widowers seek the marriage of a young girl, thus aggravating the shortage of young single girls.

After the marriage ceremony, the husband leaves the men's house and moves with his wife usually to his father's or brother's house. Typically, the newly married couple has difficulty in being at ease with each other, since they are not accustomed to being together as young people of the same age and opposite sex. As soon as the first signs of pregnancy occur, the young couple establish their own household in the village.

Sexual intercourse during marriage is considered highly pleasurable and is performed frequently, especially during the first years of marriage. The reports on marital sex include extensive foreplay in which both husband and wife actively engage. Coital positions are typically either the woman lying on her back and her husband being on top of her face to face, or both partners lying on their sides, a position that is typically used during the late stages of pregnancy. As in homosexual relations, oral-genital intercourse is unheard of in husband-wife relations.

Married men often show bisexual behavior, having heterosexual relations with their wives and some extramarital homosexual relations with a younger boy. They typically value heterosexual relations as more satisfying, though in some cases as equally enjoyable as homosexual intercourse. Obligatory or exclusive homosexuality with no interest in heterosexual intercourse is unheard of. So is transvestism.

Heterosexual relations are typically very satisfactory with no occurrence of ejaculatio praecox, frigidity, or other forms of sexual malfunction. Women become less interested in having sex after having borne several children. Marital intercourse then becomes less frequent. Before colonial administrators began to interfere, concubines were sometimes brought from other islands. They would have sexual relations with one or a group of married men in sequential partnerships. These girls were well accepted by the wives who considered them as their adopted daughters, and raised any children that might have been born to them while they were having sexual relations with the women's husbands. The concubine served also as a substitute sexual partner during the times of sexual abstinence which were required during menstruation, during a brief period after suspected pregnancy, to avoid twinning, and for one month after delivery of a new baby.

The only known method of birth control is coitus interruptus which is frequently practiced in order to allow a two-year interval between the children, and so as not to endanger the wife's life because of too many pregnancies and deliveries during a short time.

The role of a concubine did not conflict with the role of the wife. The concubine typically slept in the men's house and had no rights in the family dwelling. She was not allowed to prepare food for the husband which was the prerogative of the wife. She had generally no rights and could be sold any time. Usually, the career of a concubine ended in her becoming a wife herself by being sold to an inhabitant of another less wealthy island.

Summarized according to the categories of sexual partnership listed above, East Bay traditions are as follows: The people usually marry partners of approximately the same age and developmental physique, and according to a matching system decided upon by their kin. For the wife, the relationship is typically constant and with only one man. For the husband, there may be a plurality of partnerships extending from the partnership with his wife to extramarital homosexual partnerships of disparate age. In very rare cases, the husband takes a second wife, so that the marriage becomes polygamous, or quasipolygamous with a concubine.

Adult sexual relations are usually in private. Sometimes children sleeping close to their parents observe them having coitus. They are then instructed not to look. However, sexual matters are discussed in the family with complete frankness, and children of five or six years are rather completely knowledgeable on sexual matters.

This is a society with an institutionalized phase of sex segregation and homosexuality among prepubertal and pubertal youths, adolescents and young men. The outcome is heterosexuality or bisexuality with no obligatory homosexuality, no transvestism, and an absence of other sexual deviances.

Gender-Dimorphic Traditions in Sexual Partnerships among the Pilagá

The Pilagá Indians live near the Pilomayo River in the Gran Chaco of Argentina. Their gender-dimorphic traditions in sexual partnerships sound familiar, in comparison with those of our own society, insofar as the Pilagá do not rear their boys for an institutionalized phase of homosexuality. They sound unfamiliar, however, insofar as the Pilagá have no taboo on the rehearsal of adult sexual activity in the play of childhood. In this respect, they unambivalently prepare their children for adult heterosexuality.

Information on the Pilagá was collected by Henry and Henry (1944) in a small village of 127 inhabitants, 37 of them children under fifteen years of age. For about three months of each year, when the wild fruits and fish on which they depended became scarce, the villagers suffered semistarvation.

The data on Pilagá childhood play and sexual partnerships are here organized according to the same schema of variables used in the preceding four sections.

As reported, sexual relations are formed usually between people of the same age. Juvenile sex play up to the age of five years includes play between children of the same sex. Boys masturbate and play with each other sexually openly in public. Girls masturbate against one another in public.

From age five on, sexual interactions are typically between children of the opposite sex. Girls lie down with little boys of their own age, and the two may go through some of the movements of coitus. Forms of heterosexual coital play, along with masturbation, continue until age twelve.

There is no taboo on heterosexual activities among young adults. A partner may be from the same or another village. Young women usually have several partners before they get married. The plurality of relationships before marriage is sequential rather than contemporaneous. The duration of premarital partnerships appears usually to be transient and does not have to follow any particular rules of class or kinship.

Men outnumber women by far and have a difficult time finding sexual partners. Thus, they are generally more eager than women to get married. No Pilagá child is allowed to be born without a father, so that any pregnancy before marriage must be aborted. Contraception is not in use.

Women not only have the upper hand in the choice of sexual partners, but also of a husband. In the choice of a husband, kinship rules have to be obeyed. These rules, related to the incest taboo, forbid marriage between two people from the same village, since all inhabitants in one village consider themselves relatives. Thus, a woman chooses her husband from another village. The married man moves and settles among his wife's people in her village. In their wives' families, the husbands take the place of the young men who move away into other villages when they get married. Men are the fishermen in the family and thus the main supporters. During the time of pregnancy, the wife has to move to her husband's village and family. Both marital partners dislike leaving their own people to live either permanently or for a short time with the other partner's family. The emotional bond of marriage does not compensate for this dislike of leaving one's own people. Generally, the Pilagá live in large households comprised of several families, each recognizing itself as a family unit with private property rights.

In spite of the unfavorability of the sex ratio for men and the woman's upper hand in partner choice, the status of women is inferior in many aspects of their lives. Women are considered weak and of less value. Female infanticide had earlier been practiced. The Pilagá women are even deprived of a belief that they share in conception, since it is believed that the man's ejaculation projects a complete homunculus into the women, which grows in the woman, until ready to come out.

The marriages are as a rule monogamous, since the Pilagá women do not tolerate any co-wives, partly owing to the fact that a husband with two wives would have to divide his time to live in two different villages, except in the rare event of marrying two women from the same villge.

Regarding privacy of sexual relations, the adults have sexual intercourse at night, without any attempt at concealing it. The only strict restriction on sexual interaction exists from the sixth month of pregnancy until the baby can walk. The Pilagá believe that intercourse during pregnancy will kill the baby. Women also do not nurse two of their own children at once, and they believe that, if a child is weaned before it can walk, the child will not eat and will, therefore, die.

Institutionalization of gender-dimorphic behavior in heterosexual partnerships even in the play of childhood does not, among the Pilagá, have an adverse effect on their adult sexual lives. Quite to the contrary, there is no evidence of any sexual psychopathology.

Gender-Dimorphic Traditions in Sexual Partnerships among the Yolngu of Arnhem Land

The Yolngu are the Aboriginal people of the central north coast of Australia. They have in the last half century come in from their nomadic, hunting, and gathering life to live in small seashore settlements where the first generation of children can go to school. The information here presented was gathered in one of these settlements, Galiwinku, Elcho Island (Money, Cawte, Bianci, and Nurcombe, 1970).

The sexual tradition in Yolngu culture is a heterosexual one in which children grow up knowing their adult heterosexual roles and occasionally rehearsing them in play. The restrictions imposed on them are not on sexual behavior itself, but on who may be the partner not only in sexual activity but even in general conversation.

Two generations ago, in their walkabout life, the Yolngu built no houses, owned no other possessions than what they could carry, and wore no clothes. Today only the infants and young children stay naked, and do so at least until they toilet train themselves, or later. Many arrive at the preschool unclothed, and boys and girls all go under the shower there together, without paying attention to nudity. No Yolngu child is able to stay unaware of the anatomical difference between the sexes.

Young children, at around the ages of four to six, might sometimes be seen as they lie down to take a nap, making the thrusting movements of sexual intercourse. For example, a group of children might be having their nap in the preschool, when a boy presses against his neighbor, thrusting. Or two young children might be together, around the campfire where the family sleeps, and enact the thrusting of intercourse. The culturally appropriate response of older people is to laugh, and to consider the activity as cute. Children usually do not see adults have intercourse, as the adults seek privacy in the bush or in the darkness. The young children may learn by imitating children older than themselves, who learn from still older children who make a sport of spying on teenagers who may make illicit partnerships in the bush.

The criteria of sexual pairing follow a rigid set of totemic-kinship rules after a child reaches the age of eight or nine years, which is the time when a boy has his circumcision ceremony. The system of rules dictates which boys and girls may or may not talk together, and who might be eligible to marry one another. But marriages are decided by the even more implacable rules of the promise system. It is decided even before birth who should be a child's mother-in-law. For the boy, this woman is usually his mother's brother's wife. Her daughters will be his promise girls and, the system being polygamous, they all will come to him, after attaining the age of menarche, as wives. When a man dies, his wives traditionally become the wives of his brother, though today some insist on remaining alone with their children.

During the middle childhood years, children may sometimes engage in sexual play. Heterosexual play is unlikely, and so is homosexual play between boys. The sexual play between girls is not genuinely homosexual, for it occurs as an improvisation in a game of house. When the time comes for the mother and father to have intercourse, then one girl improvises a penis with a piece of stick, and puts it in the vagina of the other. This kind of rehearsal seems to be a cultural imperative in support of the promise system which requires that a young teenaged girl be able to perform in coitus with a man whom she may possibly never have seen before, who could be three or four times her age, and with whom she will never have the experience of falling in love. Should a girl be taken prepubertally by her older promise man (in lieu of a bride price), then sex with her would be confined to his training of her vagina in digital masturbation ("finger-dala"), until after the age of menarche. Only then would penile intromission begin.

In former times infants might be pacified by fondling of their genitals, but this practice is not obvious today. Self-masturbation in childhood is seldom heard of, and quite possibly does not occur in young adulthood or later. It is only jokingly acknowledged and not observed in teenaged boys, and apparently does not occur in teenaged girls.

Young people have love affairs which create many problems, for the lover is always someone else's promise boy or promise girl. The man to whom a girl is promised may take revenge, which in the old days meant the death of his rival by spearing. In this way the culture institutionalized love and death, reduced the population of males, and maintained a balance of females that stabilized the system of polygamy.

For young men who have no wife and no promise girl, the culture is inadequate in providing alternatives. Possibly his older brother may allow him to establish a partnership with one of his several wives. In former times there also were infrequent ceremonial celebrations (kunapipi), lasting several days, during which there was a relaxation of sexual rules, so that everyone, men and women, had a chance of having intercourse.

The promise system is not holding up well in today's era of acculturation, nor is the system of polygamy; but no alternative has yet been arrived at. In the past, the system obviously did hold up, for the society did not become extinct. How well a woman adjusts to polygamy today, over and beyond the fact that she adjusts to copulating and breeding within the system, is difficult for a male investigator to ascertain. There is a taboo against women talking women's talk with men. However, it appears that some women do have a joyous sex life with their husbands, and others do not. The sexual problems of Yolngu women were essentially the problems of sexual apathy, frigidity, or joylessness, and the despair of having more children than their health, often chronically impaired by anemia caused by untreated hookworm, permitted them to cope with. There were no other ascertained instances of psychosexual pathology or sexual behavior disorders in females.

The male counterpart of sexual apathy and frigidity in the female, namely, apathy, impotence, and/or premature ejaculation, did not present itself as a problem. To all intents and purposes, these complaints do not exist among Yolngu men, unless in association with pathological depression in rare cases. The men also did not complain about the burden of too many children. On the contrary, they were buoyantly aware of the fact that, thanks to the high birth rate and low mortality rate of life on the mission station, the Yolngu are no longer doomed to the threat of extinction that before World War II seemed so imminent. Men have no direct responsibility for child care, but fathers permit babies an indulgent amount of physical proximity when they are resting together with their infants, and they are solicitously attentive to them.

Among adult men, the reported incidence of any form of sexual behavior pathology was extremely rare. There was no reported or observable incidence of effeminate homosexuality among grown men, nor of homosexual preference of partners among noneffeminate men. Sexual activity between two males was occasionally reported, but only in connection with prepuberty and adolescence. The older boys involved were socially rebellious in various ways. They were as open in reporting this activity as any other play activity. Their game was one in which a partner, usually a younger boy, would acquiesce to taking a feminine coital position in interfemoral, but probably not anal or oral intercourse, for the reward of nothing more than being accepted by the older boys who held prestige in his eyes.

Summarized according to the schematic categories employed for the cultures already presented, gender-dimorphic traditions regarding sexual partnerships among the Yolngu do not sanction love affairs between young people who are age concordant. There are no sanctions against sexual partnerships with whites, but whites are too few for interracialism to become an issue. Marital partnerships may be either age concordant or discordant, with the man being even four times older than the adolescent girl. Marital partnerships are regulated by rigidly strict rules of totemic kinship or class known as the promise system, and they are polygamous. A wife should have no other partnership than with her husband, except at the time of ceremonial festivities which are now dying out. Marriages cannot be dissolved. When her husband dies, the wife becomes the wife of his brother. Partners copulate in private. Infants see one another nude. Children's play may include rehearsal of copulation, though childhood sex is an unostentatious feature of the culture. Apart from its sporadic incidence in the play of some rebellious young adolescent males, homosexual partnerships do not occur. When girls play mothers and fathers, one may play the father, using a piece of stick as a penis substitute. The sexes are clearly differentiated by clothing (shorts or trousers versus dresses); men have haircuts and almost all of them shave. Sexual partners do not know about contraceptive devices.

The straightforward attitude of the Yolngu toward nudity and copulatory play in young children leaves them with no confusion about their own reproductive destiny and sense of identity as male or female. It is here that one may look for an explanation of the freedom of Yolngu people from paraphiliac behavior disorders of any type. Their experience of the social environment in the postnatal phase of gender-identity differentiation evidently does not include the contingencies that foster the development of paraphiliac tendencies, even if a prenatal compliancy or disposition for such should exist.

Comment

The two cases of sex reassignment presented in this chapter demonstrate that gender dimorphic patterns of rearing have an extraordinary influence on shaping a child's psychosexual differentiation and the ultimate outcome of a female or male gender identity.

Dimorphism of rearing need not be rigidly in conformity with the expectations and rules of our own culture of how girls and boys should be reared. Indeed, the five examples of different societies demonstrate that the rearing patterns can widely vary from ours, in particular in the categories of sexual partner interaction. Multiple sexual partnerships may be substituted for monogamy. Openly accepted homosexual and heterosexual play in early childhood, and even an institutionalized phase of homosexuality in adolescence are compatible with a self-sustaining, predominantly heterosexual adult society, with less evidence of individual sexual pathology and disturbance of gender-identity differentiation than in our own culture.

Despite great variability between cultures in the prescription of gender-dimorphic behavior in childhood, adolescence, and adulthood, the existence of gender dimorphism of behavior is itself invariant. The options are not limitless. In the final analysis, culturally prescribed (or prohibited) gender-dimorphic behavior stems from the phyletic verities of menstruation, impregnation, gestation, and lactation. These verities are procreative imperatives, so to speak, in the design of any culture's definition of male and female roles, if that culture is to maintain its membership and survive. They specify that, regardless of peripheral options and alternatives, a well-defined, gender-dimorphic complementarity constitutes the nucleus—the procreative nucleus—of any system of behavior between the sexes. Children growing up in a culture differentiate a gender identity free from ambiguity if the adults of that culture, especially those closest to them, transmit clear and unambiguous signals with respect to the procreative nucleus of gender dimorphic behavior, no matter what the signals with respect to peripheral options may be.

8

GENDER IDENTITY DIFFERENTIATION

Terminology

Gender identity (as already defined in Chapter 1) is the private experience of gender role; and gender role is the public manifestation of gender identity. There is no single term to signify gender identity/role, which is a semantic handicap. Nevertheless, "gender identity" can be read to mean "gender identity/role," unless the context signifies otherwise. It is important to avoid the logical and conceptual fallacy of juxtaposing identity and role, because they are actually facets of the same entity. A good example of this fallacy is the verbal chimera that defines one type of male homosexual as "having a masculine identity juxtaposed against a feminine role, that is a man who gives a masculine impression except that he relates erotically to a male, not a female." Actually, such a person has an identity/role that is partially masculine, partially feminine. The issue is one of proportion: more masculine than feminine. Masculinity of identity manifests itself in his vocational and domestic role. Femininity of identity appears in his role as an erotic partner; it may be great or slight in degree, and it is present regardless of whether, like a woman, he receives a man's penis or, also like a woman, he has a man giving him an orgasm. It goes without saying that the ratio of masculinity to femininity varies among individuals. It may conceivably vary also in the same individual at different points in the life history.

Psychosexual Frailty of the Male

Gender identity, nonetheless, differentiates generally so as to be rather remarkably fixed in adulthood. Typically, it differentiates as primarily or exclusively masculine in boys, and feminine in girls. Possibly, however, differentiation may be unfinished as either completely masculine or completely feminine, but ambiguous instead. It is probably impossible for gender identity to be totally undifferentiated. The same is all but true for the embryonic anlagen of the reproductive anatomy, for in the case of anatomy, arrestment of development as a male is synonymous with development as a female: arrestment of female development results in no genitalia at all. The only rear-end orifice may be a primitive anogenital one, that is to say, a cloaca, or there may be no opening at all, plus multiple internal deformities.

Stated in nontechnical terms, the lesson of embryonic anatomy is that it is easier for nature to make a female than a male. The familiar embryonic and fetal rule is that something must be added to produce a male. Quite possibly, the same paradigm may apply also to gender-identity differentiation, though there is as yet no conclusive proof of this hypothesis. Such evidence as there is comes from sociological and clinical surveys of the comparative incidence of gender identity disorders. Whereas under certain conditions, such as group sex encounters, it seems easier for women than their husbands to have homosexual contacts, more men than women have homosexual relations on an exclusive, full-time, obligative basis, according to present evidence. There is a widespread convergence of data to support an estimated ratio of three or four obligative homosexual males to one such female. The disparity may be even greater. A similar ratio emerges among transexuals who apply for hormonal and surgical sex reassignment.

Homosexuality and transexualism represent incongruities of gender identity. Transvestism is similarly incongruous, but only episodically, during the period of cross dressing. There is also an element of fetishism in male transvestism, insofar as the transvestite's penis is impotent and nonejaculatory, if denied the fetishistic stimulus of female attire. Dependency of orgasm on a fetish object occurs to all intents and purposes exclusively in males, and not in females.

Fetishism, like homosexuality, transexualism, and transvestism, constitutes a paraphilia, but one in which incongruity of the sex of the partner need not necessarily be involved. Most fetishes are woman-related—often items of underwear apparel. The majority of the paraphilias are consistent with heterosexuality. They qualify as unconventional or bizarre augmentations or distortions of gender identity. For example, in exhibitionism, a man's penis is able to erect and ejaculate only if his erotic arousal has first been evoked by the shock and flight of an unknown woman to whom he illicitly exposed his penis. The Peeping Tom, or voyeur, in order to be aroused, is compelled to spy on women who do not expect his presence as they undress. The sadist is compelled to subject an erotic partner to bondage and discipline; the masochist needs to receive it. The rapist assaults his sexual partners, and the lust-murderer slaughters them. A certain few masochists arrange for themselves to be murdered. The undinist or urophiliac depends for his arousal on being urinated upon, or drinking urine. The coprophiliac is similarly dependent on feces. The necrophiliac is enslaved to corpses, the zoophiliac to animals. The scatological telephone caller reaches orgasm by talking "dirty" to an unknown party; the narratophiliac needs to be told erotic tales, and the pictophiliac responds maximally to the printed image. And so on.

The majority of the paraphilias are found as distortions exclusively of man's gender identity, not woman's. Thus they provide still further evidence that nature has more difficulty in differentiating the gender identity of the male than the female. Nature makes more errors in the male. A clue to the explanation can perhaps be found in the fact that the paraphilias of women are not only infrequent but also restricted to the haptic sense—the feel and touch of another woman in homosexuality or the feel and touch of a pet in zoophilia—rather than to the sense of sight or smell. Feel and touch require body contact, which are essential to woman's arousal, whereas man is more responsive to distant stimuli, especially visual stimuli, to initiate erotic arousal. Woman's arousal may also be linked to taking or stealing love or pregnancy substitutes, namely, in kleptomania.

Phyletically, it would appear that, in the human species, nature has ordained the man rather than the woman to be the one who is erotically attracted from a distance. In the birds, it is the other way round. The plumage, and possibly the courtship song, and the courtship dance, attract the female. In many species of mammals, not the visual but the olfactory stimulus (pheromone) is the attractant, and it is the male that is attracted to the female. In man, the sense of smell may play a role, as it has recently been shown to do in the rhesus monkey (see Chapter 11; Herbert, 1970; Michael, Keverne, and Bonsall, 1971), if not for all members of the species, then for some of them. Men who are greatly aroused by cunnilingus, as some are, are possibly responding to vaginal odor.

Pheromones notwithstanding, it would appear that nature has ordained the visual stimulus to be the distance-activator of erotic arousal in mankind, and specifically in man. There is a logic to nature's scheme, for the penis is reproductively useless to the woman unless it erects. The penis could, of course, be permanently erect; or the woman could be endowed with an automatic erection stimulator, applicable on demand. Fondling of the penis to some extent serves this purpose, but not invariably. An important part of nature's scheme does, indeed, seem to be that the man knows that he is ready and capable of erotic performance when he is visually "turned on." Then he signals his erectile competency to the female, who may, or may not, be ready to take advantage of it.

The significance of the visual image in the erotic life of the male is spontaneously made evident to the pubertal boy in the imagery of his wet dreams and masturbation fantasies. The pubertal girl has no experience corresponding to a wet dream. Kinsey's statistics showed, in fact, that women's dreams which incorporate orgasm increase with experience and age through the twenties and thirties, whereas in males they are maximal at the onset of adolescence (see also Chapter 12).

The images of an adolescent boy's wet dreams and masturbation fantasies cannot be commanded at will. They have an autonomy of their own, and present themselves uninvited, much to the chagrin of many a boy who finds himself confronted by images of a paraphiliac nature. He knows that they are socially condemned, and he is mortified by them at the same time as he is rewarded by them as the harbingers of the ecstatic feeling of orgasm.

Biographical Origins of Gender-Dimorphic Imagery

The erotic imagery of puberty is the capstone, so to speak, of the edifice of gender identity. It authenticates what previously was evident, and confirms gender identity as being masculine, feminine, or ambiguous, and as being distorted or not by paraphilia. This imagery is not, however, inaugurated by the hormones of puberty, whether in boys or girls, but simply activated to be more vivid, frequent, insistent, and associated with genitopelvic arousal and orgasm. The origin of images that demonstrate their erotic arousal power at puberty lies earlier in the biography.

In certain cases of paraphilia, it is possible to recognize a connection between the stimulating erotic image and an earlier biographical event. The earlier history may be retrieved only retrospectively, as when, in a particular case, an adult transvestite recalled being punished as a delinquent beginner at school by being forced to put on a girl's dress and to sit next to a girl. His mother, he remembered, later used the same punishment, this time mortifying him by walking him in the street where his friends could ridicule him. Still later she used him as a dressmaker's model for fitting a sport's costume being made for his girl cousin. On that occasion he experienced an enjoyable feeling of excitement, his first awareness that he had, in fact, an addiction for female clothing.

Retrospective biography is notoriously subject to selective editing of memory. Therefore, there is no way of knowing that the young boy didn't invite punishment at school in order to wear a girl's dress. As recalled, the biography could even be completely confabulatory. Yet, there is additional evidence of the mother's implicit collusion and penchant for transvestite males in that, two decades and several boyfriends later, she found the man who had become her second husband asleep in her underclothes.

Another case, briefly alluded to in Chapter 1, avoids the problem of the falsification of recall, for the biography here was documented at age six and again at age sixteen. The boy at age six was awakened, startled, by the presence of his teenaged babysitter lying on him, ejaculating between his thighs. Lacking the necessary sexual knowledge, he could construe his experience only as possibly a would-be murder. Appropriately counseled, he appeared to have escaped psychic trauma. At sixteen, however, he reluctantly managed to request further help. He defined his anxiety as a fear of not having a normal relationship with his girlfriend. His masturbation imagery included an obsessive theme, namely of reenacting the experience of age six, so as to reconstruct exactly what had happened to him. He rejected the girlfriend who wanted him; and he kept importuning the one who denigrated and rejected him—as though to guarantee a self-fulfilling prophecy that he would fail to establish a genuine heterosexual love affair, thus leaving open the door to homosexuality.

Developmental documentation in a biography like this one notwithstanding, there is always a question as to whether the original incident was in some way solicited by an already effeminate little boy. Such a likelihood is reduced in this case by reason of the fact that the teenaged baby-sitter disclosed that he had done the same thing with another still younger child, a girl.

Another degree of confidence in a biography is reached when its special features are not fortuitous in occurrence or timing, but are prospectively predictable. The biographies of many hermaphrodites provide examples, such as the following from the biography of a genetic male hermaphrodite reared as a girl. When this child was born, it was not realized that there was no vaginal opening. By age thirteen, she had no breast development and no menses, but had pubic and axillary hair and had grown tall. The voice was deep, but not remarkable in comparison with the mother's. The hair of the upper lip was darkening and becoming visible. These signs, on the occasion of a general health check-up, eventually led to the diagnosis. The treatment was removal of the undescended testes, female-hormone replacement therapy to induce feminizing puberty, and surgical feminization of the genitalia.

The girl knew that her clitoris was large and wanted it reduced. She wished her breasts would develop, and disliked the hair on her lip. She did not use the concept of masculinization in speaking about herself. Her point of view was that of a girl who had not yet feminized.

Behaviorally, she revealed only three elements in her biography that might be conceived of as unfeminine. First, she had a tomboyish preference for the outdoors and horse-riding rather than sedentary and domestic pursuits, though no more so than many farm-bred girls. Second, she liked the idea of infant care, and expected to raise up a family by adoption; but her spontaneous preference was for babies at the toddler age, rather than as helpless newborns whom she considered she might not handle correctly. Third, she had experienced erotic arousal and clitoral erection from pictorial stimuli, in a manner typical for a boy; but the stimuli were appropriate to a girl, namely, the cute boys in the clothing advertisements of the Sears, Roebuck Catalogue. She had not reached the boyfriend and dating stage. She had experienced no erotic attraction toward girls, and believed that to be not for her.

In this case one has evidence that, whereas the erotic-arousal images of early puberty were independent of genetic and gonadal sex, and also of pubertal hormonal sex, they were in agreement with the biography as determined by rearing. Possibly a prenatal androgenic effect from the fetal testes may have programed the brain to be sexually responsive to visual images, in a way more typical for a boy than a girl, but the life-history determined that the images would be those of boys. What the erotic arousal-potential of these pictures will be under the influence of estrogen remains to be seen. In the case of the patient's sister, older by two years, feminizing hormone did make a difference.

This older sister has the same hermaphroditic diagnosis, except that her clitoris was never enlarged. Before gonadectomy, and while still under the influence of her own androgens, this girl had discovered that she could be erotically and genitally aroused not by pictures but by explicitly sexual and "spicy" narratives. The clitoris would erect, and she might masturbate. Now, under the influence of estrogens, she does not have a clitoral erection and does not masturbate. Her erotic reaction is to "feel warm all over," a reaction that she values neither more nor less than the former one, but equates with it.

Matched Pairs of Hermaphrodites

Informative as they are, even large numbers of case biographies of genetic male hermaphrodites reared as girls do not give the final and conclusive answer as to the postnatal effect of the sex of rearing on gender-identity differentiation. By themselves alone, these biographies might lead one to the hypothesis that the very ambiguity of the hermaphroditic condition predisposes the child to differentiate a feminine identity. For this reason, matched pairs of hermaphrodites, concordant for diagnosis but discordant for sex of rearing are particularly instructive.

Matched pairs of hermaphrodites demonstrate conclusively how heavily weighted is the contribution of the postnatal phase of gender-identity differentiation. To use the Pygmalion allegory, one may begin with the same clay and fashion a god or a goddess. Certain conditions must be met:

(a) It is absolutely prerequisite that the parents have no doubt or ambiguity as to whether they are raising a son or a daughter. Uncertainty, if it exists at the time of birth, must be resolved in such a way that the parents follow the same train of reasoning as the experts who guide them. They then reach the same decision, instead of having to accept an instruction on faith, with no guarantee whether it is correct or in error.

(b) The sooner that the first stages of corrective genital surgery are initiated, the better. Parents need the reassurance of the baby's sexual appearance. They cannot raise a baby as a girl, despite ovaries and a uterus internally, if it has a penis externally—which can happen. Conversely, they cannot raise as a boy a baby that has a urogenital opening in the female position and a phallic organ no bigger than a large clitoris. Relatives and baby-sitters are equally nonplussed and, moreover, gossipy. When the limitations of surgical technique require delays between the progressive stages of surgical reconstruction, the prognosis needs to be given to the parents and, eventually, to the child himself or herself.

(c) At the usual age of puberty, and in concordance with statural growth, the gender-appropriate sex hormones should be administered, estrogen for the girl, and androgen for the boy. Girls with breasts too small can have them enlarged with a silicone implant; and boys without testes can have silicone prosthetic testes implanted.

(d) In age-graded steps, a hermaphroditic child should be kept diagnostically and prognostically informed with suitably simplified concepts and explanations. Ideally, this information will be interconnected with the ordinary sex education of childhood. For example, knowledge of motherhood by pregnancy versus motherhood by adoption will be familiar in advance of prognostications of fertility. Never make prophecies, only probability statements: even the most distance ray of hope should never be extinguished! Moreover, all lay people know examples of unfulfilled medical prophecies, and today's prophecies may be tomorrow's fallacies. For example, the sterility of castration today, may be the fertility of an implanted ovum tomorrow. Children respond with trust when they are entrusted. Prepared with the truth, they rehearse in their fantasies a future that will not bring the anguish of surprise and disillusionment—even a difficult future like the one that will require an artificial penis for vaginal penetration. Uninformed of his medical situation, a child makes guesswork inferences on the basis of what is done to him, or her, and of what is so easily overheard in clinics and examining rooms. Adults claim that they withhold information to protect the child, whereas actually they only spare themselves from their communicational ineptitude and anxiety.

When the foregoing conditions have been met, then it is to all intents and purposes predictable that each member of a matched pair of hermaphrodites, discordant for sex of assignment and rearing, will be discordant also for gender identity. Even if the prediction is not universally valid, then it is frequently so and, in each instance, with remarkable completeness.

In those instances where the prediction falls down, it is common to find a history in which uncertainty as to the sex of the baby at birth was transmitted to the parents and never adequately resolved. Parents whose minds are in doubt about their baby's authentic sex tend to monitor the child's behavior with supervigilance, looking vainly for signs to resolve their doubt. The versatility of childhood behavior leaves them in confusion, not sure whether to reward behavior traditionally concordant with assigned sex, or to discourage it on the chance that other behavior, discordant with assigned sex, should more legitimately be encouraged. In consequence they transmit mixed signals to the child and, above all, are not able to adapt themselves to a girl with tomboyish traits, or a boy who is an unassertive, noncompetitive loner.

Hermaphroditic children who eventually decide that they were wrongly assigned, and request a reassignment, typically have a biography of uncertainty as to their sex of assignment. The biography includes such items as a change of name and declared sex, without change on the birth certificate; overt advice to the parents that the "true sex" will not be evident until puberty; and discordance between the declared sex and the genital anatomy which is allowed to remain surgically uncorrected in childhood.

Hermaphroditic children who make sex reassignment requests may do so, irrespective of genetic and gonadal diagnosis, and they may want to change from boy to girl, or girl to boy. The statistics actually available (Wolf, 1968; Money, 1969) are skewed to an unknown degree. They cannot be taken at face value, because hermaphroditic individuals requesting reassignment are typically those for whom the sex of original assignment was improvised on the basis of an inadequate diagnostic evaluation at birth. When no testes are palpable, neonatally, because they are not present in a female hermaphrodite, or are undescended in a male hermaphrodite, then there is more chance of an improvised assignment as a female than a male. Provided the external genitalia are not surgically corrected, as easily happens under conditions of improvised diagnosis, then the child is likely to grow up with either an ambivalently or incongruously differentiated gender identity. Then, when the diagnosis is finally established correctly, so great may be the tyranny of the gonads in the mind of a physician, that it renders him incompetent to pay attention to the coital capacity of the phallic organ, or to the importance of gender identity. In consequence, he is likely to veto sex reassignment from girl to boy if the gonads are ovaries, and to demand it if they are testes.

Until further evidence might prove otherwise, it thus appears that the prejudices of physicians skew today's hermaphroditic sex reassignment statistics in favor of a change from girl to boy, and in male rather than female hermaphrodites. It would not have been necessary to belabor this point except that some writers still do not understand it (Cappon, Ezrin, and Lynes, 1959; Diamond, 1965; Dewhurst and Gordon, 1969; Zuger, 1970). Their writings become instrumental in wrecking the lives of unknown numbers of hermaphroditic youngsters, by authorizing or denying sex reassignment.

Three Matched Pairs of Biographies

The three pairs of cases herewith presented are chosen because all six are concordant for diagnosis but different in biography. In each case the diagnosis is genetic female with the andrenogenital syndrome. At birth the genitalia were ambiguous. In each pair, despite the sameness of genetic, gonadal, and fetal hormonal sex, one has a masculine the other a feminine gender identity.

FIRST MATCHED PAIR

In the first pair (Figure 8.1), the diagnosis was established early enough to permit the suppression, by hormonal regulation with cortisone, of accelerated statural growth and premature, masculinizing puberty during the years of childhood.

The child raised as a girl was actually announced as a boy at the time of birth, because of the appearance of the genitals (figure 8.2). The correct diagnosis was established by the age of two months and a sex reannouncement was decided upon. The parents were counseled on how to negotiate a sex reannouncement within the family and the community (Money, Potter, and Stoll, 1969), which they accomplished successfully. Today it is known that the first stage of surgical feminization (Figure 8.3) could have been safely carried out without delay, but at the time it was delayed as a precaution against a surgically induced crisis of adrenal insufficiency, until the age of two years. Thereafter, the child had an unremarkable childhood, medically, except for taking a daily maintenance dosage of cortisone pills. At the age of thirteen breast development began. The menses failed to appear on time, as is occasionally the case in the adrenogenital syndrome (Jones and Verkauf, 1971) and did not begin until age twenty.

During childhood, the child developed behaviorally as a girl with tomboyish activity interests, in the fashion now considered typical for children with the adrenogenital syndrome (Chapter 6), though not so as to become conspicuously different from other girls of her age. In teenage, academic and career interests had priority over dating, romance, and going steady. There was no romantic inclination toward either boys or girls, but rather a projection into the future of the boyfriend and married stage of life. Otherwise, everything about this girl was very attractively feminine to all who interviewed and knew her.

The second member of the first matched pair (Figure 8.1) was given an improvised diagnosis at birth and pronounced a male with a hypospadiac phallus and undescended testes. Three stages of surgical masculinization ended in failure, as urine backed up into the internally opening vagina with ensuing infection. At age three and a half, the correct diagnosis was established and the case was referred to Johns Hopkins. At this time the child was terror stricken at being once again in a hospital. He said that a nurse would cut off his wee wee; and that his baby sister had had hers cut off. But his big brother in the Air Force would bring him a new wee wee. His terror abated when, with plastic clay and water, he was shown how an imperfect penis could be repaired.

It was decided to allow the boy to continue living as a boy. The appropriate surgery was done, and during childhood cortisone therapy corrected the abnormal activity of the adrenal cortices and permitted statural growth to be normal. At the age of puberty, masculinization was induced by means of androgen therapy. Artificial testes were implanted in the empty scrotum (Figure 8.3).

The boy's family life, as he approached teenage, was tortured. His parents fought. The father was incapacitated by multiple sclerosis. The wife won points by reminding him that he was not the father of this particular child, and the boy himself heard what she said.

In teenage, the boy was an academic underachiever, and he tended to seek the company of quasi-delinquents where he could achieve status of sorts as a rebel. He was accepted by the other boys as one of them. He was not overly aggressive. Psychosexually, the significant finding was that all of his romantic feelings and approaches were toward girls, despite his trepidation at the prospect of attempting intercourse with too small a penis and prosthetic testes that could be recognized on palpation as not soft enough.

SECOND MATCHED PAIR

The criterion that separates the second (Figures 8.4 and 8.5) from the first matched pair of children with the adrenogenital syndrome, their gender identities respectively concordant with assigned sex and rearing, is that hormonal sex in both children of the second pair was, at age twelve, discordant with gender identity. The girl was masculinized, and the boy feminized. The boy's female chromosomal and gonadal sex were also discordant with his gender identity.

The boy was aged thirteen at the time depicted (Figure 8.4), and had to his disgust manifested breast growth since the age of eleven. Diagnostically, he was still believed at age eleven to be a genetic male with the adrenogenital syndrome, though a rather atypical case since the testes were not present in the scrotum, and the urinary opening was slightly misplaced away from the tip of the rather small phallus. He had been on treatment with cortisone since age 3½ years. The gonads being in fact ovaries, the therapy with cortisone permitted them at age eleven to secrete estrogen in the fashion typical for a female at puberty, and hence to induce breast growth. Menstrual bleeding had not yet begun when the boy was seen at age thirteen. The correct chromosomal status (46,XX) had been ascertained at age twelve, and soon thereafter the boy was referred for a decision as to whether to attempt or avoid a sex reassignment.

The decision was against a reassignment, and for the same reason as it would be for the vast majority of thirteen-year-old American boys. His mother said: "He has a sister, and they are completely different. He does not think like a girl, and he does not have the same interests. Right now, the one thing that made me very sure, is that he has a girlfriend. And that to me was a relief, because that was just the clincher that he wasn't a girl." The mother had some months earlier been told the diagnosis. For the father, the boy was very much a son, and they shared many evenings, weekends and vacations with rifle and rod. The boy's other recreational interest, shared with a boyfriend, was motor-bike racing in the dry river bed. He gave an authentic biographical account of the early phase of teenaged romantic attraction, and had a particular girlfriend. He experienced erotic arousal, which included the slow secretion of genital moistness, from being with her, and also from girlwatching. This finding was all the more significant in view of the fact that adrenocortical androgen production was low, on account of suppression with cortisone. Subsequent replacement therapy with testosterone as well as cortisone, following gonadectomy and hysterectomy, would eventually lower the threshold of erotic arousal and increase its frequency and genital carry-through, in masturbation, for instance. Meantime, masturbation was reported as nonexistent, though not morally disapproved. Phlegmatic by temperament, the boy had at first assumed that he would have to get used to having a chest with breasts on it. "I was very overjoyed," he said, when first hearing of the possibility of mastectomy; "I really couldn't wait until I could get here." He is due to return soon for his first follow-up examination in person since the termination of a feminizing hormonal puberty and its replacement with androgenization.

With respect to discordant hormonal sex, it is equally remarkable in this pair of cases that hormonal feminization did not feminize the boy's masculine gender identity, and that the great excess of premature hormonal masculinization in the girl did not masculinize her feminine gender identity. She was twelve years old at the time depicted (Figure 8.4). Like other girls in her untreated predicament, she reacted to the masculinization of her body as a deformity and wanted to be rid of it. Hormonal therapy with cortisone was begun at age twelve. It suppressed adrenocortical androgen secretion and released the ovaries to secrete estrogen. Feminine body development then ensued. She became an attractively good-looking young woman. Narrow hips and mildly short stature remained unchanged, as the epiphyses of the bones had already fused under the influence of precocious masculinization. These two signs alone remained as reminders of the past, except for a small amount of coarse facial hair, requiring removal by electrolysis. The voice was husky, but so used as to be not mistaken as masculine on the telephone.

Surgical feminization at age twelve entailed exteriorization of the vaginal opening and removal of the enlarged clitoris. The capacity for orgasm was not lost. The proof came fifteen years later, upon the establishment of a sexual relationship and marriage. It is not unusual for romance to blossom late in the treated adrenogenital syndrome in girls. In this particular case, there seemed to be an additional impediment, characteristic of girls who mature masculinized and with an uncorrected genital deformity. Even after good surgical and hormonal feminization of appearance has been achieved, such a girl is diffident and fearful of rejection—as though the old body image will not fade and be replaced by the new one. Inchoately, the girl acts as if her first lover will magically decipher her old body image and know that she used to be some sort of freak. Surmounting the barrier is a protracted business, and is achieved when intercourse in a love affair is finally ventured, with success.

THIRD MATCHED PAIR

The criterion that separates the third pair (Figures 8.6 and 8.7) from the other two matched pairs of patients with the adrenogenital syndrome is sex reassignment, requested by each member of the third pair (Money, 1968a). The special feature of the pair is that they elected reassignment in opposite directions, the one from boy to girl, and the other from girl to boy (Figure 8.7), at the ages of twelve and eleven, respectively. Both also illustrate the principle that indecision of sex assignment lays the groundwork for ambivalence or discordance of gender identity with respect to sex of ostensible rearing. In neither case were the parents given a clear directive as to the sex of their genitally ambiguous-looking newborn baby. Above all, nothing was done about surgical correction of the ambiguous genitalia.

The mother of the child reassigned from boy to girl recalled being advised at the time of birth that the child should be given a boy's name, but that it might be necessary to change later. By the age of eight precocious statural growth and pubic hair led to a complete medical workup and the establishment of the diagnosis of genetic female with the adrenogenital syndrome. A proposal of sex reassignment was offered to the mother and the child. In the hospital, as at home, the child was afflicted with elective mutism specific to anything that had to do with sex differences, including clothing. Unable to communicate with his doctor, he failed to keep counseling appointments and became lost to follow-up for nearly four years. Then the case came to the attention of the school authorities and was referred anew.

Elective mutism on sexual matters had persisted and made two-way conversation impossible on sexual topics. Therefore, the child was allowed to listen, with the mother present in the first two sessions, while simple concepts regarding diagnosis and optional prospects regarding love, intercourse, and fertility were explained. The child's own vernacular and four-letter words were used so as to maximize his understanding. The specified goal was to achieve communication so that a decision could be made, once and for always, regarding hormonal treatment, surgical repair, and the sex of living.

After the fifth weekly session, the child left a slip of paper, folded over and over into a square lump, on the arm of the chair where he had been sitting (Figure 8.8). It reads: "Dear Doctor, I do not want to be a boy. I want to be a girl just (like) my sisters."

There had not been too many preliminary clues as to what the child's decision would be. Play interests and activities at home had not shown a clear gender preference. He dressed as a boy in sometimes unmended and ill-fitting clothes shared with brothers. Socially, he tended to keep to himself. Sometimes his gait and demeanor, usually acceptable for a boy, changed to become feminine.

Figure 8.6 shows the patient a few weeks after cortisone therapy induced the beginning of breast growth, and shortly before admission for corrective genital surgery. Public appearance in the clothing of the female sex was timed by the patient herself to coincide with hospitalization, the hair having been allowed to grow longer beforehand. She decided to forego plans to leave home on vacation, in order to start life as a girl in a new town. Instead she elected to return to the same special class for underachievers, because she liked her schoolteacher. She was proud of her new status. She found her tongue in self-defense, no longer electively mute, when she took an in-law's delinquent brother to court for trying to force her to prove herself in sexual intercourse. She modeled her behavior rather explicitly on that of a sister one year older. She got married a year later than this sister and wanted a pregnancy like her sister's. What she thought was pregnancy turned out to be pseudocyesis, true pregnancy perhaps thwarted as a result of irregularity in remembering to take cortisone.

The second patient in this sex-reassignment pair (Figure 8.6) was registered on the birth certificate as a boy. Because affected by the salt-losing subvariety of the adrenogenital syndrome, the baby needed emergency hospitalization. The correct diagnosis was then established. During 2½ years of nearly continuous hospital care, the baby had a girl's name and went home as a girl, though the birth certificate was not changed. Unaccountably, corrective surgery was postponed. After intermittent treatment with cortisone, the local physician wrongly advised discontinuance of cortisone therapy. The parents had a fatalistic philosophy that their child was meant to live the way the Creator had made her.

As expected in the absence of cortisone therapy, childhood growth accelerated, with precocious and strongly masculinizing puberty. The phallus matured precociously to its full adult size. Though the urethral tube was not completely fused, by manipulating the loose skin around the urethral opening the child could manage to stand to urinate. By age eleven, the child had the appearance of a mature boy of fourteen or fifteen (Figure 8.6) except for short stature (4'7") due to premature fusion of the epiphyses of the long bones and except for the braided hair style.

Except for sometimes being obliged to wear dresses to school, the child managed most of the time to wear boys' clothing, despite the privations of rural poverty. Then she looked like a boy with a girl's haircut, which is how she was known and spoken of in the neighborhood.

Thanks to the school nurse, the child was returned to medical attention, this time to The Johns Hopkins Hospital. Like the other child in this matched pair, this child also was afflicted with elective mutism, both at home and in the hospital. Otherwise friendly and cooperative, she grasped at the idea, presented in a parable adopted from the note of the other child in this matched pair (Figure 8.8), of communicating by means of drawing or writing. Because of extreme educational impoverishment and underachievement, writing was a problem. But it was surmounted in a document (Figure 8.9) that is a masterpiece of linguistic power in three-letter words. Figure 8.9 is actually two pages photographed together, one written when only the father, and the other when only the mother was in the room. Each is signed by the parent present, as a token of willingness to accept the child's decision. The occasion was one of tense drama, while the first page was produced for the father, as there was no way of knowing whether the child would have the guts to confront her parents with her own decision, in the face of their acceptance of things as they are, and their uncertainty as to whether doctors really knew what they were talking about, or were experimenting with the child.

Among professionals, there were some who had moral and religious misgivings about removing ovaries under any circumstances. Eventually, however, the decision in favor of sex reassignment was surgically implemented, with a very successful result (Figure 8.7). The ideal in hormone therapy is for the child to take both cortisone and testosterone. If for financial or other reasons medication should be omitted, however, then the adrenals' own excess of androgen will maintain effective virilization.

The correctness of sex reassignment for this child was confirmed in part by his ability as a boy, no longer electively mute, to give a brief interview with a microphone before 200 people. Academic and social rehabilitation have been consistently positive. A little later in teenage than for perhaps most of his contemporaries, the boy began dating at age fifteen. His romantic attraction is exclusively toward girls. He is exclusively masculine in appearance, demeanor, and behavior.

Chromosomes, Hormones, and Gender Identity

The foregoing three matched pairs of hermaphrodites, and many others like them, concordant for diagnosis and discordant for gender identity, wreck the assumption that gender identity as male or female is preordained by the sex (XX, or XY) chromosomes. Clearly it is not.

The three pairs also prohibit the assumption that gender identity is automatically preordained by prenatal hormonal history. One would like to have quantity and timing of prenatal hormones held constant, as they can be in experimental animal manipulations. Meantime, the relative constancy of findings in matched pairs of human hermaphrodites lends credence to the thesis that prenatal hormonal influences influence various personality traits that, though not the exclusive preserve of either sex, are traditionally regarded and valued as sexually dimorphic. These traits may interact with postnatal social influences that shape gender identity. Prenatally induced tomboyish traits, for example, may make it easy for a genetic female to have not simply a tomboyish version of a feminine gender identity, but, if postnatal circumstances so conspire, to differentiate a transexual gender identity and want a sex reassignment. The same might happen in reverse for a genetic male.

Like hormonal status prenatally, hormonal status after birth does not have a preordained influence on the masculinity or femininity of gender identity. The evidence from hermaphroditism is confirmed by that from adolescents or adults who undergo spontaneous changes in sex-hormone balance, as from a hormone-producing tumor. Thus a boy who grows breasts wants them removed. He does not want to change his status and live as a girl, though he may worry as to whether fate may be turning his body, though not his mind, into that of a girl. Likewise, in reverse, for the girl who grows a beard and gets a deep voice and body hair. Nonetheless, it is true that such hormone-induced changes constitute a potential threat to a person's gender identity. The greater the mystery of what to expect, the more threatening the hormone-induced change. Thus, the adolescent boy who begins to grow breasts has no way of predicting what might happen next, until he is told. The younger the child who undergoes discordant hormonal body changes, the greater the likelihood of an interaction effect with the still maturing gender identity. Nonetheless, extreme discordance between postnatal hormonal sex and gender identity does occur, the prime evidence being from hermaphroditism.

The ultimate test of the thesis that gender identity differentiation is not preordained in toto by either the sex chromosomes, the prenatal hormonal pattern, or the postnatal hormonal levels would be undertaken, if one had the same ethical freedom of working in experiments with normal babies as with animals. Since planned experiments are ethically unthinkable, one can only take advantage of unplanned opportunities, such as when a normal boy baby loses his penis in a circumcision accident. We have under long-term study two such children, both reassigned in infancy and given the first stage of surgical reconstruction as females. One of these children is now of school age (see Chapter 7), and her behavior as a little girl is in remarkable contrast to the little-boy behavior of her identical twin brother.

Parallel Between Gender Identity and Native Bilingualism

A bilingual child encounters two systems of language in tonality, vocabulary, syntax, grammar, and idiom. They are encountered as sound waves. They are processed in the brain as independent, nonoverlapping communication systems, each with its own boundaries. This remarkable brain work in establishing boundaries is made easier if each person in the bilingual child's environment uses only one language in which not only to initiate talk, but also in which to listen and respond. It is confusing if both languages are used by one or more of the people who talk, listen, and respond to a child. The child's language development is then slowed down, and he tends to get elements of the vocabulary, idiom, and syntax of both languages scrambled together in his speech before, belatedly, he gets each separated and coherently organized within its own boundaries. By contrast, a child who participates in two nonoverlapping language environments learns each rather rapidly and effectively. To illustrate: an American infant growing up in Russia with parents unilingual in English has no option but to speak and listen in English at home with his parents, whereas at play and in school with his unilingual age mates he has no option but to speak and listen in Russian. By contrast, the child of Russian immigrants in the U.S. whose parents and other people at home speak and listen to him in both Russian and English, is likely to confuse and mix the two languages in the early years of his own linguistic development. Then later, unless there is a unilingual Russian member of the household, such as a grandparent, whom the child likes to talk to, he is highly likely to quit speaking in Russian, in favor of English, the language of the majority in the neighborhood and at school, though he may to some degree retain the capacity to listen to and comprehend Russian. Should an American immigrant child from Russia favor the Russian language to the extent of neglecting the English of his playmates and school peers, he would indeed be a peculiar child. It is even peculiar for such an immigrant child to retain a Russian accent and to neglect or disregard the sound of the spoken English of his peers.

With respect to gender-identity differentiation, the ordinary infant is exposed to what, by analogy with bilingualism, may be called bigenderism. In the same way that the bilingual child encounters two sets of language stimuli requiring two sets of responses, so the ordinary child receives and responds to two sets of gender stimuli, one the behavior of females, the other the behavior of males. The child's response to one set is to imitate or identify with, and to the other, to reciprocate in a complementary manner.

An actor can establish an identity as a character on the stage not simply by learning his own lines, but only when he knows the lines of those who will share the stage with him. By analogy, a child establishes his (or her) gender identity by the dual process of identifying with a person, commonly the parent of the same sex, and complementing with another, commonly the other parent of the opposite sex.

The rules of male-female complementarity in behavior vary according to ethnic location and history, but the fixed pivot around which all rules vary is that women menstruate, gestate, and lactate, and men don't. Secondary to this pivotal difference are others. Thus, women have breasts and a feminine smell; they do not have whiskered faces, Adam's apples and deep voices; and they are not called he or him. It is vice versa for men.

One of the remarkable findings of studies of transexualism as well as of hermaphroditism is that a mother does not need to be a genetic female who actually menstruates, gestates, and lactates in order to be a psychologically adequate mother surrogate to an adopted child. Provided she looks, feels, talks, and behaves like a mother, she may have been born a genetic male who received subsequent surgical and hormonal treatment to agree with her behavioral development as a female. In the case of a hermaphrodite, the assigned sex may have been female from birth onward. In the case of a transexual, the original assignment would have been as a male, with a sex reassignment in young adulthood to agree with the behavioral conviction of femininity and a feminine gender identity.

Conversely, it is possible for a person who once was capable of menstruation, gestation, and lactation to be an adequate father figure after the hormonal, surgical and legal transformation of a sex reassignment, concordant with a masculine gender identity. The male-to-female transexual passes as a woman. So also the female-to-male transexual passes as a man. Except in the intimacy of a physical examination, he has the physical appearance of a man. In public, he has the social presence of a man, so convincing that no reader of this sentence would think to question it unless forewarned. The adopted child of this same person responds to this man as to a daddy in a way indistinguishable from that in which any child might respond to the male parent. It is the visible appearance and the behavior of the father as a man that counts, and not his genetic or gonadal sex. Even his coital handicap, provided his wife has adjusted to the use of an artificial penis, has the same irrelevance to his paternal behavioral role as it would in the case of a genetic and gonadal male who lost his genitalia in war.

From the point of view of the child, visible and behavioral sex supersede genetic and gonadal sex in his or her own experience of gender-identity differentiation. To secure a child's correct gender-identity differentiation, it is important to establish in that child's earliest experience that the implications of the phyletically prescribed elements of gender dimorphism are not, as they may otherwise appear to be, optional. Then male-female overlap with respect to culturally or historically defined aspects of sex-different behavior is inconsequential to the child's own gender-identity differentiation.

It doesn't matter if father cooks the dinner and mother drives the tractor. Cultural and historical variations of the masculine and feminine social and vocational roles are acceptable so long as there are clear boundaries delineating, at a minimum, the reproductive and erotic roles of the sexes.

The traditional content of the masculine and feminine roles is of less importance than the clarity and lack of ambiguity with which the tradition is transmitted to a child. It is difficult and confusing for a young boy, for example, if his mother or father is in the unlucky position of despising the penis as the organ of coitus, so that either parent surreptitiously conveys to him the message that he would be even more adorable if he didn't have a disfiguring appendage to his abdomen. Correspondingly, in another family, a parent may convey a similar surreptitious message to a daughter of the ignominy of a vagina, menstruation, and pregnancy. There are, of course, many other ways in which a child may be subtly robbed of his or her pride of gender.

When the models of gender identification and complementation have unambiguous boundaries, then a child is able to assimilate both schemas, the same way that a bilingual child assimilates two languages, the users of which are clearly demarcated and nonoverlapping. The analogy with bilingualism is closer than it seems, if one considers those cases of the children of immigrants who learn to listen and to talk in the language of the new country, but only to listen in the language of the old country. The parental language is enveloped with shame and indignity. In the brain, it is negatively coded: Not for vocal use! The vocal chords and organs of articulation cannot even speak it without an accent.

The two gender schemas are, in the development of the ordinary child, similarly coded as positive and negative in the brain. The positive one is cleared for everyday use. The negative one is a template of what not to do and say, and also of what to expect from members of the other sex. This theme is further developed in Chapter 12.

Unfinished Gender-Identity Differentiation

There is, as yet, no systematic catalogue of knowledge as to why some individuals fail to differentiate a unitary or monistic gender identity. One may postulate a factor of vulnerability or predisposition to gender-identity error on the basis of a cytogenetic error, an error of fetal hormonal secretion, an error of genital morphology, an error of hormonal puberty, an error of social programing, or an error of brain function. In all cases, the final common pathway is obviously in the brain and mind of the person concerned. The more prospective case studies (as compared with retrospective case studies that are kept on record), the better. The following data are taken from one such record.

The case is one of a genetic male with a micropenis that in adulthood approximates in size the distal-half of the thumb (Figure 8.10). The testes are vestigial, possibly totally atrophied and resorbed. Though lacking its own androgen, the body has become well virilized by means of androgen replacement therapy begun at age 13½. Masculine physique and function are maintained by injections of long-lasting testosterone enanthate, 200 mg every three weeks. In a medical examination nothing is unusual until the genitalia are exposed. The following summary is from his file.

During childhood, he took advantage of the offer of self-demand psychologic consultations, and requested one return visit annually. At age ten he began to retreat from play with boys, a change which he explained away as inconsequential. I was not satisfied. Therefore, I resorted to a personalized projective test in the form of a narrated parable, drawn from clinical experience. The parable was of a boy with a micropenis who had dreamed that perhaps God had intended him to be a girl. In fact, he had actually dreamed of changing to be a girl.

With all of the calm of a ten-year-old who had just learned that his talking doctor had nonexplosive ears, the listener then responded that he also often thought about changing his sex. He knew something of Christine Jorgensen's case through the news media. He had already made up his mind, however, that he would not bother with a change of sex, unless he could be guaranteed to have children by his own pregnancies.

The upshot of this interview was that the boy elected to try local application of an androgenic ointment (0.2 percent testosterone propionate in a water-miscible stearin-lanolin cream base) to the penis in order to induce its pubertal growth ahead of time. Fortunately, there was no problem of androgen insensitivity. The penis enlarged, with some growth of surrounding pubic hair, but no other bodily signs of puberty. The morale enlarged even more.

In early teenage, I arranged a program of sex education which included complete and frank discussion of how other people had compensated for a micropenis with manual and oral stimulation, and with the use of a prosthetic penis. The subject of sex change fell by the wayside. At the age of nineteen, I specifically referred to it again in inquiring about masturbation imagery. Approximately 25 percent of the time the fantasy would be of having sex as a girl; and 75 percent of having sex as a boy with a normal-sized penis.

At around the same time, the boy began writing verse and short stories, the verse in French and the short stories in English. Insofar as one can classify writing by the sex of the author, the French verse was feminine, and the English prose masculine in both content and style.

Two options of language were being opened, so to speak, to match two options of gender identity. It is almost a foregone conclusion that English and masculine will predominate over French and feminine in the long term, as they do at present.

Meanwhile, the boy's sex life resembles that of a college teenager, except that he gets severely depressed and is more diffident than most boys, because of his genital defect, about actually venturing beyond heavy petting to attempt coitus.

From within the confines of our sex-restrictive culture that generally discourages children from expressing sexual ideas or having sexual experiences, it is rare to get such articulate evidence of gender-identity differentiation actually taking place during childhood. The case illustrates that the process of differentiation is not automatically preordained but is, indeed, developmental and dynamic, and that its completion may be disrupted, inhibited, or delayed in a child confronted with ambiguous or conflicting evidence as to his status as a boy or girl.

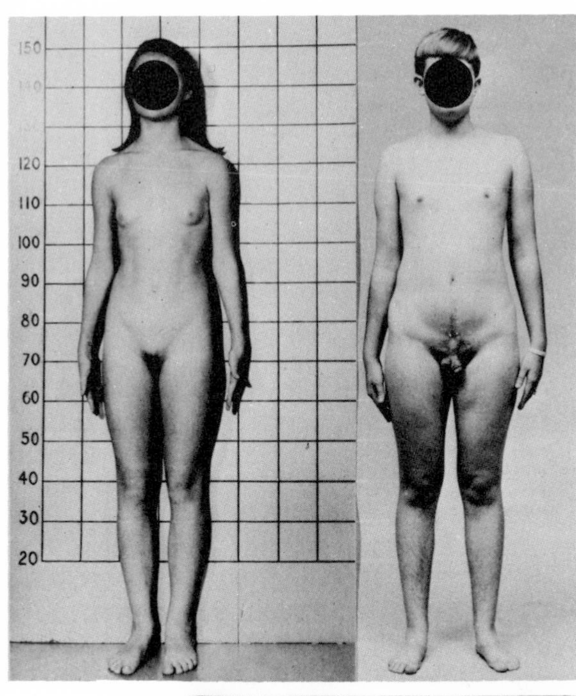

Figure 8.1. Early treated, matched pair of patients concordant for diagnosis of hermaphroditism in a genetic female with the adrenogenital syndrome, but discordant for sex of rearing, surgical and hormonal treatment, and for gender identity differentiation. Ages as photographed are 14 years 6 months (girl) and 15 years 1 month (boy).

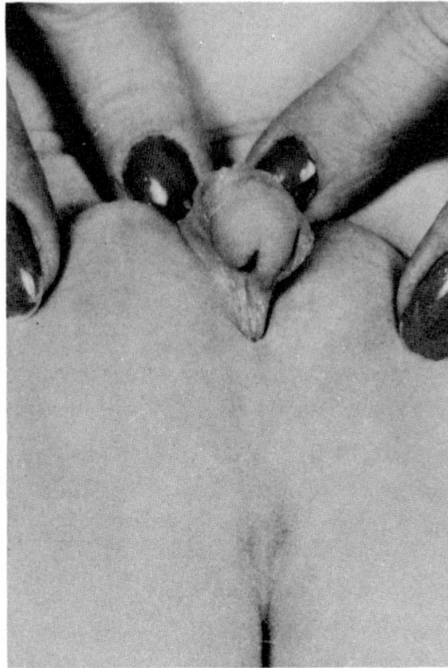

Figure 8.2. Neonatal appearance of the genitalia of the girl of Figure 8.1. The appearance of the boy of Figure 8.1 was similar.

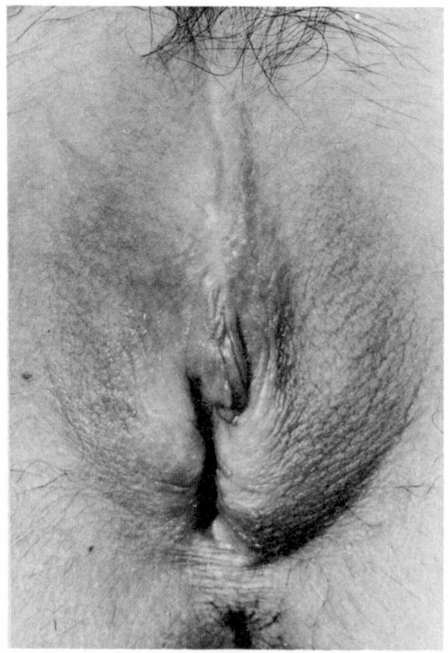

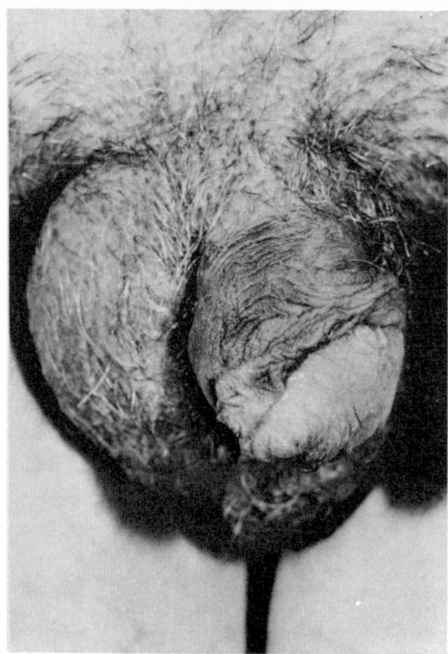

Figure 8.3. Postoperative appearance of the genitalia of the patients of Figure 8.1. Prosthetic testes have been inserted into the scrotum of the boy, for cosmetic appearance.

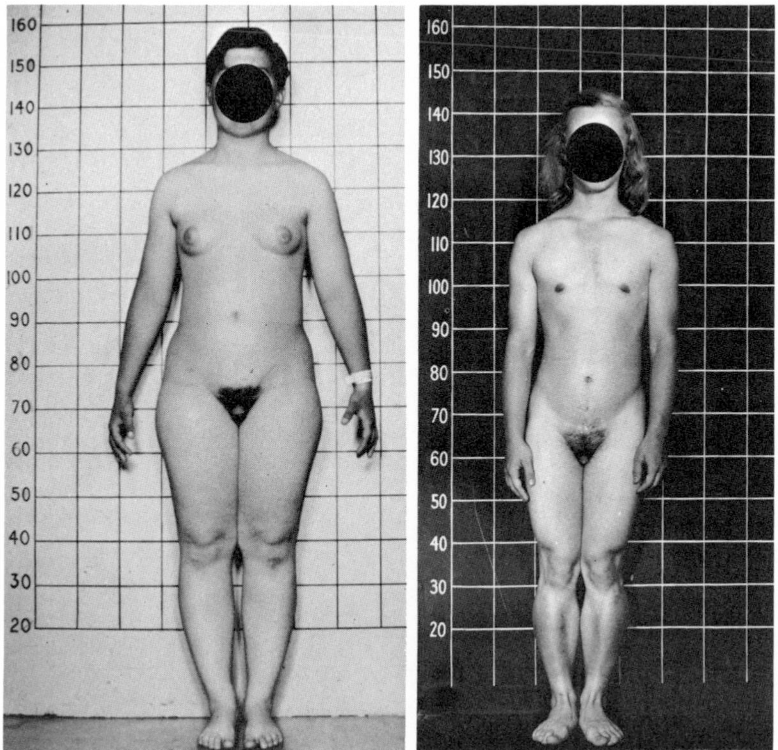

Figure 8.4. Late treated, matched pair of patients concordant for diagnosis of hermaphroditism in a genetic female with the adrenogenital syndrome, but discordant for sex of rearing, hormonal status at the age of puberty, and gender identity differentiation. Hormonal status was eventually corrected to agree with identity and surgical feminization of the genitalia was effected for the girl. The boy's penis needed no genital surgery ever. Ages as photographed are 12 years, 3 months (girl) and 13 years, 0 months (boy).

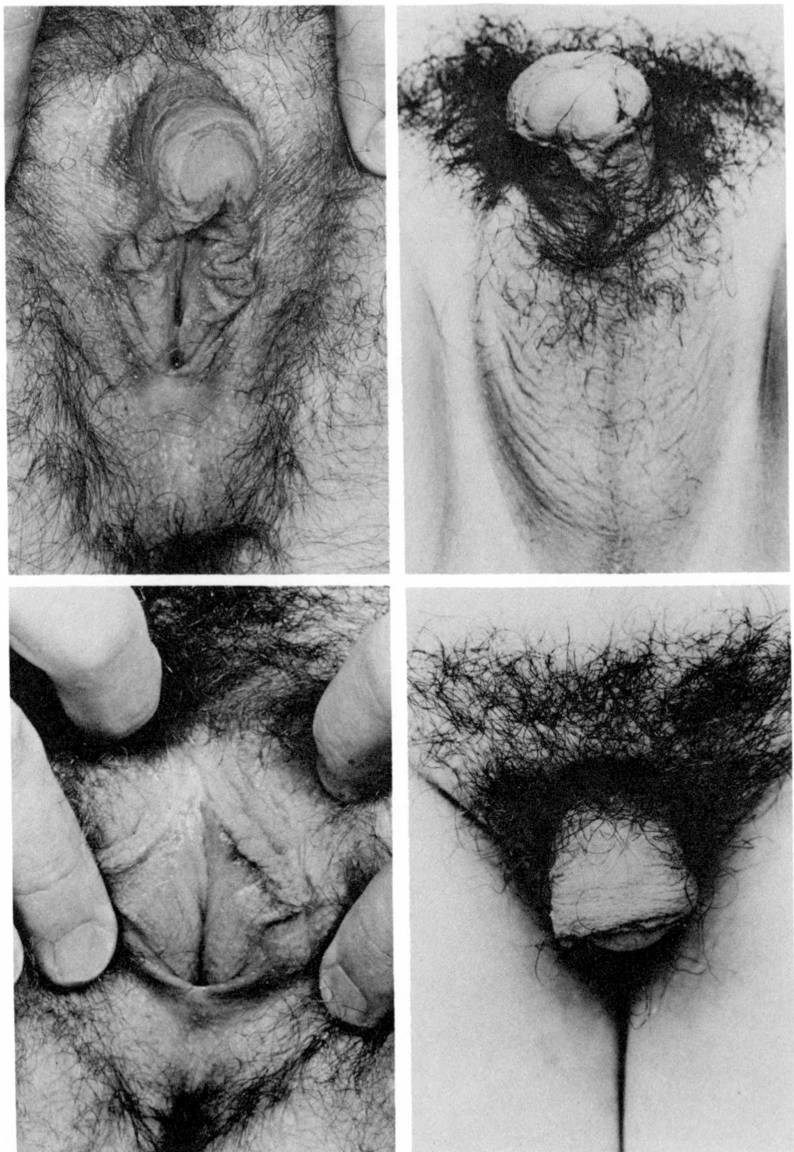

Figure 8.5. Pre- and postsurgical appearance of the genitalia of the girl in Figure 8.4, and two views of the genitalia of the boy, showing that the penis was sufficiently well formed to not need surgical correction.

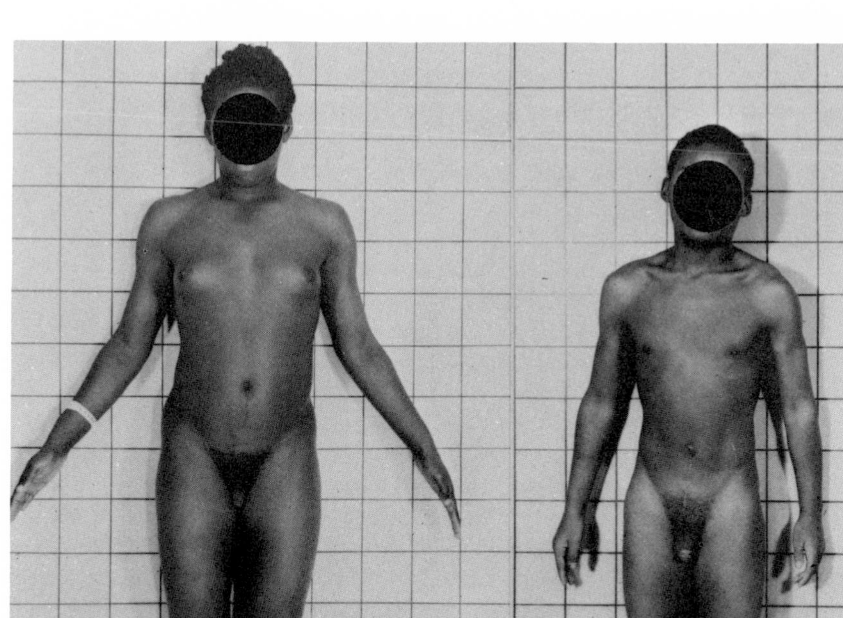

Figure 8.6. Matched pair of patients concordant for diagnosis of hermaphroditism in a genetic female with the adrenogenital syndrome, both with a childhood history of neglected surgical and hormonal treatment. Though discordant for announced sex, they were concordant for rearing insofar as it was equivocal. Each eventually resolved on a sex reassignment, one to be a girl, the other a boy, and was given appropriate surgical corrections and hormonal therapy, as illustrated, concordant with gender identity. Ages as photographed are left, 12 years, 8 months and right, 11 years, 7 months.

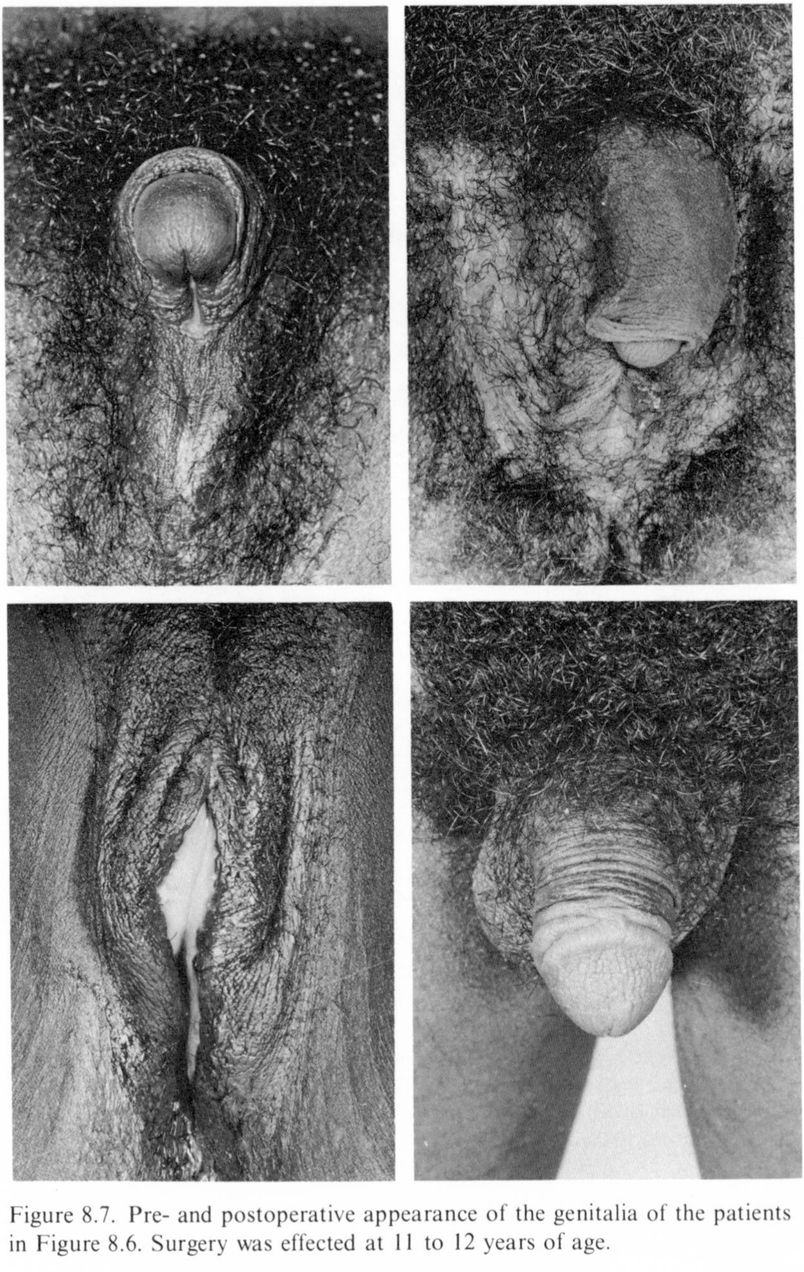

Figure 8.7. Pre- and postoperative appearance of the genitalia of the patients in Figure 8.6. Surgery was effected at 11 to 12 years of age.

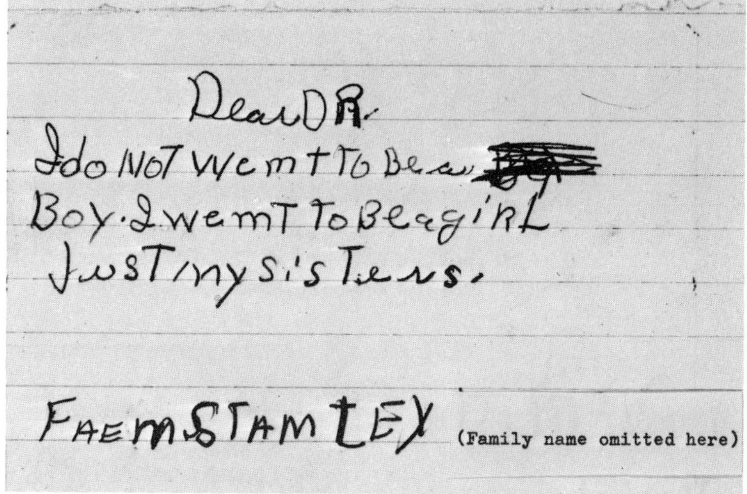

Dear DR.
Ido NOT wemt To Be a Boy. I wemT To Be a giRL
JusT my sisTers.

FAEm STAmLEY (Family name omitted here)

Figure 8.8. Unsolicited declaration of desire for sex reassignment given by the boy-to-girl patient in Figure 8.6 in order to circumvent the elective mutism that inhibited vocal communication on sex-related topics.

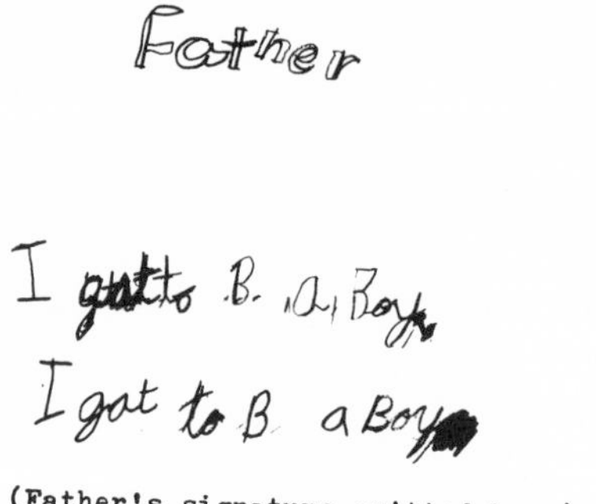

April 20 1966,

Father

I gutto B. a Boy

I got to B a Boy

(Father's signature omitted here)

April 20, 1966

Mother,

I gut to Ba Boy.

I gut to B a boy.

(Mother's signature omitted here)

Figure 8.9. Separate messages for, and signed by each parent, written upon request in their presence by the patient of Figure 8.6 who wanted sex reassignment as a boy. The wording was spontaneous. Elective mutism inhibited vocal communication of the messages.

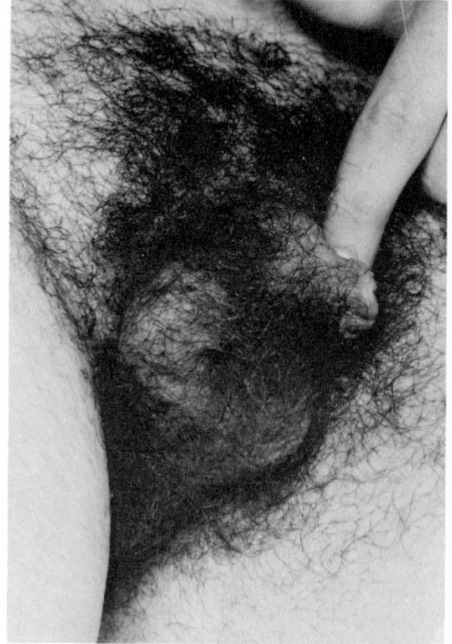

Figure 8.10. Genital appearance in late teenage in a case of congenital microphallus. The structure of the penis is more skin than corpora, but erotic feeling is present. Erection and ejaculation are maintained by hormone therapy since the scrotum contains prosthetic testes, implanted for cosmetic appearance.

9

DEVELOPMENTAL DIFFERENTIATION

Core Gender-Identity Differentiation and Imprinting

In those cases of hermaphroditism in which a too hasty decision was made in declaring the sex at birth, one has a degree of freedom to decide on a change during the first year to eighteen months of life, but this freedom progressively shrinks with each month of subsequent age. The age of establishing conceptual language is also the age of establishing a self-concept. This self-concept is by its very nature gender-differentiated. It is often referred to as the core gender identity (Stoller, 1968).

Establishment of core gender identity is obviously a process of learning, insofar as it takes place in social interaction. Establishment of language also is a process of learning. But the establishment of vocal, syntactical, conceptual speech is possible only in the human species: it first requires a brain that has been phyletically programed to be able to acquire speech. Then it requires that this brain interact with other members of the species who have a history of using a language. This interaction of brain and sound waves (or actually of the brains and sound waves of at least two people) is by phyletic decree, programed to take place at a specific and sensitive period in the juvenile life cycle, if it is to be optimally effective. Then the establishment of language is remarkably rapid, and, above all, remarkably ineradicable.

Learning in animals that conforms to the following four criteria is of the type known as "imprinting": 1) a responding nervous system and a special set of stimulus signals must meet; 2) they must meet at a sensitive developmental period; 3) bonding of signals in the brain at the sensitive period is rapid; 4) such bonding is tenacious and long-lasting.

The process of imprinting was first fully elaborated by Konrad Lorenz (see review by Schutz, 1968) in studies on birds. The essence of the first demonstrations was that one may, during a critical time period, induce newly hatched mallard ducklings or greylag goslings, to follow a squat-shaped moving object or member of another species as if it were the mother. It then remains imprinted to this surrogate mother, to the neglect of a replacement from its own species.

Subsequently, the adult sexual behavior of these birds was affected by the earlier imprint. For example, a mallard duck raised with geese would be attentive only to a goose, not to a member of its own species, as a sexual mate. The same male duck, if exposed only to other male mallards upon hatching, would thenceforth be fixated exclusively on a male as a potential mating partner. A characteristic of the behavior of the homosexual pair is that both react sexually as though the other were a female. Both go through the movements and rituals of the male, neither taking over the part of the female. The two of them thus repeat the routine preludes to copulation, without ever achieving the full copulatory act. The relationship of a homosexual pair proved to be stable, lasting for years, if not until the death of one partner.

A homosexually imprinted duckling did not necessarily mate with a partner to which it had actually been imprinted as a hatchling. Another representative of the class, namely males, to which it had become imprinted would be adequate to elicit the response. Had the original imprinting been to a goose, then mating would be generalized to the class, geese.

The pervasive power of the early imprint-stimulus is evident not only in the choice of a mate, but also in the fact that a homosexually imprinted duck, in attempting to mount ducks others than its mate, would try to force other males, not females, into the crouching position. The power of the early imprint stimulus is also evident in the partial homosexuality that may occur if male ducklings are reared in the company of males only, except for one female, the mother. When older, and released into the company of other ducks, some of these segregated males formed homosexual mating partnerships. Others showed transient homosexual behavior with a sibling or other male mallard, but eventually established a permanent heterosexual partnership. When homosexually-imprinted male ducks were kept in pens with wild adult males, the latter did not become homosexually imprinted and resumed their normal heterosexual mating behavior once they were free again.

Female mallard ducks did not show the same early susceptibility as males to either homosexual imprinting, or cross-species imprinting. Irrespective of their early imprint history, in maturity they would respond to the male with typical female courtship behavior. Possibly, their courtship response may have been released, in part, by the strong color stimulus of the adult male's plumage (Schutz, 1965).

There is room for argument as to whether it is correct to apply the term, imprinting, to human beings as well as to birds. However, it is the concept, not the term, that is important, and there seems every good reason to distinguish the acquisition of language and core gender-identity from other, more transient learning, such as memorizing the summer bus schedule. The distinction makes sense in view of the fact that errors of core gender identity are notoriously resistant to change. This resistance can be used to great therapeutic advantage in such an instance as when one assigns the female sex to a newborn genetic male with agenesis or traumatic loss of the penis. With an appropriately timed program of surgical and hormonal correction, the baby's core gender identity will then differentiate as female.

Once the core gender identity has differentiated, an imposed change of sexual status will not automatically be followed by a corresponding change in gender identity. Rather, an imposed change places an obligation on the mind and the brain to dissociate from future recall all of the preceding biography. Some people are able actually to retrieve and independently authenticate memories dating from as early as the second half of the second year of life. Actual retrieval is not the only criterion of memory, however. Speed and perfection of relearning are others. Thus, the child whose native language was lost at the age of two in favor of another will surpass his classmates, at a later age, in learning his former language.

Progressively with age after around eighteen months, the child of above-average to average cognition and intellectual function has progressively increasing difficulty in accommodating to the discordance of an imposed change of sex. The degree of difficulty varies with the degree to which the gender identity had already become differentiated as unitary versus ambiguous or dualistic. The greater the discordance between the gender identity that should be differentiated according to the newly decreed sex and the gender identity already differentiated in the sex formerly decreed, the greater the risk of failure to make the transfer, and the greater the risk of attendant psychopathology. The latter may represent covert sedition and sabotage, in the form of defiant and negativistic behavior against the parents who sanctioned the change. Alternatively, it may represent self-sabotage, in the form of developmentally regressive behavior, intellectual underachievement, and partial loss of recall.

By the ages of twelve to eighteen months, if not earlier, parents have so completely habituated themselves to having a daughter or a son, both in their relationship to the baby and to their relatives and friends, that they need an expert's counseling and guidance (Money, 1968b) if a sex reassignment should prove desirable or obligatory. After the age of eighteen months, parents need still more frequent help. Even when this help is extended to the child, the problems of cognitive discordance may be incapable of resolution without some lasting residual signs of psychosexual impairment relative to reassigned sex.

By the age of three to four years, it is typically as difficult for an hermaphroditic child as it would be for an ordinary child, or an adult for that matter, to negotiate an imposed change of sex. In other words, though not essentially lethal in its long-term implication, the change is incompatible with a concordant change of gender identity. It is not predictably free from the complications of life-long psychosexual impairment which may, indeed, be severely disabling.

Gender Dimorphism in Early Mother-Infant Interaction

Behavior of the newborn is individually variable, especially in terms of sleeping versus waking, motility versus resting, contentedness versus fussing, feeding versus starving, and thriving versus cachexia. Though such variations occur independently of sexual dimorphism, they are not necessarily independent of people's stereotype of what to expect regarding behavioral dimorphism on the basis of sex.

Rhesus monkey mothers are said to inspect the genitalia of their neonates, perhaps to identify the sex. In human beings, so strong is the stereotype and the expectancy of sexual dimorphism of infant behavior that, in our antinudist society, a newborn's sex is publicly declared by the color-coding of blue for boys and pink for girls, long before an infant has enough hair for a boy's or a girl's haircut, or enough excretion control to make different styles of pants functional. Even strangers are left in no doubt as to what gender-dimorphic vocabulary, or stereotypes of gender-identity behavior to employ. From earliest infancy onward, a baby's social experiences are inevitably gender-dichotomized.

Lewis and coworkers (Kagan and Lewis, 1965; Goldberg and Lewis, 1969) found a correlation between gender dimorphism in mother-infant interaction at age six months and infants' behavior at thirteen months. They observed sixty-four mothers and their infants, half boys and half girls, together under standard conditions. When the babies were six months of age, more mothers of girls than boys obtained high scores for frequency of touching their infants. The same disparity held for vocalizing and breast feeding.

When the babies were thirteen months old, the statistical trend was for boys who had earlier had more tactile contact with the mother to touch her more often than those who had had less. Girls followed the same trend, except that girls who had been touched less compensated by more frequently trying to touch the mother than did their male counterparts.

These findings are significant in showing the early age of onset of a gender-feedback effect, in the behavioral interaction of parent and infant, whereby the behavior of each reciprocates from stimulus to response vis-a-vis the behavior of the other. Such an early onset of a feedback effect in gender-dimorphic behavior guarantees perpetuation of the cause-effect riddle of whether the chicken or the egg came first—the parents' gender-dimorphic expectancy, or the infants' gender-dimorphic activity—if one studies only randomly sampled, normal children.

The answer to the riddle most probably is that interactional feedback is essential from the beginning, and is phyletically ordained to be so. Child-parent interaction is as inevitable to the development of behavioral sexual dimorphism as is anlagen-hormone interaction to the development of sexual morphology, and both are part of the phyletic scheme of things.

The riddle of behavioral etiology notwithstanding, at the age of thirteen months the behavior of the babies studied by Goldberg and Lewis could be statistically classified as gender dimorphic on some of the criteria employed. For example, when boys were put down from their mothers' laps, they more often delayed their first return than did girls. Once the children ventured afield, boys made fewer interim returns to the mother. Then, when tested by being set down by the mother, with a light wire-mesh barrier between mother and child, the boys as a group spent less time crying, or standing at the center of the barrier, and more time at the ends of the barrier, trying to push their way out, than did the girls.

Studies of Gender Dimorphism in Play

Exposed to a collection of toys, the same boys and girls studied by Goldberg and Lewis did not yet, at thirteen months of age, show clearcut gender-dimorphic toy preferences. Boys more than girls, however, did manifest a preference for activity, as in banging toys.

By age two, children show a preference for playmates of their own sex (Koch, 1944). By age three, children begin to recognize gender-appropriateness of toys: Miller (1946) found children of three aware that it was inappropriate for boys to be playing with dolls. Using dolls dressed as male and female, Rabban (1950) asked children to select one like and one unlike themselves. He found that, at age three, both boys and girls were likely to be inconsistent as to whether or not the sex of the doll and their own sex matched. By age four, however, conceptual generalization from doll to self, on the criterion of sex, was well nigh complete. It was not quite so complete at age four when the criterion was whether the children wanted to grow up to be a mother or a father. By age five or six, with boys tending to be ahead of girls, both sexes were conceptually accurate in both of Rabban's tests. They correctly matched the sexual status of dolls, themselves, and themselves as future parents.

Rehearsal of masculine and feminine roles in the play of childhood generally is, prior to the age of four, independent of the sex of the child according to Murphy (1947). Sex-appropriate matching of masculine roles for boys, and feminine roles for girls, in the role rehearsals of childhood play, begins at age four or five, with boys tending to be ahead of girls in establishing exclusively sex-differentiated play rehearsals.

By age six or seven, a child's gender-appropriate play preferences are strongly enough established that they can be elicited even obliquely, from pictorial illustrations of gender-related toys and accessories, according to Brown (1957). Brown found that children tend to choose between matched pairs of illustrations concordantly with their own sex, even though not specifically requested to do so. Boys tended to be more uniformly masculine in their preferences than girls were feminine. There were too many discrepancies, however, for the procedure to be precise in individual evaluation.

From around the same age of six or seven years, children also demonstrate the primacy of their own gender identity by representing their own sex when instructed to draw a person, the sex being deliberately not specified in the instructions (see Table 1 in Money and Wang, 1966). Boys who draw males outnumber girls who draw females. The exceptions are too numerous for the procedure to be an infallible guide to an individual's gender identity.

The gender preferences of play regardless of their origin in early childhood are expanded and reinforced in the gender-dimorphic games and play of later childhood. Thus they may generate or contribute to various skills or abilities differently distributed between males and females. Girls, when they play house, for example, construct what might be called a domestic nest for their baby dolls. Boys are more interested in forts and tree houses which are places of refuge and escape.

Boys, more than girls in our culture, to take another example, intercept a moving ball in their games. Thereby they build up experience not only in visual-motor coordination, but also in judgments of distance, speed, and trajectory, all of which may contribute to the fact that males ultimately outnumber females in superiority of spatial, mathematical, and mechanical ability. The practice and growth of these abilities through play may take place, however, as a sequel to a prenatal, perhaps hormonally determined sex difference in directional and spatial sense. In many mammals, it is the male who establishes territorial rights by marking boundaries with odiferous substances, pheromones. The specialized glands that secrete these pheromones are regulated, in the mature animal, by androgen. Marked boundaries delineate the eating and breeding territory of an individual pair in some species, or of a troop in others.

Territoriality is less prominent in the human male than in various lower species, but some signs of it are evident. Boys rather than girls are youthful explorers, fort-builders, and scouts, and boys are the ones who form gangs or troops that set up territories, dare rivals to trespass, and attack them if they do.

Dimorphism in the Erotic Rehearsals of Childhood

Eroticism and sexuality in our culture are nowhere more strongly subject to ambivalence and taboo than in childhood. Hence it is difficult to find or collect systematic information on dimorphism of erotic and sexual play in childhood. Society, afraid even of ordinary sex education in some school districts, is afraid also of investigations of childhood sexuality. One's career might be imperiled simply by showing pictures of sexual activity to children. Sexual studies in childhood are assailed as on the one hand, a violation of the age of so-called sexual innocence, and on the other, as an incitement to the lurking demons of original sin. Meanwhile, childhood sexuality remains the arcane subject of unconfirmed doctrine, projection, and conjecture; and childhood sexual play continues as the unadmitted practice of children everywhere.

The cultural sex taboo affects some children so that they literally are denied an early chance to know the genital difference between males and females. Conn (1940) found that half of a group of children aged four to six were unable to verbalize their knowledge of the difference of the sex organs. Another 17 percent, though known to have seen the difference, failed to put it into words. In the eleven to twelve age group, only 14 percent failed to specify the difference. In another study of boys aged five to six, Katcher (1955) found that only 50 percent correctly identified a picture of the female genital.

These findings about either inhibition or ignorance concerning the genitalia are of significance insofar as they are culturally specific, not universal (see Chapter 7). They are significant also in that they are at variance with what is known about infantile sexual knowledge in the play of subhuman primates. The often-quoted work of Harlow and his associates at Wisconsin (Harlow, Joslyn, Senko, and Dopp, 1966), on the rhesus monkey, offers rather conclusive proof that the rehearsal of part-functions of the copulatory act, notably mounting and being mounted, with pelvic thrusting, excluding intromission, in the juvenile play of both sexes, is essential to successful copulation and breeding in adulthood. Isolated monkey babies of either sex, deprived first of mothering and then of play with other juvenile infants, grow up unable to breed.

It is known from ethnic studies in human societies not characterized by restrictions on childhood sexual play (Chapter 7) that human primates also rehearse mounting and thrusting (minus intromission) in play, at around the age of five. To prevent or forbid this kind of play, as happens in our own society, may very well have a deleterious effect on gender-identity differentiation, and may even foster errors of this differentiation. Common sense dictates that there is less chance of future ambiguity if all children know early the copulatory and reproductive function of the sexual organs—and if they are also able to take this knowledge for granted with all other children and adults.

In the years of middle childhood, between the ages of approximately seven and puberty, the sexual play rehearsals of the earlier period continue and are likely to include play attempts at intromission. Whether or not the prototype of orgasm may occur is arguable, and in any case is peripheral to the activity itself. At this same stage of development, the involvement and erotic personal attachment of falling in love are not yet ready to express themselves. In traditional terminology, these are the developmental years of the latency period—a misnomer. It is not an age of latency with respect to sexual play. But such play between the sexes is sporadic. For much of their play time, boys and girls segregate, as though to consolidate their gender identities and roles, free of mutual contamination. Latency means, if anything, that love affairs do not occur in connection with sexual play. A girl may have a secret crush on a "cute" boy, and a boy may give more than passing attention to a pretty girl, but genuine falling in love is a later phenomenon. Falling in love is timed on a biological clock that is generally coordinated with hormonal puberty, but not invariably so. Cases of precocious and delayed onset of hormonal puberty show that the correlation is not perfect (see Chapter 10).

Dimorphism in the Romantic Rehearsals of Childhood

Falling in love is inextricably bound up with sentimental romance, and neither are clearly separable from sexual eroticism. Yet, for the purpose of delineating the developmental differentiation of gender identity, it is imperative not to mix or confuse them. The first authentic experience of falling in love is a characteristic adolescent phenomenon, and is associated with the adolescent experience of leaving the parental nest to achieve independence. Earlier developmental play-rehearsal of sexual positioning does not necessarily have far reaching connections with romantic attachment; and rehearsals of the romantic role in childhood do not necessarily ever relate to playmates who share sexual games.

Romantic rehearsals is a term faut de mieux. It refers to those behavioral manifestations of childhood development that have to do with preparations for relationships between the sexes that will eventually have love-affair and erotic overtones.

Before gender dimorphism enters into romantic rehearsals, gender-neutral foundations are laid in haptic and cuddling relationships, and also in oral and feeding relationships. The oral phase of development is familiar in Freudian doctrine and its derivatives; but the haptic phase of touch, clinging, and cuddling was for the most part overlooked until Harlow's work with nonhuman primates brought it to attention. The anal phase of development, Freudian theory notwithstanding, is less related to sex than it is to phyletic developmental mechanisms, in certain mammals, for urinary or fecal marking of territorial boundaries, versus the covering of excreta.

Freudian theory, formulated prior to more recent evidence from hermaphroditism concerning the differentiation of core gender identity, had no provision for differentiation of psychosexual development as male or female until the genital or Oedipal phase, beginning at round age five. In point of fact, neither Freudian theory not its derivatives address themselves expressly to the process of psychosexual differentiation as compared with psychosexual development. The female, by Freud's account of her, is a male *manqué*, which she should not be.

By age five, the so-called Oedipal age, little girls are in fact very much gender-differentiated as little girls, and little boys, correspondingly, as little boys. They have achieved this differentiation through their relationship of complementation to members of the opposite sex, and of identification with members of the same sex, especially those who live in the same household. The contingencies of approval for both complementation and identification are not the exclusive province of either sex. Thus, a mother approves the gender-appropriateness of her daughter's responses toward not only herself, but toward the father also. The father reciprocates. The same applies, correspondingly, to a son.

In most children's lives, the parents are the primary identification and complementation figures. The mother-baby feeding bond in the newborn period, probably universal in mammalian species, ensures an especially close tie with the mother, except when it is pathologically absent or weak. Nonetheless, even the mother of gestation can be replaced by a surrogate, and so may the father of fertilization. Moreover, before many months of age, a baby is ready to begin to generalize from mother to other women and girls, and from father to other men and boys in the domestic environment. It is even possible that, in a home with one parent absent and no member of the opposite sex present domestically, the remaining parent may, by reason of complementation, be able to substitute for the parent in absentia. Mostly, however, it would seem preferable for children to have models of both sexes in the domestic environment against whom to pattern their gender-dimorphic complementation and identification. Children often show their need for finding their own surrogate for a missing parent, attaching themselves in a manner reminiscent of the way a homeless puppy or kitten will follow a stranger and adopt him as a new master.

Many if not most studies to date by developmental and social psychologists on "sex-typing" and "sex-role differentiation" are founded on identification theory alone. Insofar as complementation theory is not incorporated into the design of studies, then relevant phenomena may have been overlooked, and the findings and conclusions are thereby vitiated. Herein lies one reason why most of the literature on developmental gender-dimorphic behavior is still very weak. Another weakness is that identification, as learning, is commonly assumed to be diametrically opposed against innateness of sex differences, whereas the both actually interact.

In the life of a five-year-old, it is neither complementation nor identification alone that is important, but the reciprocal consistency with which both are responded to by mother and father, or anyone else of either sex. Here lies the true lesson of developmental relationships that are conventionally labeled Oedipal. Difficulties or complications lie ahead for the child whose one parent transmits one set of directives for that child's relationship with him or her, while the other parent transmits a discordant set of directives for the same relationships. An extreme of this dilemma is often seen, quite unequivocally, in the children of a divorce.

The ideal is for a child to have parents who consistently reciprocate one another in their dealings with that child. Then a five-year-old daughter is able to go through the stage of rehearsing flirtatious coquetry with her father, while the mother appropriately gives reciprocal directives as to where the limits of rivalry lie; conversely for boys.

From three to six, more or less, is the developmental stage when children can be outrageously flirtatious and seductive, impersonating mannerisms of parents, older siblings, television actors, or whoever. At this same time they are likely to play-act love affairs with preschool and kindergarten playmates, replete with fantasy plans for a wedding, honeymoon in Paris, ranch in Wyoming, and such like.

Some time after the age of six, children go through a developmental stage in which modesty and inhibitions are the watchwords. Even in a nonprudish household, bathroom privacy is demanded—the same child perhaps bouncing naked from the bathroom to the bedroom to retrieve forgotten clothing! This is the developmental stage of establishing moral standards and restraints, especially those of the culture rather than the family. Sexual play, if it occurs, is likely to be secret and private, in obedience to our cultural taboos. Talk of even fantasies that are sexual or romantic is likely to be evaded with an adult, even under auspicious circumstances, and even if guilt and anxiety are minimal.

In the years of later childhood and preadolescence, most children are in a developmental phase of consolidating their own gender identity. Sporadic sex play may continue, though without the distraction of how to relate to a romantic partner of the opposite sex. The exceptions are likely to be children whose previous romantic rehearsal went awry, and who have romantic trouble ahead.

As they grow older, some children lose their distrust of adults, in our culture, but only if these adults prove that they definitely can be trusted. With preadolescents and adolescents, most adults react not in terms of themselves at that same age, but in terms of how well they can impersonate their own parents when they, their children, were preadolescent and adolescent. Hence the generation gap gets perpetuated for yet one more generation.

Adolescence and Dimorphism of Eroticism

Hormonal puberty is a time when the motors of sexual drive, but not of gender-identity differentiation, are set in high gear. Gender-identity has already been effectively differentiated, plus or minus errors, ahead of time; puberty is the time for it to declare itself. A boy most typically gets the declaration in the imagery of his erotic daydreams, nocturnal wet dreams, or masturbation fantasies. A girl, since girls typically do not have orgasm dreams in adolescence and are less likely than boys to masturbate, will more likely be presented with erotic imagery in romantic day-dreams, perhaps in elaboration of an actual experience, a love story, or a romantic movie.

Either a boy or a girl at puberty may experience a discordance between the ideal of gender identity that he, or she, wants as normal, and the actual, biographical truth revealed in imagery. Thus, a boy may be dismayed to be confronted by imagery, perhaps in dreams, of a homosexual, sadistic, voyeuristic, or other paraphiliac type. If so, he usually has no mandate to be able to disclose his imagery to his parents, or others to whom he usually has turned when needing help. Since he cannot, by any act of decision, change the imagery of his dreams and fantasies, he has no choice but to live with it, and probably, one day, put it into action in real-life experience. A girl is caught in the same trap; but girls have fewer varieties of nonconventional imagery than do boys, the most common probably being fantasies of being a courtesan or prostitute, or of being a homosexual lover. Parents and other adults usually do not know how much of the "difficult" behavior of adolescence is actually in response to problems arising from erotic imagery inconsistent with the ideal gender identity.

Some adolescents are confronted by an extremely insistent sex drive, and a vivid, frequent erotic imagery demanding to be put into action. Others are more low-powered. Rarely, low power may signify erotic apathy or inertia, as found, for example, in some cases of failure of hormonal puberty, and in most cases of XXY (Klinefelter's) syndrome. Usually, however, low power in sex drive and erotic imagery cannot be etiologically explained, only described as an inhibitive tendency. High-powered sex drive is equally without adequate explanation. It does not correlate with increased hormonal levels. It is not known whether factors in the social or physical environment may be important. The possibility of a social-stimulation factor is suggested by the experiments of Vandenbergh, Drickamer, and Colby (1972) which show that female mice become sexually mature earlier if reared in the presence of the pheromonal odor of mature males. There is a possible human counterpart, insofar as college girls who live in proximity in a dormitory tend to synchronize their menstrual periods, perhaps because of an odiferous or pheromonal signal (McClintock, 1971).

People with a strong erotic inhibitive tendency are not necessarily unusual in other ways. They may be looked upon simply as late bloomers. Others may be unusual in that their inhibition covers over a discordant or paraphiliac trait in their gender identity, which will not show up until later teenage or adulthood. For example, it is not too uncommon to come across a person, man or woman, who went through all the motions of teen-aged dating and perhaps marriage, but in a rather perfunctory way as compared with other people. Then, later, he or she has, or makes an opportunity for a homosexual relationship, and then realizes how perfunctory the heterosexual relationship had been. The same discovery may apply to other, more unusual varieties of sexual expression.

Such a delayed discovery of one's erotic potential may lead to the belief that the change was caught, like an infection, from the example of the first experience, or from reading. This belief leads to the idea that some people are sex degenerates, going on from one depraved form of sex to another, sampling everything. The truth of the matter is that each person's erotic preference or turn-on has rather fixed boundaries and, once established, is remarkably stable throughout life. The exclusively heterosexual person, for example, cannot turn on for a homosexual relationship, nor the exclusively homosexual for a heterosexual one. The bisexual person, whose ratio of preference may be 50:50, or 10:90, or any other proportion, usually retains his bisexual potential, whether or not it is manifested in action.

The kind of person who is likely to experience a delayed turn-on to a formerly suppressed erotic possibility has not been well studied, nor have the circumstances that will elicit the change. Calhoun (1962), in experimentally overcrowding rats, found that lack of life space released atypical sexual behavior, especially in the males. They became marauders, making sexual attacks on females and homosexual attacks on less dominant males; and they also cannibalized the young. Among human beings, the sexual effects of crowding have not been systematically studied.

Some human beings respond to a traumatic emotional event with a sexual change, as in a case of the sudden emergence of transvestism (Money, 1967a). Depression itself is accompanied by sexual apathy. The long-term effect of incarceration may release otherwise inhibited erotic potential, notably in homosexual release. As some people experience it, marriage itself might be perceived as a long-term incarceration.

Sexual apathy in a marriage is illustrated, for example, by a simple case of infidelity in a highly-achieved man of forty who had formerly thought of himself as exclusively monogamous. The main points in the sex history were: prudish but wholesome upbringing in a large family where sex was officially taboo; late puberty at around fifteen; no recall of wet dreams or erotic daydreams; infrequent erections; no masturbation until age twenty-four; no heavy petting until mid-twenties and then rarely; no intercourse until married in late twenties; intercourse a couple of times a month; trouble obtaining a complete erection; three children; attempted infidelity while away on business foiled by impotence; wife also had a new partner while alone at home; and wife then resolved not to be shortchanged by her husband's sexual inadequacy any longer. Brief counseling of the husband led to greater sexual adequacy and erotic enjoyment than previously in the marriage.

There is no good etiological explanation for such a sex history, and especially not for the fact that improvement in coital frequency was delayed until age forty-three. Depressed people have slow sex lives, but an obsessive personality, as in the present instance, does not necessarily entail depression. Nor does it entail a hormone deficit, or a chromosome anomaly.

Falling in Love

Along with sex histories, love histories also vary at adolescence. One extreme is represented in the schizoid or schizophrenic temperament. Such a person may have a secret, one-sided love affair, being unable even to declare it, or unable to accept a negative response. Instead, he or she languishes with a broken heart, carrying an undying flame for the impossible, for years. Another extreme is that of the Don Juan (in females the nymphomaniac), psychopathic type who is able to establish only transient love affairs, intense and persuasive, but on a come today, gone tomorrow basis.

The phenomenon of falling in love can be analyzed as an imprinting phenomenon (Money, 1960a). The critical period for this imprint initially is in adolescence, though it is not simultaneous with the advent of hormonal puberty, as can be seen in cases of precocious hormonal puberty (see Chapter 10). For some adolescents, the first manifestation of falling in love may be subject to inhibition and delay, dependent on sociocultural expectancy, opportunity, and individual variation. A large part of individual variation seems to be determined by the individuality of prior life experience. Personal idiosyncracy of ability to respond to certain characteristics of a love object may be so persistent that only love objects possessing the characteristics can be responded to as releaser-stimuli. Evidence of this specificity is to be found in cases when a second lover or mate resembles in appearance and personality one who was discarded as unsatisfactory.

One of the social limits imposed on sexual partnerships and, by implication, on falling in love, is that which forbids the pairing of a couple who bear a certain relationship to one another by class, caste, totem, tribe, or kinship. In its most generalized manifestation, this limitation has long been known as the incest taboo. The incest taboo is usually thought of as referring to a veto on sexual relationships between people of close genetic relationship. Its origin has been the subject of much theoretical conjecture and speculation. A recently completed investigation (Shepher, 1971a, b) throws entirely new light on the issue involved by showing that it is apparently impossible for people to undergo the experience of falling in love with one another if they have been brought up in intimate proximity from birth until the age of five, even if they are genetically totally unrelated. Shepher studied all 2769 marriages in the second-generation offspring of the kibbutzim of the three major kibbutz federations of Israel. Not a single marriage took place between any two people who had grown up uninterruptedly together in the same infants' dwelling for the first five years. In one kibbutz, where all the amorous relationships of the young people could be ascertained, there were also no known love affairs between partners who had been so closely reared together. In fact, there was evidence to the contrary, namely, that early proximity made subsequent love affairs impossible to occur. Individuals needed no effort to prevent love affairs, or to suppress them, for they simply did not occur. Nor were there any traditions or community attitudes against such love affairs. Moreover, in infancy, the children who lived together had sometimes engaged in sexual play together, and there was no official policy, overt or covert, against it. Evidently the intimacy of close proximity, including sexual play in infancy, left an imprint that precluded the subsequent establishment in adolescence of a new, falling-in-love imprint.

There is still today an unfulfilled need for experimental study of those characteristics of a love object that are more or less potent releasers of the falling-in-love response. Visible features of the loved one seem to have a position of special prominence, as can be demonstrated in relation to men who fall in love with women who are reassigned, male-to-female transexuals (Money and Brennan, 1970). It is possible to fall in love at first sight and at a distance. It is even possible to fall in love with a person represented at second hand, as a movie star on the screen. The head and face only may be a sufficient stimulus to trigger a falling-in-love reaction. Of the remainder of the body, the hips and torso are potent stimuli, as is the chest. No part of the body is by itself indispensable as a releaser-stimulus, however. For mankind in general, there is flexibility, and different societies have developed cultural emphases on one or the other part of the human frame as having greatest allure. In societies like that of the Aboriginal Australians where complete nudity was the tradition, the naked body of and by itself alone did not have falling-in-love allure, apart from motions and gestures that might have an erotic implication, or apart from the erotic mood and disposition of the viewer at a particular time. In societies where the body is covered, the part deemed alluring may be exposed to encourage falling-in-love responses in others, or covered to discourage them. In the latter case, uncovering may then be used as an invitation or gesture of allure, in a manner reminiscent of the way in which a rhesus monkey entices the male by presenting her rear end to him. Thus, the Moslem woman's uncovering of her face may be as alluring as the American girl's display of her legs and thighs.

The response, released when falling in love has been successfully triggered off by an appropriate stimulus, has been celebrated in the declamation of love poets over the ages. There is an intense prepossession with the loved one, and his or her every perceptible feature and action may become the trigger of minor raptures. This prepossession tends to be jealously possessive and brooks no interference from a competitor. It excludes the possibility of simultaneously falling in love with a second person, though not of having sexual companionships with another, or others. The lover wants to be with the partner all the time, to touch and fondle in close tactile contact, and to have sexual intercourse, even though held back by moral inhibitions.

The state of being prepossessed and engrossed in love may be of gradual or sudden onset, and is enhanced if the other person responds in like fashion. The stage of maximal prepossession is of variable duration, after which it wanes. There seems to be no constant time interval before the great intensity of falling in love goes on the wane, though the maximum period is probably around two years. Thereafter, when waning does occur, the couple may lose interest in one another, or they may find themselves in a calmer, more steady relationship of love and affection in which each remains powerfully sexually stimulated by the other.

Our own cultural tradition is confused and inchoate with respect to its directives to couples whose love wanes to the point where they lose erotic interest in one another. On the one hand, they receive the cultural directive that they must stay together for better or for worse, and for the sake of the children. On the other hand, they receive also the opposing cultural directive and example of obeying the dictates of a new love affair leading into what may become serial monogamy. In the more recent era, there is also the new tradition of consensual adultery and group-sharing of partners. It is said that the man is more likely than the woman to be inconstant and have plural love affairs, but there is no conclusive evidence in this respect, other than that the tradition of the double standard condones such behavior in men more than their wives or girlfriends.

Falling in love is not a one-time thing. The couple whose love has waned and left no mutual erotic interest may each be able to find a new partner with whom to fall in love all over again. The spurned lover, with rare exception, is able to fall in love with someone else, and the widowed spouse may do likewise. After the first big experience of falling in love in adolescence, however, and especially in a couple who have kept together, an extramural sexual affair is likely to be less a falling in love than a different kind of agreement to have fun with one another. It is wrong to call such an affair purely physical, or a yielding to animal passions, as is the common parlance. It has its own special emotional bond, even though it may not qualify as a total and complete manifestation of falling in love.

Falling in love and its vicissitudes are one aspect of sexual behavior that would appear to be not too greatly gender dimorphic. In other words, men and women go through pretty much the same experience. Falling in love is, perhaps, not only Nature's way of guaranteeing the mating of the species, but also of keeping the couple together long enough for sexual affection to be joined by parental affection, and thus of ensuring the proper care and protection of the young.

Individual preferences and rejections among mating partners have been reported for the rhesus monkey (Michael, 1968; Herbert, 1968, 1970) and beagle dog (Beach, 1970). Such preferences do not depend simply on the cyclic hormonal status of the female, nor on the hormonal status of the male. They are genuinely a matter of individual preference and are durable over time. Beach has records of preferences lasting for six years in the beagle. There is no corresponding phenomenon, to be looked upon as the prototype of being attracted to a partner in a love affair, in laboratory rodents. Rodent mating behavior is more completely predetermined by hormonal status alone.

In the higher primates, personal-partner preference may come even closer to a prototype of falling in love: it is said of the gorilla (D. Hamburg, personal communication) that the dominant male sometimes may take his favorite partner, at the ovulatory phase of her cycle, into the jungle alone for a few days—for a honeymoon, so to speak.

Lifelong devotion as mating partners is characteristic of some birds, including among others the jackdaw and greylag goose (Lorenz, 1952) and the Adele penguin.

Sexual Intercourse

Dimorphism of behavior in the act of sexual intercourse between man and woman is just about everybody's specialty, and yet there are virtually no experts in this aspect of human behavior, its errors and corrections.

The lack of experts is a product of the prudish taboos of our cultural heritage. Until Masters and Johnson (1966) publicly declared their breaking of the taboo, for medical and scientific purposes, of watching people copulate, it was as morally illicit to be a sexual observer as it had been, in the sixteenth century, for Vesalius to dissect a human cadaver and establish the science of anatomy.

At the present time more is known about the determinants, manifestations, and variations of the copulatory patterns of rats, dogs, and monkeys than of man. However, there are some answers that can be given to some of the most commonly expressed uncertainties and questions. One question commonly asked is: what is normal? The norm is literally the example set by the middle group of people, the 68.27 per cent between the extremes; but they do not represent either the mode, or the acceptable. Specialists in sexual counseling usually allow people great freedom in what they do sexually, provided neither partner imposes what is objectionable to the other, and provided violence and personal injury are avoided.

Many couples enjoy oral-genital sex and body licking, and some like anal sex. A few agree to mate-swapping or group-sex, but many more have a silent understanding that adulterous affairs will be more or less open secrets. The same applies to homosexual adultery, whether involving the husband or the wife. A marriage is likely to break up when one of the partners has a hangup on unconventional or far-out sex which is too flagrant and too easily leads to arrest and trouble with the law, especially if a third person might be involved. Such a hangup interferes with erotic ecstasy, without which mutual sexuality does not exist. Erotic ecstasy usually entails orgasm, but orgasm is not a sine qua non of enjoyment in every sexual experience. The experience can sometimes be less tumultuous but highly enjoyable. Never to have an orgasm, however, is being cheated of one's birthright. The person who never has an orgasm is usually a woman, because anorgasmia in males, though it occurs, is very rare. Coital anorgasmia is a phobia of sorts: in either females or males, it is often not present when the vagina or penis is finger-stimulated or mouth-stimulated, but only when the sex organs, male and female, are together.

Simultaneity of orgasm in oneself and one's partner can be mutually rewarding and exciting in the extreme, but it is not necessary to aim for it as the ideal of every act of intercourse. Moreover, the female often is able to pass from the initial excitement phase through the plateau phase of sexual arousal toward not a single climax in the orgasmic phase, but two or a sequence of them, prior to the phase of complete resolution (Masters and Johnson, 1966). The male, by contrast, more usually enters the resolution phase after but one climax in the orgasmic phase. His erection subsides and then resumes, if he will be capable of another orgasm. Even for a youth who will be capable of more than one orgasm in a given copulatory period, the shortest refractory period between one orgasm and the next is in the order of twenty minutes. However, if he can hold his erection long enough without ejaculating, his partner may have her repeat orgasms with only a few minutes in between.

The frequency of sexual relations is optional. Three or more times a day, except on special occasions, is rare, and is usually an imposition on one of the partners, just as a handwashing compulsion is an imposition on the hands. Intercourse less than twice a week during the years of sexual vigor in young adulthood and middle age is likely to be a negative imposition on one of the partners, or an indication that, for one or both, nonsexual activities are overcrowded into their lives. If at all possible, it is better not to have sex crowded out of one's life.

The use of an effective method of birth control is optional, acceptable, and indeed desirable, despite conservative opinion to the contrary. It is desirable also for unmarried teenagers who begin their sex lives, far more desirable than is illegitimate grandparenthood for their parents. The various methods of birth control do not interfere with genital feeling or orgasmic ecstasy.

Should contraception fail, legal abortion is an acceptable alternative. A girl should prefer an early abortion by the very simple suction method, prior to the end of the second month of gestation. The procedure is then the equivalent of inducing the period, and has none of the hormonal or sentimental accompaniments of terminating a new life.

There is no incontrovertible need, in today's birth-control world, to postpone the onset of one's sex life too long. Contrarily, there is absolutely no need to begin it too soon. The onset is personal and optional. Each adolescent must make the decision conjointly with his or her ability to depart the home nest and to establish erotic autonomy.

10

PUBERTAL HORMONES: THE BODY AND ADULT REPRODUCTIVE STATUS

Introduction

After the very active period of sexual differentiation in fetal life, sexual dimorphism of body development is relatively in abeyance during the childhood years of growth, prior to the onset of puberty. Then, under the influence of pubertal hormones, dimorphism becomes the foremost feature of adolescent growth and development. Dimorphism of hormonal influences on the body is the main focus of this chapter, and influences on behavior, of the next—with overlap whenever needed.

Growth of the body in childhood is not quite so sexually neutral as it once was thought to be. From birth onward, girls are slightly ahead of boys in bone age.[1] Until age five, boys are slightly bigger than girls, but the difference is insignificant. After the age of five, and until just prior to the onset of the female pubertal growth spurt, at around the age of eleven, sex differences in nearly all measurements except those of the head are trivial. Then girls take a temporary lead over boys as they enter their earlier puberty.

[1]Data on pubertal growth are based on Tanner, 1962, 1969; and Marshall and Tanner, 1968, 1969, 1970.

Timing of Puberty

The biological clock of puberty is programed in the brain, especially in the old brain or limbic system. The final common pathway is by way of the hypothalamus (Ramaley and Gorski, 1967), through which the pituitary gland is programed to secrete gonadotropic hormones (see Chapter 4, footnote 1) which, in turn, program the secretion of sex hormones from the gonads—from the ovaries in the female and the testes in the male.

Since the mid-1960s, a radioimmunoassay technique has been developed to measure the gonadotropins FSH and LH in blood plasma and urine. It is now known that there are low levels of gonadotropins in the blood of children as young as at least five years of age. The rise toward postpubertal levels appears to antedate the clinical signs of puberty, especially in boys, according to experimental data available to date: the rise commences between the ninth and tenth years of age (Johanson, Guyda, Light, Migeon, and Blizzard, 1969; Raiti, Johanson, Light, Migeon, and Blizzard, 1969; Raiti, Light, and Blizzard, 1969). The menstrual cycle in females is associated with a cyclic pattern of gonadotropin release, whereas in males there is no such cycle (see Chapter 4).

There is as yet no scientific explanation of the timing mechanism of the biological clock that initiates puberty, and therefore no explanation of why puberty may be too early, too late, or on time. In pathology, it is known that lesions in the brain in the vicinity of the pineal gland, or of the pituitary gland and adjacent hypothalamus, may accelerate or delay pubertal onset; but such knowledge is more anecdotal than explanatory. Functional changes in the pineal (Wurtman, Axelrod, and Kelly, 1968) or the pituitary also may affect the timing of puberty. Initial causes notwithstanding, the final common factor in the onset of puberty is the release of sex hormones from the ovaries or testes. It is routine laboratory knowledge that puberty in normal animals may be experimentally prevented by prepubertal removal of the gonads (ovaries or testes). Adult maturation, minus fertility, may subsequently be reinstated by injection or ingestion of the sex-appropriate hormones.

Puberty may also be induced prematurely by sex-hormone injections. In the intact animal, normal adult hormonal functioning eventually ensues, once exogenous hormonal treatment stops. In the case of prior castration, the animal requires hormonal replacement therapy throughout maturity, at least until old age, if normal adult sexual functioning (minus fertility) is to persist.

Normative statistics (Marshall and Tanner, 1969, 1970) for the onset and progress of the developmental signs of puberty can be given only approximately. The various signs of development make their appearance insidiously and cannot easily be dated precisely, except for first menses or first ejaculation. In girls, the age norm for pubertal onset is around the age of eleven, with first menstruation at age thirteen. It is within normal limits, however, for the first menstruation to occur at eleven or fifteen years of age. The first sign of puberty is usually the budding of the breasts, though the appearance of pubic hair may precede it. The growth spurt in height keeps in close synchrony.

In boys, the norm for pubertal onset is around the age of thirteen, if one uses as the criteria the beginning of penile enlargement, the beginning growth of pubic hair, and the beginning of the growth spurt in height. However, these changes are typically preceded by initial enlargement of the testes and scrotum a year earlier, by which criterion the age norm for pubertal onset in the male is twelve. It is within normal limits for male puberty to have its onset two years earlier or later than the ages specified by either of the foregoing two criteria. The sequence of events of puberty in the male is fairly regular, beginning with testicular and scrotal enlargement. The appearance of pubic hair may then precede penile enlargement or coincide with it, in synchrony with the growth spurt in height. About two years after it begins, the growth spurt is all but complete, and the penis is full grown. The voice change, accompanying the enlargement of the larynx and formation of an Adam's apple, has begun, but is not complete. The first ejaculation might have occured within a year of the onset of the growth spurt, subject to individual variation in the frequency of nocturnal emissions and/or masturbation and other sexual activities. The spread of pubic and body hair is genetically determined and is subject to age changes throughout life. Axillary hair may precede the growth of pubic hair, but typically follows it by two years, at which time facial hair also begins to grow. The appearance of moustache and beard requiring shaving may be delayed for another three to five years, however, dependent on racial stock.

The age of puberty has been becoming progressively lower for at least the last century and a half, judging by the evidence of records preserved in Europe and the United States. Figure 10.1 (Tanner, 1962, p. 153) shows a progressive decrease in the age of first menstruation from seventeen, in 1833, to thirteen today. Such a consistent, long-term tendency is known as a secular trend or change. No explanation for it is entirely satisfactory. Today it applies to all parts of the world. Nutrition and public health may play a role, since there has been a parallel increase in childhood growth and in average adult height. Support for a nutritional explanation may be found in the recent discovery that the timing of the pubertal growth spurt, and then of the onset of menstruation, correlates with body weight (Frisch and Revelle, 1970). Girls whose puberty is mildly early, on time, or mildly delayed all have the same weight when they begin their growth spurt and

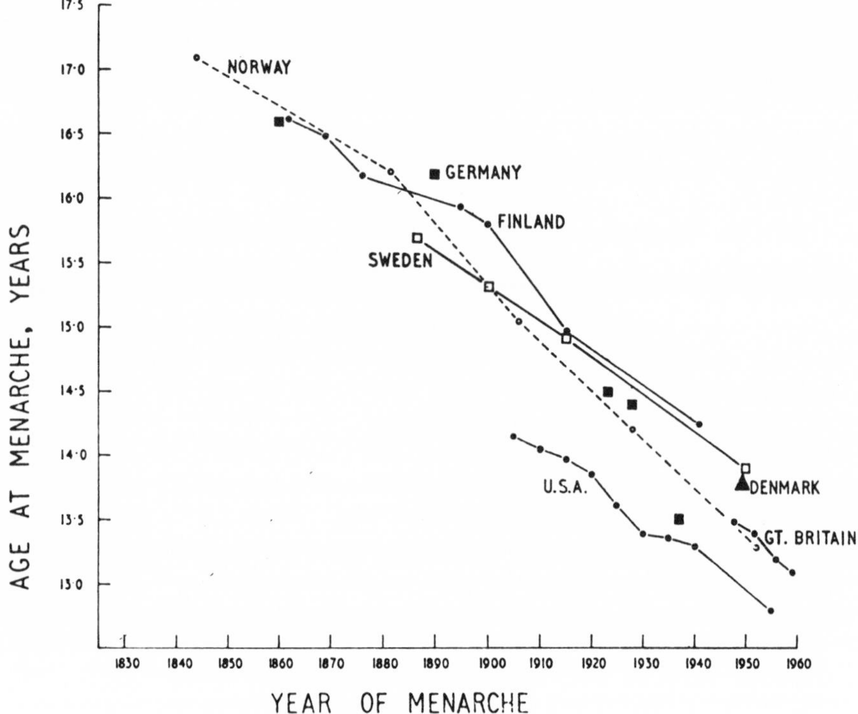

Figure 10.1. Graphic representation of progressive lowering of the age of menarche since 1830. Reproduced from Tanner (1962).

their menses—which suggests that there may be a signal relayed from the metabolic system to the hypothalamus and pituitary regarding pubertal timing.

Politically, socially, and psychologically, the significance of the secular trend toward a lower age of puberty has scarcely been recognized in terms of appropriate changes in the legalities and customs affecting teenagers and their domestic, academic, vocational, and sexual behavior. The newly accomplished lowering of the voting age may eventually have some effect.

Physique Age, Chronologic Age, and Psychosocial Age: Precocious Puberty

Quite apart from the secular trend toward a lowering of the age of puberty, there is also a rarely occurring condition of precocious onset of puberty (pubertas praecox). The error in timing may be so great that the onset of puberty coincides with birth. Between four and six years of age, or later, is more likely. More often in the male than the female precocity is secondary to a brain or glandular lesion, though in either sex it may be idiopathic or spontaneous in onset. Idiopathic precocity is so named because there is no abnormality other than the precocious timing of pubertal onset and the premature attainment of somatic maturity, and the beginning of aging. It may be either sporadic or familial. If familial, it may affect only sisters, or brothers, or both.

In animals, precocious puberty can be easily induced by the injection of sex hormones. In human beings there are no therapeutic occasions or reasons to administer sex hormones prematurely. Only when precocious puberty occurs naturally, therefore, is there an opportunity to study the phenomenon in man.

The psychologic consequences of precocious puberty lie first in the discrepancy between chronologic age and physique age (Money and Alexander, 1969; Money and Walker, 1971). In the early period of precocious pubertal onset, physique age is advanced by reason of secondary sexual development and the adolescent growth spurt in height and bone maturation (epiphysial closure). The dental age remains closer to the chronologic age. The mental age, measured on an intelligence test, also remains closer to chronologic age, though the level of IQ will depend partly on how much the academic age has been advanced by planned acceleration at school, and how much the social age has been advanced through companionship with older children.

The social, or psychosocial, age in sexual precocity lies somewhere between chronologic age and physique age. A six-year-old girl who has fully developed breasts and menstruates, and who has the same height as twelve-year-olds, is not able to enter into all the activities and interests of the twelves or older. She does not have their repository of social know-how, nor their shared background of knowledge. The hiatus between chronology and physique is too great to be bridged. At age six, the maximum amount of attainable acceleration in social age is probably between two and three years. By age ten or eleven, however, a precocious girl may be easily able to belong socially with developed adolescent girls as old as thirteen plus, and boys of fifteen plus.

Whatever the eventual compromise between chronologic age and physique age, younger precocious children are likely to experience their difference from their age-mates as a form of freakishness. Their being different is in some way destructive to self-esteem and the self-image. In the late preteen or early teenaged years, when their physical maturity is matched by a sufficient degree of social maturity, precocious girls and boys may begin to have romantic or love-affair feelings toward someone in the young adolescent age group. Then they are likely to be beset by doubts, and by fear of ridicule or rejection, lest the older partner discover their true age, inexperience, or history of having been deviant in developmental physique. One possibility is a too easy acceptance of an exploitative copulatory relationship; another is a too easy attraction to a partner who is overburdened with a personality disability of his or her own; and a third is to be essentially a loner, romantically, through teenage and the early twenties. In our own experience with long-term follow-up of precocious puberty, early sexual experience, including breeding and marriage, has been extremely infrequent in both males and females—the timing has been perhaps even a little later than might be found in a sample unselected for precocity.

Erotic age, as judged by dating and sexual experience, does not develop automatically in parallel with physique age (nor hormonal age) in sexual precocity. It belongs with other aspects of psychosocial age in that its acceleration is subordinate to the individual's history of social experience. Erotic age as judged by romantic or sexual imagery in daydreams and dreams is somewhat different than erotic age as judged by dating and sexual experience: the content of imagery can be erotic without necessarily pertaining to dating or coitus.

For example, the young precocious boy may have masturbation fantasies or ejaculation dreams, featuring imagery of women's breasts or scantily clad women, months or years in advance of his knowledge of genital intercourse. The content of his imagery seems to be dictated by the extent of his cognitive experience of sexuality and his everyday knowledge of sexual differences. It is, indeed, desirable that his sex education be so timed that his erotic imagery can very early become authentic imagery of intercourse. In this way he is spared the risk of an erotic fixation and the possible development of a paraphilia. For example, a precocious boy of six whose erotic imagery is focused exclusively on brassieres is in danger of becoming a brassiere fetishist; and another boy whose early experiences are in homosexual play with an older teenager is in danger of becoming an obligative homosexual with a hang-up on having an older person as a partner. It is possible for a precocious boy to have imagery of intercourse without having a compulsion to have the actual experience—exactly as is true in most early adolescent males. The uninformed, on the basis of their ignorance, often believe that sexually precocious children will be sexual maniacs, behaviorally. They are not. They are as much capable, with suitable sex education and guidance, of monitoring and regulating their behavior as are ordinary adolescents of similar family and social background.

Young precocious boys are more likely to disclose their erotic imagery in the earliest years of their precocity than later in childhood. They then go through a period of being closed-mouthed during what corresponds to the so-called latency period in normal boys. During this period, they consolidate moral conceptions of right and wrong in sexual behavior in their society, including conceptions of privacy.

All children, like all other infant primates, are quite uninhibited about the sexual play rehearsals of infancy, unless they are conditioned otherwise. Left to their own devices, they sooner or later go through binges of sexual modesty. Modesty, in our society, is strongly reinforced. It may, however, have phyletic origins in the need for copulatory secrecy, since the copulating couple is all too vulnerable to attack. Such a conjecture notwithstanding, the behavior of male precocity reinforces the evidence from sexual play in normal childhood to suggest that the latency years have been wrongly named. Privacy rather than latency would seem a more appropriate term. Additionally, these preadolescent years constitute a period when sexuality is sporadic and experimental, rather than reiterative as it is in adolescent masturbation, or persistent as it is in an adolescent love affair. In childhood, more time is devoted to consolidating one's own gender identity than to complementing that of the other sex.

The sexually precocious boy, despite his adolescent hormonal and libidinal levels, has something in common with his pubertally normal counterpart in having a period of childhood when he is not girl-crazy, and does not fall in love. The earliest genuine love affair we have encountered in a precocious boy was at age twelve. One may conjecture that the biological clock controlling the brain's mechanism or program for falling in love is independent of the clock that initiates the pituitary-gonadal mechanism of hormonal puberty. There is some further evidence, in cases not of pubertal precocity but of pubertal hormonal failure, to support this inference: some teenagers whose hormonal puberty fails do have love affairs before they are given hormonal replacement therapy (Money and Alexander, 1967).

In precocious girls, the ability to fall in love would seem to occur a couple of years earlier than in boys, namely around the age of ten. In our own group of cases, the youngest conception took place at age ten, the baby's father being fifteen. The girl lived in an urban neighborhood where early teenaged pregnancies were not exceptionally uncommon, and where the maternal grandparents rather than the father took responsibility for the baby. The love affair was short-lived. Among the other girls in the group under study, there were no other known examples of falling-in-love until the age of finishing high school or later, and no other pregnancies.

During childhood, after the age of eight and in advance of any actual teenaged love affair, some of the precocious girls had fantasy romances. Some had them much later than others. These fantasies did not include imagery of erotic body stimulation, either mutual or one-way, and did not include imagery of intercourse. In this respect, precocious girls and boys show some of the same difference in erotic imagery reported by people with normal puberty (Kinsey, Pomeroy, Martin, and Gebhard, 1953, Ch. 16). This difference is examined further in the next chapter.

Children with precocious puberty, after they live through the early period of discrepancy between chronologic and physique age, settle down to a teenage and adulthood in which they are physically inconspicuous except for shortness of stature—a sequel of early, rapid bone maturation. The speed of aging is not known. Reproduction is normal. The chance of having a sexually precocious child is dependent on variable genetic factors and is usually unlikely. Parental behavior is normal. Adults with a history of sexual precocity are capable of careers with beyond-average achievement.

Physique Age, Chronologic Age, and Psychosocial Age: Delayed Puberty

In delayed puberty, the gap between physique age and chronologic age is the converse of what it is in precocious puberty. The challenge for the sexually infantile child is to keep psychosocial age as close to chronologic age as possible, and not to decelerate or regress to the social level of physique age. The challenge is more difficult if, at the expected time of puberty, the child is abnormally short—that is, if height age as well as hormonal age are in arrears. It is difficult enough to be accepted by one's peers in adolescence when one looks sexually immature, but doubly difficult if one looks dwarfed as well.

The double difficulty of delayed puberty and dwarfed stature occurs particularly in three syndromes: chronic hypopituitarism, reversible hypopituitarism, and Turner's syndrome. The first two occur in both sexes, and Turner's syndrome occurs in morphologic females with agenesis or dysgenesis of the gonads (see Chapters 2 and 6).

In chronic hypopituitarism, the primary defect lies in the pituitary gland and its activation from adjacent nuclei in the hypothalamus. The defect may be a tumor, a postsurgical sequel of tumor removal, an accidental trauma, or an idiopathic functional failure. The symptoms of hypopituitary dwarfism depend on how many of its hormones the pituitary fails to produce. Among the failures are: growth hormone, thyrotropic hormone (to stimulate the thyroid gland), adrenocorticotropic hormone, ACTH (to stimulate cortisone release from the adrenal cortex), and, at puberty, gonadotropic hormones (to stimulate sex hormone release from the ovaries or testes). Missing hormones can be easily and cheaply substituted, except growth hormone. In chemical structure, growth hormone is a complex protein molecule. It has been successfully synthesized, but will be in short supply until commercially producible. The human organism can utilize only human growth hormone. The total available supply must presently be extracted from the pituitary glands of human cadavers.

When a hypopituitary dwarf is fortunate enough to obtain investigative treatment with human growth hormone, the prognosis is encouraging, but not ideal. Adult height tends to level off at around five feet. More disappointing is the effect of pubertal treatment, when needed, with either gonadotropins or the sex hormones directly, for complete maturity of appearance seems not to be possible, especially in boys. The face does not undergo full change from its juvenile dimensions to those of adulthood, and the beard is niggardly, if it grows at all. The sex organs change from the juvenile to the adult state, though in boys the penis may remain small. Libido, in both sexes, is variable in the strength of its manifestation, and there may or may not be a manifestation of romantic interest and a love affair.

The program of hormonal management, with its necessary priority on growth, may require that hypopituitary teenagers wait until late teenage before puberty is hormonally induced. On the criteria of both height and sexual maturation they are, therefore, on the outside looking in, so far as the social activities of all their contemporaries are concerned. The effect of their long separation from full-fledged participation in age-group affairs may leave a permanent personality scar, so that they settle for spinsterhood or bachelorhood, even if they have the chance to meet short-statured partners of the opposite sex. It is not possible at the present time to differentiate such a personality effect from a possible hormone-resistant, low-level libido.

Hypopituitary girls have an advantage over boys insofar as they have cosmetics, fashion wigs, and padded bras commercially available to help overcome their immaturity of teenaged appearance. However, it is the self-concept, reinforced by actually having one's own breasts and menstrual periods, that is more important than external appearance alone.

Dwarfism with complete hypopituitarism, including gonadotropin deficiency, involves infertility, except for the rare chance of successful treatment with newly available human gonadotropin. This treatment is necessary for ovulation in females, even though standard cyclic sex-hormone therapy may have induced cyclic menstruation.

Reversible hypopituitary dwarfism is a rather mysterious condition, the detailed etiology of which is far from having been worked out (Powell, Brasel, and Blizzard, 1967; Powell, Brasel, Raiti, and Blizzard, 1967; Patton and Gardner, 1969). Its defining features are: failure to grow, failure to sleep (Wolff and Money, 1972), and failure to make growth hormone while the child lives in the place of regular domicile, with reversal of all three failures when the domicile is changed to the hospital, convalescent home, or other (foster) home. Growth hormone levels change from near zero to normal within a few days of admission to the hospital. In some cases the home and family situation where growth fails is manifestly deleterious, whereas in others it is difficult to point the finger of blame. The majority of cases brought to medical attention for failure to grow have been infants and young prepubertal juveniles. A few, however, have been beyond the expected age of puberty, and still prepubertal. They demonstrate a relationship between growth hormone and sex hormone, still not scientifically unraveled. One boy of sixteen, for example, had the size and development of a boy of eight. Away from his home environment, where he was an authentic example of the battered child, grossly mistreated, isolated in a closed closet, and deprived, he began to grow, and soon entered physiologic puberty. He had had no schooling. His speech was defective. He had a very long way to go in order to catch up to other teenagers in psychologic age and intellectual maturity. Yet his erotic knowledge was not too far in arrears, for from the locked closet in which he spent many months of imprisonment during his lifetime, he had been able to peep on his parents' varied sexual activity.

Girls with Turner's syndrome share some of the psychodevelopmental problems of girls with chronic pituitary dwarfism. If both are untreated, Turner girls are likely to grow a little taller, probably no less than 4 ft. 6 in. and not much more than 5 ft. In Turner's syndrome, growth hormone is not particularly effective, but patients may gain one to two inches in ultimate adult height if estrogen-induced epiphysial bone closure is delayed until later teenage, and preceded by a growth-promoting treatment with a weak and poorly virilizing androgen such as Anavar® (oxandralone). A major developmental problem of girls with Turner's syndrome is, therefore, that of continuing social maturation during the waiting period before their pubertal appearance and menstrual periodicity is hormonally induced. Psychologically, it is a taxing delay, even though a girl desperately wants all the inches she can gain. She needs someone to turn to for professional counseling and advice, when the going gets tough. Eventually she is capable of a normal sex life and motherhood by adoption. Her chief problem is to locate short men with one of whom she can fall in love.

Girls as well as boys may be affected by the pubertal delay of hypopituitary dwarfism, and girls alone have the gonadal agenesis of Turner's syndrome with its cytogenetic anomaly. Girls also share with boys the possibility of pubertal delay, secondary to long-term medication with high doses of cortisone, for the control of other diseases like ulcerative colitis or nephrosis; or as a direct consequence of the untreated early phases of various rare conditions like Cushing's syndrome and Addison's disease. By and large, however, delayed puberty is more common in boys than girls. In the female, problems of the onset or regularity of menstruation outnumber problems of the actual onset of puberty.

Boys of normal stature whose puberty is delayed beyond the usual age of fifteen may have a simple problem of timing delay—that is to say, they will eventually advance into puberty and attain adult height, if left untreated. They may or may not have other signs of developmental impairment, including mild birth deformities and, occasionally, low IQ. Other boys prove to have complete pubertal failure, secondary to a failure of pituitary gonadotropic function (hypogonadotropinism) that will eventually require hormonal substitution therapy, most usually with testosterone, to induce adolescent maturation and prevent excessive, eunuchoid lengthening of the limbs. There is one fairly rare condition, Kallmann's syndrome (more rare in females), in which a hypothalamic-pituitary-gonadotropic deficit can be implicated early in the diagnostic workup, by reason of an associated deficit in the sense of smell. The deficit may amount to complete anosmia. Though the evidence is not yet final, it seems likely that youths with Kallmann's syndrome tend to be hyposexual and to be late in falling in love and marrying (Bobrow, Money, and Lewis, 1971).

Another source of pubertal failure in boys of normal stature lies not in a timing delay, nor in hypothalamic-pituitary malfunction, but in the gonads themselves. They may be missing, having completely atrophied, or be partially atrophied and nonfunctional. In some cases the testes have been seen at exploratory surgery in childhood, during an attempt to bring them into the scrotum, only to disappear in complete atrophy by middle teenage. It is believed that their atrophy is brought about by an autoimmune reaction whereby the body becomes immunized against one of its own organs and develops antibodies that destroy it. For boys with anorchia or hyporchia, testosterone replacement therapy is always essential. They may also be given prosthetic silicone-rubber testes for cosmetic purposes. Hormonal virilization in these cases is excellent, which is by no means always true in cases involving pituitary deficit.

Regardless of the etiology of pubertal delay or failure, it is preferable not to leave a boy untreated after the fifteenth year. Otherwise the gap between prepubertal physique age and chronologic age imposes an undesirable handicap on psychosocial maturation. If only a timing delay is suspected, then a trial period of 3 to 6 months on either the gonadotropin,

FSH (follicle stimulating hormone), or on testosterone will have a priming action that stimulates the testes to their own adolescent activity. If the testes fail to respond, or fail to continue their response, then the trial treatment becomes diagnostically valuable as having indicated the probable need for long-term testosterone replacement therapy.

The relationship of pubertal delay to erotic function in boys of normal stature is partly a function of diagnosis. Whereas all are at a disadvantage with respect to physique age and participation in dating and teenaged affairs, some have more difficulty than others in keeping up with their age group. One has the impression that boys in whom pituitary malfunction is involved have a greater likelihood of difficulty in this respect. Some boys have romantic imagery and fantasies while still hormonally prepubertal. Some are girl-watchers and a few even have full-fledged sexual affairs. One anorchic boy had married at age 19 and had sexual intercourse routinely before his prepubertal condition was discovered, at age 21, when testosterone therapy was instituted (Money and Alexander, 1967). Such a case is the exception and not the rule, however. Many boys with delayed puberty are indifferent with respect to sexual urge and sexual activity, including masturbation, until they receive testosterone. In some cases of hypogonadotropinism, there is a large residue of indifference even after testosterone therapy.

Hormonal Dimorphism

Because sex differences have traditionally been conceived of as dichotomous and absolute, it was assumed in the early days of sex-hormone research, at the beginning of this century, that females produce only female sex hormone, and males only male sex hormone. The sex hormones were named accordingly. In actual fact there is overlap, and the hormones of both sexes are present in men and in women. The hormonal difference between the sexes is not a matter of either-or, but of proportion between estrogens (the feminizing hormones), androgens (the masculinizing hormones), and progestins or gestagens (the pregnancy hormones).

All three of the sex hormones, gestagen, androgen, and estrogen are closely related in chemical structure, and all three have several structural variants (which may or may not be biologically active). The pattern of hormonal synthesis in the body is from progestin to androgen to estrogen. For all three, the site of production may be the ovary or testis, or the cortex of the adrenal gland.

Circulating sex hormone levels in blood plasma may be measured directly from blood samples. In special cases, and for precision purposes, the blood sample may be taken from the vein leaving the testis, or ovary, or adrenal cortex. Alternatively, hormone levels may be estimated approximately and indirectly from their residues, or metabolic breakdown products, in the urine. The technical obstacles to obtaining an accurate measure of biologically active plasma estrogens, androgens, and gestagens circulating in the bloodstream are considerable. Satisfactory techniques of measurement, based particularly on the method of radioimmunoassay, were developed only as recently as the latter half of the 1960s. Measurements to date (C. Migeon, personal communication) indicate that testosterone level in the male is ten times higher than in the female. Androstendione, a weak androgen, is slightly but significantly higher in the female than the male, and dehydroepiandrosterone is the same in both sexes. Estrogen level is more difficult to report, because of the magnitude of its fluctuation with the menstrual cycle. One stable comparison is between normal males and post-menopausal females. In both, the levels of estradiol may be as low as between approximately one seventh and one ninth, respectively, of the level in normal menstruating women at the peak of their cyclic estrogenic production (Korenman, Perrin, and McCallum, 1969). Progesterone measurements in the male are low, as in the nonprogestinic phase of the female's menstrual cycle, and not easily measurable by today's techniques.

In the normal male, the influence of male sex hormone overrides that of female sex hormone normally produced in the male body. The reverse holds true for females, except that the growth of pubic and axillary hair is attributed to adrenal androgen. Also, as women age after the menopause, androgenic influence becomes more obvious in deepening of the voice and growth of facial hair.

Heterotypic Use of Estrogen

Experimentally it is easy to demonstrate a heterotypic or incongruous sex-hormonal effect in animals by administering estrogen to males and androgen to females. In man, there must always be a therapeutic or iatrogenic rationale to treatment with hormones that normally produce effects typical of or appropriate to the opposite sex. Alternatively, there are pathological conditions in which the effect of spontaneously produced heterotypic hormones can be studied. Whether iatrogenic or pathologic in origin, heterotypic hormones have their effect on the mind either indirectly through changes they induce in the body, or directly through changes induced in the nervous system and brain. The latter are dealt with more in the next chapter than in this one.

Estrogen injected into human males replicates what has been found experimentally in animals. In human beings, there are three conditions under which genetic and gonadal males receive estrogen. One is in the case of birth defect of the genitalia when the individual has been reared as a girl and needs estrogen to feminize at puberty. The second is in cases of male-to-female transexualism. The third is in cases of cancer of the prostate gland, when estrogen is used to help suppress the malignancy.

The most complete estrogenization of the genetic male is obtained when the hormone is used before masculine puberty has had a chance to exert its own effect. This condition is met when a genetic male baby is assigned at birth as a female (see Chapter 7). Such a baby is born with congenital absence of the penis or with a micropenis that is or is not hypospadiac (Figure 10.2) and too miniscule to permit reconstruction as a functional organ of copulation. In such a case, the first stage of feminizing surgery to correct the external appearance is usually performed in the first weeks of life. Surgical creation of a vaginal cavity is better left until later, nearer to the time when the vagina will be kept open by use in intercourse.

The testes, which may or may not be descended, are usually removed at the first operation. Their removal is primarily to prevent their secreting male sex hormone at puberty. It also guarantees against the risk of cancer in later life, for when the penis is severely deformed, there is a high chance that the testes also will be defective, sterile, and prone to develop malignancy in adulthood.

A child given the foregoing type of treatment at birth grows normally, physically and psychologically, as a girl, without further surgery or medication during childhood. Special psychologic counseling of parents and child in connection with sex education is needed to prepare the girl for estrogen substitution therapy at the age of puberty, for motherhood by adoption, and for vaginoplasty later in teenage. Estrogen substitution therapy is timed to coincide with the social age of puberty—a little later if more height is needed, and a little earlier if the girl is growing too tall. The result is a perfectly feminized body, indistinguishable in morphology and appearance from that of a genetic female with her own ovarian puberty—though menses, of course, are lacking. Figure 10.3 shows what can be achieved, even in a case in which the male gonads were not removed until age eleven, after they had already begun to secrete male sex hormone.

The effect of medication with estrogen for male transexualism and for prostatic cancer is more limited than in the foregoing type of case, since masculine secondary sexual development will have already taken place. The visible effects are enlargement of the breasts; a tendency to feminine deposition of subcutaneous fat; reduced oiliness of the skin; reduced facial acne, if present; and an arrest of masculine balding, if it has begun. Beard and body hair do not disappear, but the hairs tend to be less wiry, and more slow growing. Needless to say, these changes are not appreciated by men with prostatic cancer, whereas transexuals, who want to live as women, are delighted with them—so much so that they sometimes treat themselves with estrogenic birth control pills or estrogenic skin creams.

Cancer of the prostate and its surgery interferes with sexual functioning. Unoperated transexuals, therefore, are the best source of information on the effect of estrogen on male sexual functioning. From them one learns that the penis, testes, and prostate gland regress in size. In the testes, spermatogenesis in the seminiferous tubules ceases, and androgen production in the Leydig cells is reduced to zero or near zero. Prostatic secretion fails, so that there is no ejaculate, even if there is an erection, which is itself unlikely. Transexuals find their loss of potency gratifying, for, unlike regular men, they want to escape from all reminders of the penis and its functioning. For them estrogen is an erotic tranquilizer. Estrogen given to heterosexual men with cancer does not cause them to have homosexual desires. Their heterosexuality remains unchanged except for diminution of libido and loss of potency, both of which they regret.

Heterotypic Use of Androgen

The effect of exogenous androgen on females is similar in animals and man. In the human species, there are three conditions under which genetic and gonadal females are given a strongly masculinizing form of the hormone, usually testosterone. One is in cases of genetic females, born with ambiguous genitalia, reared as boys, and needing hormonal masculinization at puberty. The second is in cases of female-to-male transexualism. The third is in cases of cancer of the breast, when androgen is used to help suppress the malignancy.

As in the counterpart case of pubertally induced feminization of the male, the most complete masculinization of the genetic female is achieved when the hormone is used before feminine puberty has had a chance to exert its own effect. The specifications for such treatment are that a female hermaphrodite had a large enough phallus at birth to have been perceived as a male hermaphrodite and reared as a boy. Then, at the age of puberty, with the appearance of breasts and urethral (menstrual) bleeding, the diagnosis is belatedly established, but not soon enough for the boy's sense of psychosexual identity to be changed to female. Surgical and hormonal corrections are therefore directed toward masculinization. Such cases are extremely rare, first because cases of female hermaphroditism uncomplicated by adrenocortical virilization (the female adrenogenital syndrome) are rare; and, second, because modern diagnostic vigilance rarely lets adrenogenital cases pass unrecognized at birth, whereupon they are successfully assigned and surgically corrected as females.

When testosterone therapy is undertaken at puberty, it arrests feminine enlargement of the pelvis, prevents feminine deposition of fat, and induces masculine muscular development. Breast growth is arrested, though such glandular tissue as may have already developed does not totally regress: it needs to be removed surgically (mastectomy). Body hair grows in masculine distribution, including a beard. The voice deepens as the larynx enlarges to form an Adam's apple.

Menstruation is suppressed, though with the possibility of eventual break-through bleeding. Permanent menstrual suppression requires ovariectomy and hysterectomy, which also are advisable to prevent possible back-up of urine after the phallus is repaired for urination in the standing position. The phallus itself enlarges and becomes erectile as a penis, its erectile potency being dependent on continuing testosterone therapy (either with methyltestosterone linguets, daily, or by injection with long-acting testosterone enanthate monthly). To the extent that labioscrotal fusion had occurred prenatally, there will be a rudimentary scrotum which will become more rugose and wrinkled; it can be used to hold artificial testes made of silicone rubber.

The extent to which the prostate gland can develop under testosterone stimulation will depend on the extent to which it differentiated prenatally. Its size and the continuity of testosterone therapy will govern the quantity of ejaculatory fluid that can be produced. Orgasm will occur, regardless of the quantity of ejaculate, and may, perhaps, be successively repeated with a shorter refractory period than in the typical male.

The overall effect of pubertal androgenization of a genetic female is to produce a handsome-appearing man whose medical status cannot even be guessed at by those with whom he works and socializes, even should these others be medical and biological scientists. Somatic virilization is far more complete than in genetic male hermaphrodites who have a partial androgen-insensitivity syndrome and are partially resistant to androgen at the cellular level.

Testosterone virilization of the female transexual (Figure 10.4) is similar to that described in the foregoing, except insofar as the adult female pelvic bone structure cannot be reduced, and the breasts do not disappear except under surgery. The amount of facial and body hair growth is individually variable, but may be masculinely complete. Eventually the hairline may recede, as in most men. The voice deepens. Feminine subcutaneous fat depots change, so that the contour of appearance becomes more masculine. The skin, especially of the face becomes more oily, and may for a while show adolescent-type acne. Perhaps because of such skin changes, there is an overall appearance of looking more youthful, at least for a time, than the chronologic age—which also happens in reverse, in the feminization of the male.

The clitoris enlarges under the influence of testosterone, and its corpora becomes more effectively erectile. The enlargement is not sufficient to give the appearance of a penis. Surgically, the clitoris can be imbedded into a skin-graft simulation of a penis, but the result is far from satisfactory. Permanent suppression of the menses requires hysterectomy and ovariectomy.

The virilizing body changes that make the female transexual feel happy are detested, but must be tolerated, by the woman with breast cancer. Cancer patients sometimes report an increase of libido under the influence of testosterone, whereby they become more actively interested in initiating sexual intercourse. They may or may not enjoy this change, dependent on its consistency with their self-image. Since transexual women tend to be fairly active sexually, such a change is not particularly evident in this group. Heterosexual women do not become homosexual under the influence of increased androgen which, within limits, affects their libido only by magnifying it.

Clinical Syndromes: Incongruent Hormonal Effects in the Male

Therapeutic masculinization of the female, or feminization of the male, is resented unless it happens to be congruent with the gender identity. Regardless of what they do to the body, exogenous hormones do not change the sense of self, sexually, nor the choice of the object of erotic desires (see Chapter 8). The same is true of developmental conditions in which the body has some feature or features of the opposite sex (Figure 10.5).

In the male, the most visible deviation from normal masculine body build is the growth of breasts, gynecomastia. A small amount of glandular growth behind the nipples and areolae at the time of puberty (adolescent gynecomastia) is so common as to be considered a normal variation, especially since the swelling eventually regresses. There are some cases, however, when it does not, and must be surgically removed: the breasts grow as large as those of a normal adolescent girl. A boy with such breasts regards them with shame, as an affliction. Unable to predict the direness of the consequences involved—cancer? turning into a girl?—he binds his chest in secret with a binding cloth, and avoids seeking help, lest he hear the worst. Of course he cannot keep the source of his shame hidden for ever, but by the time he does get directed to medical help, a great deal of psychologic mischief may already have been wrought.

There is no satisfactory etiologic explanation of adolescent gynecomastia. It may be that too much biologically potent estrogen is being produced by the testes, or is not being rapidly enough destroyed by the liver—breast enlargement may occur secondary to liver damage induced by severe starvation. Alternatively, there may be a peculiarity of end-organ response to hormone at the cellular level in the glandular tissue of the breasts. One condition known to favor an unusually high incidence of persistent adolescent gynecomastia is the XXY (Klinefelter's) syndrome. More rarely, in adulthood, gynecomastia may be the product of an estrogen-secreting tumor of the testis.

Apart from gynecomastia, there are no other clearly hormone-linked feminine traits that may occur in the male. Youths with gynecomastia do not necessarily have a feminine pelvis and fat distribution on the hips. There are some males, however, who do have disproportionately large hips. Little is known about the growth chemistry of variations in body build. Some are obviously genetic, in that they are shared by other members of the same genetic stock.

On the assumption that growth chemistry, especially hormonal, will influence not only body build but also mental attitude, some investigators have, from time to time, expended considerable effort in trying to identify indices of gynandromorphy (or androgyny). However, correlations with personality, especially with reference to bisexuality, have proved to be inconsequential. There is no correlation between body type and virility or feminity of erotic behavior or parental behavior. Also, there is no demonstrable correlation between body build and homosexuality in either the male or female (see Chapter 11).

Hermaphroditic children who, upon reaching the age of puberty, are confronted with an incongrous hormonal sex relative to their gender identity can, in the majority of cases, be helped with hormonal therapy. In some instances, gonadectomy may also be necessary. The only cases for which no hormonal therapy has yet been devised are those cases of genetic males who are unresponsive to androgens, and living as men. There are two types, both rare. One is the variant of the adrenogenital syndrome with 17α-hydroxylase deficiency that blocks the synthesis of steroids, including androgen. The other is the incomplete form of the testicular-feminizing, androgen-insensitivity syndrome. In this syndrome there is a blockage of androgen uptake at the cellular level, hereditary in origin, but biochemically as yet undeciphered. Affected individuals are able to maintain a masculine gender identity, if reared as males, despite total lack of secondary sexual masculinization, and lack of erectile capacity of the incompletely-formed, hypospadiac micropenis. Life is not easy for them, however, as one can well imagine. It would have been their great good luck had they originally been assigned as females.

Clinical Syndromes: Incongruent Hormonal Effects in the Female

The counterpart of gynecomastia in the male is hirsutism with voice deepening and clitoral hypertrophy in the female. In the adult female, such virilism may occur in response to a male-hormone secreting tumor of either the adrenal cortex or the ovary. It may also occur in the Stein-Leventhal syndrome of polycystic ovaries, amenorrhea, sterility, and hormonal imbalance. More rarely, virilism may also occur as an atypically late-appearing manifestation of the adrenogenital syndrome, in which masculinization more usually appears so early as to be evident at birth (see Chapter 6). At puberty and thereafter, an unregulated excess of the male hormone responsible for the pathognomonic virilism of the adrenogenital syndrome may also be responsible for menstrual irregularity or failure (for which, however, there are other different causes in other different syndromes), and for an otherwise unexplained failure of lactation, should lactation have been established following a successful pregnancy.

Postpubertal virilism induced by the adrenogenital syndrome of late onset can be severely disfiguring to a woman, but it is not disfiguring to quite the same excessive extent as in a woman afflicted and untreated since birth (Figure 10.6). In teenage, such an individual may have almost the appearance of a stocky muscle-man in a physique magazine.

Regardless of its etiology, masculinization of the body typically is a source of mortification to the woman afflicted. The hormonal source of bodily masculinization does not masculinize also her mind. By contrast, her mind focuses on the possibility of finding a way to be rid of the masculine stigmata which the unwanted hormone produces.

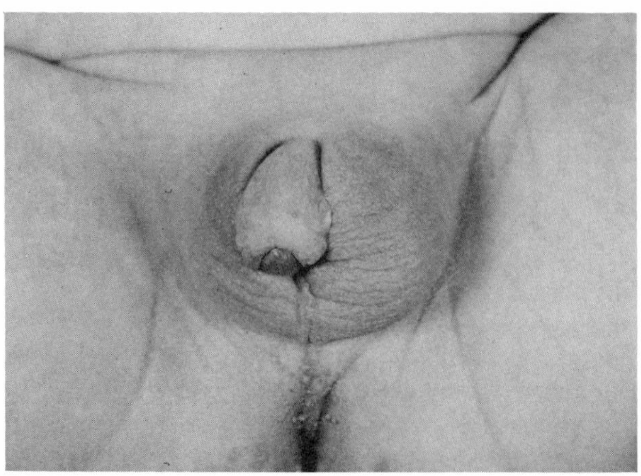

Figure 10.2. Hermaphroditic ambiguity of the genitalia resulting from failure of masculine differentiation in a genetic male.

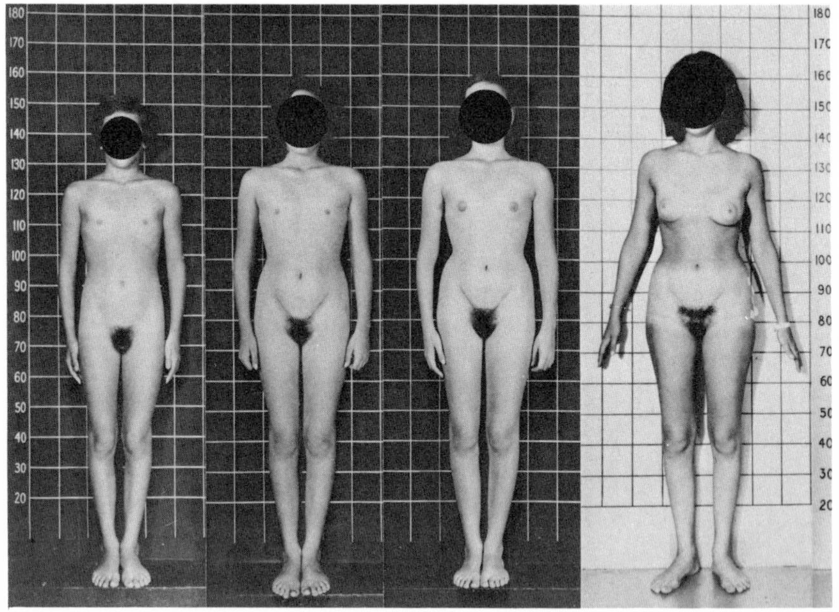

Figure 10.3. Pubertal feminization of a genetic male hermaphrodite by means of estrogen therapy. The photographs were taken at ages 11, 12, 13 and 19 years.

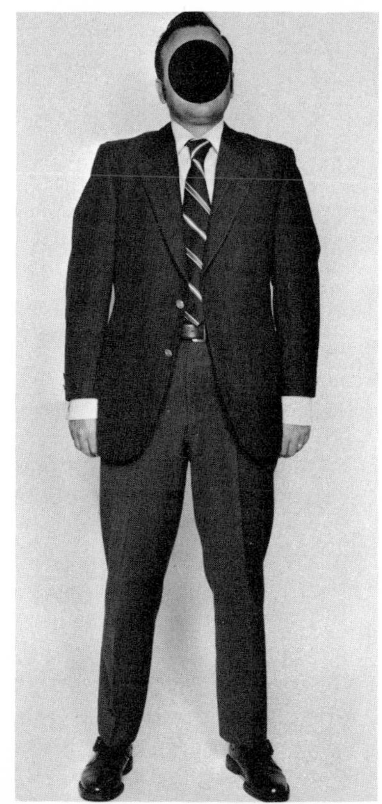

Figure 10.4. The appearance as a man of a sex-reassigned female transexual, who is accepted unambiguously in social life as a man.

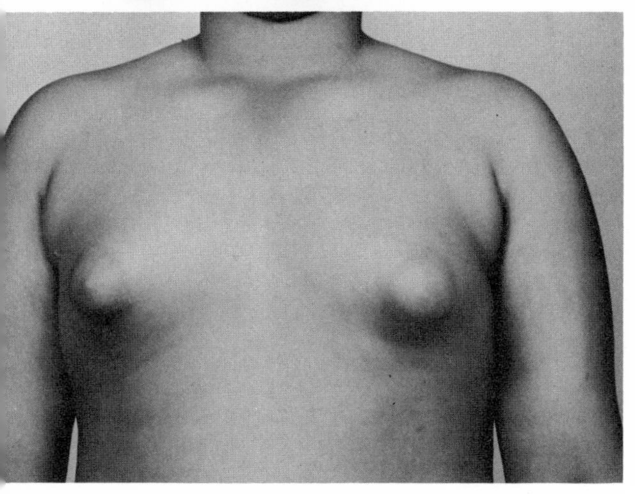

Figure 10.5. An example of idiopathic gynecomastia in a boy of 13 years, otherwise endocrinologically and anatomically normal.

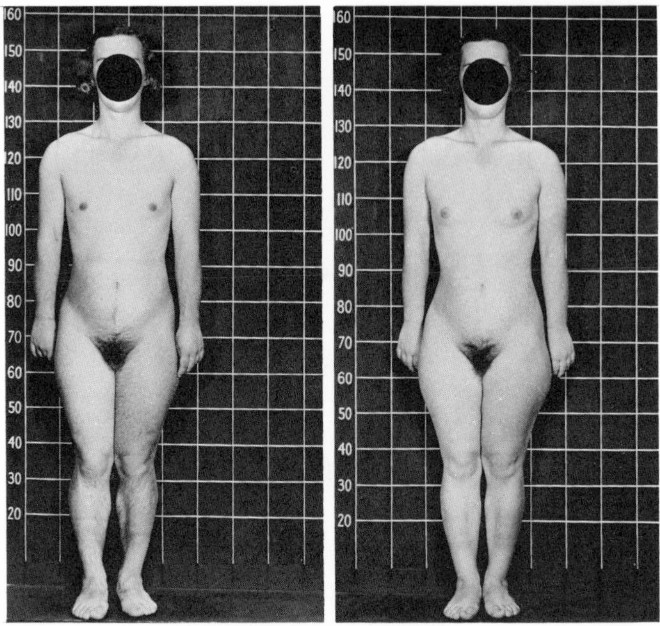

Figure 10.6. Masculinized body appearance of a teenaged girl with the untreated adrenogenital syndrome, showing the induction of feminine breast development (right) following initial treatment with cortisone which disinhibits the secretion of ovarian estrogen.

11

PUBERTAL HORMONES: LIBIDO AND EROTIC BEHAVIOR

Castration and Menopausal Effects

Mankind has known, apparently since time immemorial or at least since the discovery of animal husbandry, of the effects of castration on the mammalian male. The castration of captured enemies has long been recorded, as has the castration of youths assigned to be harem attendants. As late as the eighteenth century in Europe, boy soprano virtuosos were castrated to provide the opera with castrate sopranos for adult female roles, in an era when a stage career for a woman would have been morally vulgar. Even until the early twentieth century, there survived members of an obscure Russian sect, the Skoptsy, for whom removal of the testes, and preferably the penis also, was an article of faith and a badge of membership. Castration was part of the pseudomedical fake experimentation performed in Hitler's concentration camps, some of the survivors from which are still living as castrates on testosterone substitution therapy.

Castration is practiced in today's medicine chiefly for cancer of the testes, or as adjunctive therapy for cancer of the prostate. Rather rarely, it is also performed on transexuals who change their way of life from male to female. In some political jurisdictions, it has been possible, by court order, to castrate mental defectives and criminal sex offenders (Bremer, 1959). It is now realized, however, that vasectomy is sufficient to prevent a mentally defective youth from breeding, and that hormonal castration, which is reversible, is perhaps more effective than surgical castration, which is not, in the treatment of criminal sex offenders (Money, 1970c).

The effects of castration on the body, when it is performed on a boy before puberty, are the same as described in the preceding chapter for complete testicular failure. The eunuch retains a soprano voice and grows no beard. His arms and legs grow disproportionately long, relative to the trunk. Pubic and axillary hair grows (presumably under the influence of adrenal androgens), but, along with body hair, is feminine in pattern. There is no masculine balding. Subcutaneous fat deposits are feminine in distribution.

There is an extraordinary lack of recorded information, from the time when prepubertal castrates were easy to find, concerning their sexual and erotic capacity (see reviews by Money, 1961a and 1961b). The older authorities, often with one eye on experimental animal evidence, generally claimed that prepubertal castrates showed no libidinal behavior. However, the evidence that prepubertal boys can easily get an erection and do sometimes, in prepubertal play, effect vaginal intercourse, contradicts this claim. Moreover, it is not unheard of for a teenaged castrate-equivalent, a boy with developmental anorchia, to marry (Money and Alexander, 1967) and by his own evidence and that of his wife have regular sexual intercourse accompanied by mutually satisfying erotic feeling. For the boy concerned, there was no ejaculatory discharge. It was not possible to calibrate and compare the orgasmic feeling he reported initially with the feeling he experienced following androgen treatment—except that the two were different.

Exceptional cases notwithstanding, it is probably true that prepubertal castration, without subsequent testosterone replacement therapy, is followed more often than not by sexual apathy in adulthood. Sexual apathy is not, of course, equivalent to effeminacy. If one judges from cases of anorchia (since prepubertally castrated normal males are almost nonexistent today), then lack of testes and testicular hormones does not, per se, dispose a boy to feminine emotionality, with lack of aggressive self-assertion and easy tears. He may be overcome by self-pity as he contemplates his nonvirilizing fate, but it is also likely that he will rile against his adversity, with defiance and determination to overcome it. Yet, even if he is disheartened and weepy as a teenager, it is because he strives to be a man, not because he is homosexually effeminate in wanting to be loved as a female.

The general and clinical wisdom of the ages, based on observation of human beings and of animal experiments, has long been that the effects of prepubertal and postpubertal castration are different. The difference in the postpubertally castrated male is that his genitalia, especially internally, have matured to full size, and his mind has accumulated the memory of sexual sensation and the feeling of ejaculatory orgasm. Animal and human evidence alike show that there is not only species variation, but also a wide range of individual variation. In human males, erection and ejaculation are both dependent on the central nervous system as well as the hormonal system. Ejaculation is more hormonally dependent, and so disappears first, but may be supplanted by a dry-run orgasm with corresponding feelings. Even when the feelings diminish in their peak of intensity, they may still be rewarding, so long as the erection is still potent and responsive to erotic stimuli. The length of time before erectile potency is eclipsed, after loss of the testes, is extremely variable. Some men lose it rapidly, within weeks, and others gradually, over months or years.

The same variability that relates to loss of erection relates also to emotional changes following castration. One man may be rapidly overtaken by almost catastrophic crying spells and depressions, whereas another finds himself sliding slowly, over a period of two years or more, into a state of reduced initiative, energy, and ability to assert himself socially and vocationally among his colleagues. One injection of long-acting testosterone enanthate, or a week of oral methyltestosterone, and the deleterious effects, emotional and erotic, are completely reversed.

As difficult as it is to find untreated eunuchs who were prepubertally castrated, it is virtually impossible to find their female counterpart. The removal of ovaries is surgically far more complex than the removal of testes, and there is no customary or legal tradition for doing so. In the rare case of a medical indication for prepubertal ovariectomy, replacement hormones are administered at the expected age of puberty. The most likely instance of the persistence of infantilism until late teenage generally proves to be diagnostically a case of Turner's syndrome (Chapter 6). The growth defect of Turner's syndrome is incompatible with the eunuchoid increase in height that would otherwise accompany failure of ovarian puberty. Vaginally, however, there is the same failure of adult secretions as in castration. In both instances, if intercourse is attempted before hormonal replacement therapy and without application of an artificial lubricant, the vagina will be dry and painful.

Vaginal dryness is one of the chief sequelae of ovariectomy in adult women (Filler and Drezner, 1944; Waxenberg, 1963) and also of the menopause (see review by Kane, Lipton, and Ewing, 1969). It can be corrected by estrogen substitution therapy in small dosage, or by use of a lubricant.

Adult ovariectomy has been, and sometimes still is, recklessly included in surgery for hysterectomy. Usually it is unnecessary and undesirable and should be expressly forbidden by the patient when she signs the operative permit, particularly if she is not yet postmenopausal. Otherwise, unless she is put on replacement hormone, she will enter a postcastration menopause, with irregularities of vasomotor function, temperature, and perspiration control, emotional equilibrium, and sleep.

The symptoms of postcastration menopause are experienced by women with the androgen-insensitivity syndrome (Chapter 6), if their feminizing testes are removed after puberty and if replacement estrogen is not prescribed. Castration before puberty does not, however, induce such symptoms either at the time of the operation, or later, after the expected age of puberty. Girls with Turner's syndrome who have no ovaries do not exhibit castration symptoms if they remain untreated throughout teenage, nor if they later withdraw themselves from estrogen substitution therapy for a period of time. The same is true of hypopituitary dwarfs who have ovaries, but no gonadotropic hormones from the pituitary to stimulate the ovaries.

The equivalence of vasomotor postcastration symptoms in cases of the testicular-feminizing syndrome and in normal women, and their absence following castration in normal men, gives poor support to those who uphold the idea of a male climacteric as the equivalent of the female menopause. In normal male aging, there is a gradual quantitative tapering off of male hormone production, but no dramatic change, as in the cessation of hormonal cycling that heralds the finish of menstrual periods in the female. The older male is likely to find that his penis obliges with an erection less often than his libidinal desire would dictate, for he undergoes a slow diminution, in this respect, from the typical pneumatic-hammer insistence of the penis in early adolescence to its quietude in the eighth and ninth decades. The female may undergo a corresponding progressive libidinal quiescence, but her copulatory role is such that she possesses, mechanistically speaking, an orifice and a cavity that will awaken to their own feelings while they are in copulatory use, instead of as a prerequisite to their being put to such use, which is the way of the penis.

Hormonal Castration Effects

In everyday usage, castration means surgical castration. The alternative of hormonal castration has already been mentioned (Chapter 10) in connection with the estrogen treatment of male transexuals. Functional castration with estrogen is familiar to livestock farmers for increasing the fat and weight of carcasses.

On a limited scale, estrogenic castration has sometimes been used as an attempted method of suppressing libido and sexual behavior in habitual sex offenders whose behavior otherwise would bring them excessively long or indeterminate jail sentences. The castrating effect is reversible. But, because estrogen promotes breast growth, its use is abhorrent to most men, irrespective of the nature of their sexual compulsion and the term of their prison sentence.

Like estrogen, progesterone also has a functional castration effect on the male (Diamond, 1966). By inhibiting spermatogenesis, it induces sterility, and by inhibiting androgen secretion by the testes, it induces a reduction of sexual activity. The testes become reduced in size. All these effects are reversible. There is no breast growth.

Within the past decade, hormones other than estrogen have been found to have nonfeminizing, androgen-depleting or antiandrogenic effects (Neumann and Elger, 1966; Diamond, 1966). They are synthetic hormones and they belong among steroids, as do also the naturally-occurring sex hormones. One is cyproterone acetate, a derivative of hydroxyprogesterone, already mentioned in Chapters 3, 4, and 5. The other is medroxyprogesterone acetate (Provera®). Both of these nonestrogenizing hormones, when given to male sex offenders, have been discovered to have a favorable effect, at least in some cases, in lowering libido and facilitating better monitoring and regulation of sexual behavior so as to keep the offender out of jail (Laschet, 1969; Hoffet, 1968; Seebandt, 1968). Cyproterone acetate is said to have its effect at the cellular level by competing with and blocking the use of the body's own testosterone at the receptor sites of the target organs (Neumann, Steinbeck, and Hahn, 1970). Medroxyprogesterone is said to have its effect by lowering the plasma level of testosterone from the testes (Migeon, personal communication; Money, 1970c). Since the drug itself does not have an androgenizing effect, it thus acts as a chemical castrating agent for as long as it is administered. The effect is reversible. Its efficacy, while being administered, may conceivably be due also in part to a direct, inhibiting action on sex-organizing centers of the brain, for it is one of the progesterones that, in large enough doses, is known to have an anesthetic effect on the central nervous system.

It is probable that the beneficial effect of androgen antagonists is not simply a matter of their hormonal action alone, but also of a psychic realignment (Money, 1970c) made possible by reason of the life crisis commonly responsible for the initiation of treatment.

Medroxyprogesterone acetate administered to very young girls with idiopathic precocious puberty suppresses breast enlargement and suppresses mentruation. Since these young girls, if untreated, do not show overt sexual behavior to any significant degree, one has as yet no way of knowing whether the hormone may also reduce sexual behavior in the female. At the present time, as a matter of fact, there is no pharmacologic agent known specifically to suppress libido and sexual behavior in the female.

When androgen is given to women, it does not have a counteractive but an augmentive effect on sexual desire and the potential initiation of sexual behavior. One may, indeed, make a case for the proposition that androgen is the libido hormone in both sexes (Money, 1961a)—in woman, for the initiative phase versus the acceptive phase of her menses-cycle of erotism. (See also the section on primate experiments, below.)

Woman's Sexual Cycle

In the male, androgen is secreted by the Leydig cells of the testes either at a steady rate or, possibly, with episodic peaks related to sexual activity (Anon., 1970). The possibility of a peak derives from the evidence that the shaved beard grows faster the day before intercourse is expected following a period of forced sexual isolation and inaction. In the female by contrast, the hormonal secretions of the ovary are cyclic, in synchrony with the menstrual cycle. At the completion of the phase of menstrual bleeding, a new egg-containing follicle takes its turn at enlarging, and secreting estrogen. At mid-point in the new cycle, ovulation occurs: the follicle ruptures and releases its egg. Estrogen production then diminishes during the succeeding week, while progesterone, the pregnancy hormone (also referred to as a progestin or a gestagen), increases. It is the withdrawal of estrogen that induces the uterus to shed its unoccupied endometrial lining and to menstruate, as is evident in all cases requiring replacement therapy: it is sufficient to prescribe estrogen for three weeks on, and one week off, to induce regular menstruation. Progesterone (gestagen) is literally a gestation hormone, its initial gestational function being to facilitate nidation of the egg in the uterine wall, should it have encountered spermatozoa and have become fertilized by one of them.

The hormonal events that lead up to menstruation are not restricted to the ovaries and uterus. Because the delivery system for all hormones is the bloodstream, all cells of the body are potentially involved. This is the physiological fact that underlies the phenomena of premenstrual tension and/or menstrual cramps. Some women will frankly describe themselves as cranky, bitchy, and impossible to live with, in spite of their own best intentions, during the days of premenstrual tension. Others will not even be aware that their cycle has revolved full turn, unless they look at the calendar. And some, because of negative attitudes instilled into them in childhood, will transform a mild malaise into a major hypochondriachal illness.

There is no satisfactory explanation as to why some women are afflicted with particularly difficult premenstrual tension and irritability. The fact that they are is important, however, in any study of the female's peak period of sexual desire, because these women may feel too miserable to be bothered with sexual intercourse. These are women who are more likely to say that their period of maximum interest in sex is around the midcyclic time of ovulation.

Other women will say that their period of maximum desire corresponds with the menstrual phase of their cycle—even though they may not be able to do much about it, if they (or the partner) live with a taboo against menstrual blood.

Few studies have been done on the cyclicity of woman's sexual desire (Kane, Lipton, and Ewing 1969; Udry and Morris, 1968; review by Hampson and Hampson, 1961). These studies have produced confusing or contradictory results because they did not clearly distinguish between the quality of sexual desire that woman may experience at the ovulatory versus the menstrual phase of the sexual cycle. At the ovulatory period, her feeling of sexual desire is likely to be a desire to surrender and to be occupied sexually. At the menstrual period it is likely to be a feeling of desire to capture and envelop. The accomplishment of this desire requires taking the erotic initiative or, in the standard jargon of sex, being aggressive—which conventionally is supposed to be the prerogative of the male. The man who adheres scrupulously to the outmoded convention that a woman always is and should be erotically and sexually passive is wrong. Not only is he wrong, but he also doesn't know what he is missing—nor does the female. She too has the capacity and feeling for taking the sexual initiative. This is the feeling that seems to be enhanced if, for some or other therapeutic reason, a woman is given androgen in amounts abnormally high for a female.

The cyclic change in the nuance of woman's sexual desire, from being more receptive to more assertive, may manifest itself not only in her sexual behavior but also in her dreams. Van de Castle and Smith (1971, personal communication) studied 50 women student nurses, collecting their dreams over the course of the menstrual cycle, an average of nine dreams per person (range, 4 to 16). With reference to aggression in general, not specifically sexual aggression, they found a significant ($p < .001$) increase of dreams of aggression toward males, but not females, during the menstrual phase as compared with the nonmenstrual phase of the cycle. During the nonmenstrual phase, there were more dreams than during the menstrual phase ($p<.001$) of the female being the recipient of male aggression, but not of aggression from other females.

Friendliness toward both sexes was higher during the menstrual than the nonmenstrual phase, but only in the nonmenstrual phase were men in the dreams more frequently friendly toward a woman dreamer than were women. Friendliness initiated by other women was the same in both phases of a woman's dreams, but friendliness initiated by men increased significantly ($p<.001$) during the nonmenstrual phase.

Adding together dreams of either aggression or friendliness initiated, versus those of aggression or friendliness received, the menstrual phase emerged as the one when more interaction is initiated with either sex in dreams ($p<.001$); and, conversely, the nonmenstrual phase as the one when there is more dream interaction received from either sex, but especially from men ($p<.001$). In both phases men figure more frequently than do women in dreams as initiators or recipients of either aggression or friendliness. The additive effect reaches higher statistical significance ($p<.001$) in the nonmenstrual than the menstrual phase, which obviously is the phase when a woman dreams predominantly of encounters with men, whether positively or negatively.

Van de Castle and Smith did not make a study specifically of the approach-receive dimension in the sexual interactions represented in their subjects' dreams. The ratio of dreams with sex to total dreams during the menstrual phase was .105, and .111 during the nonmenstrual phase, the difference not being statistically significant. The total number of dreams in each phase was 114 and 352, respectively.

Human females are not alone in having two peaks or phases of sexual desire per cycle of menstruation. Loy (1970) studied free-ranging rhesus monkeys on Cayo Santiago, Puerto Rico, and found that nonpregnant females showed a phase of sexual behavior at midcycle, and another phase of similar behavior perimenstrually or during menstruation.

Primate Experiments on Hormones and Mating Cyclicity

Because of the convenience of their size, rodents have been favorite laboratory animals on which the effects of hormones on mating behavior have been tested. For those who are interested in human sexual behavior, however, these animals are not so valuable: they are an estrous species and we, with other primates, are a menstrual species. Moreover, rodents, as well as annually seasonal mammals, exhibit certain components of copulatory dimorphic behavior only if the necessary and appropriate hormones activate them. By contrast, many components of sexual behavior in the human and other higher primates are not exclusively hormone-dependent, even if hormonally influenced, for their release. The most valuable animal experiments for human beings interested in themselves are, therefore, experiments on higher primates.

Michael (1971) and Herbert (1970) and their collaborators have directed research expressly to the determinants of sexual behavior related to the sexual cycle of the female rhesus monkey. Their experiments are all carefully designed, with all the necessary cross-checks and controls, so that their findings are clear and not contaminated with doubt. Their studies make clear that the female's hormonal cycle influences not only her own behavior, but that of her male partner also. The hypothesis, namely that the male's sense of smell is influenced by odor (Wiener, 1966; Herbert,1967; Michael and Keverne, 1968, 1970) emanating from the vagina has been conclusively demonstrated by Michael, Keverne, and Bonsall (1971). They isolated the odiferous substance from the vagina, that is to say the pheromone, named copulin, which is at its peak level at the time of ovulation. It proved to be constituted of short-chain aliphatic acids. The strength or level of this pheromone in the vagina is at its height at the time of ovulation. Then, when the cells lining the vagina are cornified, the male rhesus finds the female most attractive, and he initiates sexual activity more persistently. The amount of time from first mount to ejaculation is shortened, and the mounting rate and number of thrusts per mount increases.

The rhesus male typically mounts once or twice a minute, and after inserting the penis makes up to ten thrusts in 1½ to 2½ seconds before dismounting. The number of mounts may be half a dozen or more before ejaculation occurs. After dismounting, the animals sit together and may groom each other. In her estrogenic phase, the male grooms the female more than she him, whereas at other times, she is likely to groom him more (Michael and Herbert, 1963). He is then likely to be inattentive if he has access to another female who is at the ovulatory point of her cycle, even though this female would normally be low on his list of preferred females.

Sexual preference exists among rhesus monkeys, apparently in much the same way as it does in human beings. It can be easily tested by putting two females and one male together. One becomes his favorite, and the other a lonely outcast, unless she is ovulating or estrogenized by injection while the other female is not. Though the basis of preference is known not to be hormonal, its actual basis has not been discovered. It may bear some relationship to dominance hierarchy, for when raised in a troop, an infant monkey's subsequent dominance is affected by its mother's own dominance position; and the dominance position of the mother herself reflects the favoritism accorded her by the dominant male of the group. By contrast, a monkey raised in isolation, with no mother and no playmates, is unable to be sexually receptive and to position itself correctly for coitus in adulthood (Harlow, Joslyn, Senko, and Dopp, 1966).

When a female is at her maximum attractiveness to the male, either because she is at the ovulatory phase of her cycle or because she has been experimentally estrogen treated, the male usually makes his mounts without any visible invitation from her in the form of a sexual presentation. Such signaling is not necessary to stimulate the male at this time, though it may help to arouse his interest later in the cycle.

The various experiments of Michael, Herbert and their co-workers leave no doubt that the female's attractiveness to the male is estrogen determined. If she is ovariectomized, it disappears. Likewise, if she is injected with progesterone, it disappears. At the same time, her own receptivity and interest in sex, as indicated by her standard gesture of presenting her hind end in sexual presentation, does not disappear. Obviously, sexual attractiveness and sexual receptiveness are not synonymous in monkeys (nor are they in human beings!). Herbert addressed himself to this issue and approached it specifically in consideration of the human clinical evidence that androgen is the libido hormone in women as well as men (Money, 1961a). He administered a small dose of testosterone (1 mg/day) to ovariectomized females and found that it greatly increased the number of times they presented sexually to males. The behavior of the males was unaffected. Larger doses of testosterone did not increase sexual behavior in the females, but diminished it by inducing aggressiveness in their behavior. The males did not retaliate.

The crucial question remaining was whether the female monkey's own endogenous production of androgen affected her sexual drive or receptivity (Everitt and Herbert, 1969, 1970). The adrenal cortex is the principal source of androgen in females (Baird, Horton, Longcope, and Tait, 1968). Herbert's next experiment, in collaboration with Everitt was one utilizing the drug, dexamethasone sodium sulphate (0.5 mg/kg/day), to suppress the production of hormones by the adrenal cortex. As expected, androgen levels fell, as did the levels of other adrenocortical hormones. At the same time, sexual receptivity also fell, as indicated by reduced presentations to invite the male to mount, or by outright rejection of his attempts to mount. This loss of receptivity was not responsive to any type of hormone treatment except treatment with minute amounts of testosterone (100 or 200μg/day). Receptivity was then completely restored. Moreover, treatment with testosterone before dexamethasone prevented the dexamethasone suppressive effect on sexual receptivity.

Herbert's experiments suggest that knowledge of human sexuality can be expanded by studying patients undergoing special treatments or tests—the dexamethasone test of adrenocortical function for example. Waxenberg (1963) and coworkers gathered psychosexual information on women undergoing ovariectomy first and then adrenalectomy, as part of a radical treatment for breast cancer. They found that only after the adrenals as well as the ovaries had been removed did libidinal feeling disappear.

More needs to be done also on the sense of smell in relationship to sexuality in men and women. It is known that women's smell acuity is, in general, superior to that of men, and that this superiority is lost if estrogen levels fall, after ovariectomy, for example (see review by Money, 1965a). Smell acuity also varies with the menstrual cycle. There is lesser acuity during the menstrual phase, and greater acuity at the ovulatory phase when the level of estrogen reaches a peak.

With respect to the male, one wonders whether the avid interest of some men in cunnilingus may not be related to an odiferous arousal or enhancement of sexual enthusiasm, but there is no experimental evidence one way or the other at the present time.

Pubertal Hormones and Homosexuality, Bisexuality, and Heterosexuality

The ordinary heterosexual man or woman is unable to reconcile his or her own common sense expectations with the phenomenon of an anatomic male who behaves with the mannerisms of a female, and is capable of a love affair and sexual relationship only with another anatomic male. Conversely, the same irreconcilability holds with respect to the masculine-behaving lesbian. The evidence of common sense is still further challenged, if the homosexual male or female also dresses as an impersonator of the opposite sex, and passes maritally, socially, and occupationally as a member of the opposite sex.

Impersonative homosexuality can be perhaps an obvious travesty, or else so convincing that writers of social, psychologic, or medical texts have fallen easily into the trap of reiterating a venerable shibboleth, namely, that homosexuality in one of its forms is innate and in its other form is acquired. Shibboleths, by their very nature, don't need proof. There is, as yet, no currently acceptable evidence of an innate form of homosexuality (Money, 1970b). There is also no evidence of an exclusively acquired form of homosexuality, as traditionally defined, for the so-called "acquired form" is actually a manifestation of bisexuality. Permanent or exclusive homosexuality will most likely be eventually explained as the product of interaction between prenatal and postnatal determinants.

All discussions of homosexuality become wasteful word games unless, at the outset, a differentiation is established between homosexuality defined as a behavioral act, versus homosexuality defined, by inference, as a permanent state of erotic disposition and preference. Any mammal is capable of homosexual behavior, in the sense of performing part or all of the act of mounting on a member of the same sex. In the case of males, intromission per rectum may also occur, and has been proved, in the ram, one mode of infectious sterility. This kind of behavior is widespread in the animal kingdom, though the evidence is transmitted, often by oral tradition in anecdotal accounts, rather than systematically observed and reported in writing. Mounting and smelling behavior is probably the most common homosexual behavior in the lower animals, and licking of the genitals of a same-sex partner less common than intromission between males.

Farm animals or wild animals observed in homosexual behavior are, almost without exception, also able to breed. In other words, they are bisexual. When in season, they copulate with alacrity if the opportunity provides for it. They exhibit homosexual behavior more often in childhood than in adulthood, and more often when sex-segregated than not. House-bound animals raised as pets and wild animals raised or held in captivity are more likely to show such long-term deviations from heterosexual behavior as preferential homosexuality.

Among human beings, optional facultative homosexual behavior sometimes occurs as part of the sexual play of childhood and prepuberty, or part of the sexual exploration of puberty and adolescence. Facultative homosexuality in the early years of sexual maturity may be in part a by-product of sexual segregation and cultural injunctions against boy-girl relationships. In some societies, indeed, adolescent homosexuality is a prescribed instead of a proscribed way of life (see Chapter 7). After adolescence, facultative homosexuality may be a product of enforced sexual segregation, as in prison or military service.

In our own society, the phenomenon of facultative homosexuality is nowhere better illustrated than when men or women are segregated in jail (Davis, 1969). In a men's prison, some men are of a sexual type known, in some institutions, by the nickname of "gorilla." The gorillas are men whose sexual activity on the outside is, by strong preference, heterosexual. They are not so moralistically and inhibitedly heterosexual, however, as to be incapable of achieving erection and orgasm by means of oral or anal insertion, whereas there are some men who are unable to hold an erection for oral or anal insertion. The gorillas, while they are incarcerated, therefore, seek opportunities for oral or anal sexual liaison with other male prisoners. There are certain rare institutions which permit cell-mate arrangements between such men and essential or obligative homosexual male prisoners who want to be the sexual partner of an otherwise heterosexual male. Other institutions segregate obligative homosexuals in a special tier or cell block. These are the institutions in which the gorillas earn their nickname. With no willing homosexuals available as partners, they test all newcomers of slight build to see if they have the will, the power, or the weapon (sharp objects are traded among prisoners) of self-defense. If the newcomer qualifies as timid, then he is slated to become the victim of repeated homosexual anal rape, in the shower room or in the cell block. It is perilous for him to lodge a complaint. Since the problem is frequent, the authorities do not have facilities to deal with it. A complainant is, therefore, subject to severe retribution from the gorillas against whom he has lodged a complaint.

Sexual relationships in a woman's prison are somewhat similar, except that the dominant and demanding partner, the "bull" or "stud", is one who is either lesbian or bisexual by preference on the outside and, in prison, tries to establish a relationship with a fellow prisoner who would, by preference, be heterosexual.

The male prisoner who is subjugated by the gorilla, and the female prisoner who is subjugated by the bull, do not develop a long-term pattern of homosexuality as a result of their experiences. The influence of experience in prison is, in fact, more likely to be that it exposes potentially bisexual people to the example of how to be gorillas or bulls, until they are released. Training in bisexuality of this type is, indeed, one of the indictments that may be brought against our juvenile detention institutions.

Imprisonment is not, of course, the sole source of facultative homosexuality—it is simply an exceptionally clear illustration of the difference between the extremes of obligative heterosexuality, facultative heterosexuality-homosexuality, and obligative homosexuality. The origin of these three different conditions in human psychosexuality is still without a definite explanation. The new science of cytogenetics gives no answer, for the majority of homosexuals and bisexuals have the same number of chromosomes as obligatively heterosexual people. Whether there may be not a chromosomal but a genic difference between the three psychosexual types is an open question for which no answer is available at the present stage of the development of genetic science.

The science of endocrinology also gives no clear clue as to the origin of the three psychosexual types—homosexual, bisexual, and heterosexual.

In the 1940s, there were a few studies of the urinary output of metabolites of the sex hormones in homosexuals versus controls, but the methods were crude, and the results equivocal (see Money, 1961a). Interest in this particular type of investigation lapsed until 1970, when two new publications appeared (Margolese, 1970; Loraine, Ismail, Adamopoulos, and Dove, 1970). Both used improved, modern methods of estimating sex-hormone production by measuring hormonal metabolites in urine. This is an acceptable procedure, but one that yields no precision of information regarding the level of biologically active sex hormones in the blood stream. The metabolic breakdown products of sex hormones get into the urine by way of the liver and the kidneys. Urinary levels of these metabolites often tell more about the functional efficiency of the liver than they do about the amount or type of sex hormone actually released by the gonads and the adrenal cortices into the bloodstream. Hormone release is best determined by directly measuring hormone levels in the blood's plasma.

Both of the 1970 studies claim to find different proportions of various selected metabolic products of sex hormones in the urine of homosexuals—females are included in the sample of Loraine and coworkers—as compared with heterosexual controls. Both are pilot studies with too few subjects from which to formulate any statistical conclusions with confidence. There are various weaknesses in experimental design, such as not controlling for age, nor for amount or frequency of sexual deprivation or activity, which might be important, nor for general health status. Loraine and co-workers used the dubious statistical procedure of making a t-test to compare, for example, 21 urine samples from one homosexual against 38 samples contributed by 14 different heterosexual controls.

The only safe inference to make at the present stage of history is that, if indeed there are differences between homosexuals and heterosexuals or bisexuals in urinary excretion of sex-hormone metabolites, then there is such extreme variation in the amount excreted by heterosexual controls, that the number of homosexuals tested will need to be much greater than in the samples of two, four, and fifteen so far reported. If the reported differences should hold up when larger samples are tested, then their origin and significance will remain to be explained, for they may prove to be related to homosexuality only secondarily or derivatively.

The more exact and newly developed method of measuring sex hormone levels by direct blood plasma determinations of hormones circulating in the blood stream was first applied specifically to the homosexual-bisexual-heterosexual issue in 1971 (Kolodny, Masters, Hendryx, and Toro). They found no difference in the distribution of plasma testosterone levels between a control group of heterosexual college men and approximately 75 percent of a group of bisexual and homosexual college men.

The remaining 25 percent, who ranked among the most extreme on Kinsey's six-point rating scale for homosexuality, had levels of plasma testosterone lower than those of the lowest normal controls. These same homosexual men also manifested an excess of low sperm counts, including four with no sperm count at all. It seems likely that these men, low in sperm count and plasma testosterone, may represent an as yet unidentified syndrome, perhaps of prenatal origin (see reference to Ward, 1972, below, and in Chapter 5) in which a homosexual gender identity differentiates more easily than in the population at large. If so, then the syndrome would have a parallel in the XXY and the XYY syndromes, in both of which homosexuality tends to appear rather frequently.

An earlier study of homosexual plasma testosterone levels (Migeon, Rivarola, and Forest, 1968) had as its subjects five male transexual patients awaiting hormonal (estrogen) therapy and sex-reassignment surgery. These patients may be regarded as being at the extreme of the homosexual spectrum, since they seek a partnership with a male after surgery, if not before. All five patients had plasma concentrations of the androgens testosterone, androstendione, and dehydroisoandrosterone that were within normal limits. These same five patients also proved to be within normal limits in urinary excretion of steroids measured as 17-ketosteroids, 17-hydroxycorticosteroids, pregnanediol, pregnanetriol, and estrogens. They were also within normal limits of urinary gonadotropin secretion.

Corresponding to the report of Migeon and associates on male-to-female transexuals, there is one report on hormonal levels in three female-to-male transexuals (Jones, 1972). Utilizing gas-liquid chromatographic methods, he determined plasma testosterone concentrations in the three female patients. In two cases, additional determinations were done in conjunction with gonadotropin and ACTH suppression and stimulation.

The baseline plasma testosterone concentrations were within the normal female range in two patients (0.02–0.04 mg/100 ml plasma) and in the range found in the androgenizing-ovary (Stein-Leventhal) syndrome in the third patient (0.05–0.08 mg/100 ml plasma). In no case did the baseline concentrations of testosterone approximate the normal male range, and they were not as high as the concentrations found in the testicular feminization syndrome or in female patients with a masculinizing tumor of the ovary (arrhenoblastoma). The suppression-stimulation studies generally indicated that approximately 50 percent of circulating testosterone was of ovarian origin and 50 percent of adrenal origin, a finding consistent with control studies in normal females.

There is another approach to the hypothesis of a hormonal effect on homosexuality, bisexuality, or heterosexuality in adolescence or adulthood, namely, by way of patients whose proper hormonal balance is upset by developmental malfunction or disease. For example, a boy at adolescence may undergo breast enlargement (for reasons not yet scientifically explainable) similar to that of an adolescent girl. He may wonder whether fate has destined him to turn into a female, or a half-female freak, but the very thought mortifies him, because he does not feel like a female and does not want to be one. Medically, his only ambition, judging by the majority of cases, is to be rid of the deformity on his chest, so that he can be normal as a young man. So strong is the desire to be heterosexually normal that one young man, who wanted very much not to be drafted for the Vietnam war, was totally unable to entertain the idea that, if he had had but one homosexual experience, he would be ineligible.

The converse of the estrogenized boy is the adolescent girl who virilizes because of an adrenal or ovarian malfunction or tumor. Such a girl wants only to be rid of her hairy disfigurement, and to get her menstrual periodicity reestablished. She may wonder whether fate is turning her into a circus freak. If she does, she resents the idea totally and longs to be told that she can be restored to morphologic normalcy.

The lack of a relationship between postpubertal androgen or estrogen levels and homosexuality, bisexuality, or heterosexuality is further indicated by the fact that injections of hormone are used therapeutically in vain, if the intention is to make homosexuals heterosexual, heterosexuals homosexual, or bisexuals monosexual. The effects of such injections are only that androgen, within limits, increases libido in both sexes, and estrogen has a functional castrating effect on the male (see Chapter 10).

The most likely source of hormonal difference between homosexual, bisexual, and heterosexual people, if there is one, will not be found at puberty, but prenatally. Prenatal hormonal differences between the three types, if they in fact exist, are not at present known. Nonetheless, an open mind is in order, in view of such evidence as that of Gorski and his associates (see Chapter 4) on the effect of prenatal drugs that counteract prenatal hormones. These researchers found that they could prevent the well-known masculinization of a female fetus under the influence of excess male hormones injected into the pregnant mother animal, if they simultaneously injected either a barbiturate (phenobarbital or pentobarbital), or an experimental antibiotic (puromycin or actinomycin-D). The daughter fetuses then were protected against the expected masculinizing influences of the male sex hormone injections, presumably because the second injection competed with the first and cancelled its action on the chemistry of the genetic code within the body's cells.

Nothing at present is known concerning a possible prenatal drug effect that might predispose toward the later differentiation of a homosexual as compared with a bisexual or heterosexual gender identity. In fact, very little is known about the effect on the fetus of medications taken by the pregnant mother, especially if the effect should be delayed and manifested not in anatomy but only in temperament or behavior. Conceivably, not only medications, but also foodstuffs might be implicated, or even the hormones produced by the mother's own placenta or other endocrine organs, if one builds a conjecture on the basis of the competitive-uptake, radioactive-hormone studies of Stern and Eisenfeld (1971).

The possibility that an endogenous substance produced by the mother might have a predisposing effect on the psychosexual differentiation of the offspring is given more credence than would otherwise be the case by the experiment of Ward (1972; see also Chapter 5), which showed that stress of the pregnant mother rat had a transmitted effect, presumably hormonally mediated, on the fetus, rendering the sons deficient in masculine behavior in adulthood. Not only the hormonal effect of the mother's stress may be implicated, but also a hormonal effect from brothers or sisters in the uterus, according to the evidence of Clemens (see Chapter 5). Surprisingly, a presumed hormonal effect may be transmitted from the grandmother: Wehmer, Porter, and Scales (1970) found that stress of the pregnant mother increased not only the exploratory behavior of her daughters, but also that of the daughter's offspring in the next generation.

Since there are no systematic data relative to a possible relationship, either direct or indirect, between prenatal stress, prenatal medication, or prenatal hormonal functioning and the subsequent development of homosexuality, bisexuality, and heterosexuality in adulthood, an open mind obviously is in order. Nonetheless, in view of the fact that the incidence of homosexuality and bisexuality crosses many ethnic barriers into cultures that have entirely different traditions of food, medications, and stress conditions in pregnancy, the hypothesis of prenatal effects will need to be tested very rigorously.

The concept of a prenatal hormonal component in the eventual differentiation of homosexuality is difficult to sustain also because the phenomenon of obligative homosexuality, to say nothing of facultative homosexuality or bisexuality, is by no means uniform in its manifestations. The erotic preferences and activities, and the general everyday behavior of one obligatively homosexual person (male or female) may differ so widely from that of another homosexual as the behavior of an obligatively heterosexual woman differs from that of an obligatively heterosexual man. Thus, whereas one obligative homosexual male may impersonate a female in dress, daily living, and sexual relationships with men, another may be indistinguishable among his heterosexual colleagues, except in the general context of his private life and sexual activities. The same holds true, obversely, for the obligative homosexual female.

Despite the nonuniformity of traits in the homosexual personality, there is one that tends to be shared by obligative homosexual males: as boys, they were not fighters. They avoided challenges to compete for dominance in the dominance hierarchy of boyhood. Like girls, they remained low in the pecking order of their respective childhood groups. The obligative homosexual female, by contrast, is likely to have competed for dominance as a child, and to have been weak in maternalistic play interests.

Competitive dominance-aggression and maternalism are both traits that might conceivably be subject to prenatal hormonal influences on the brain. Their presence or absence need bear no fixed relationship to psychosexual differentiation on the homosexual-bisexual-heterosexual continuum. Nonetheless, atrophic competitive dominance-aggression in a boy, or its hypertrophy in a girl may, dependent on other developmental experiences, be a contributing influence in the psychosexual differentiation of obligative homosexuality. Lack of maternalism may have a parallel influence. Though the hypothesis is an attractive one, the idea of a prenatal hormonal influence on the brain is not integral to it. Lack of dominance-aggression or maternalism, or too much of either, may equally well be conceived of as having a postnatal origin either in bodily size, health and strength, or in social contingency learning. In male rhesus monkeys, a correlation has been found between dominance hierarchy ranking, assertive aggressiveness, and blood-testosterone level (Rose, Holaday, and Bernstein, 1971). In the hamster, assertive aggressiveness is a trait of the female, the larger sex, in interaction with the male, and correlates with blood levels of progesterone, not testosterone (Payne and Swanson, 1971).

There is no more convincing evidence of the power and importance of social contingency learning in the establishment of homosexuality, bisexuality, and heterosexuality than that offered in Chapter 8 with respect to matched pairs of hermaphrodites. Such cases show that gender identity can differentiate discordantly with chromosomal sex, prenatal hormonal sex, and even postnatal hormonal sex and secondary sexual body morphology. The discordance is so complete and predictable that one can actually make therapeutic plans for its occurrence in cases of a genetic male, born with a microphallus too miniscule ever to function as a copulatory organ, who is assigned and surgically and hormonally corrected for life as a female. The same applies, for example, to the case of a normal boy who suffers complete accidental ablation of the penis in infancy as the result of a circumcision accident, and is immediately rehabilitated as a female.

These cases represent what is, to all intents and purposes, experimentally planned and iatrogenically induced homosexuality. But homosexuality in these cases must be qualified as homosexuality on the criterion of genetic sex, gonadal sex, or fetal hormonal sex. Postsurgically, it is no longer homosexuality on the criterion of the external sex organs nor of the sex of replacement hormonal puberty.

The most likely explanation of the origins of homosexuality, bisexuality, and heterosexuality of gender identity is that certain sexually dimorphic traits or dispositions are laid down in the brain before birth which may facilitate the establishment of either of the three conditions but are too strongly bivalent to be exclusive and invariant determinants of either homo- or heterosexuality, or of their shared bisexual state. The primary origins of the three conditions lie in the developmental period of a child's life after birth, particularly during the years of late infancy and early childhood, when gender identity differentiation is being established (see Chapters 8 and 9). The state of knowledge as of the present does not permit any hypotheses (many psychodynamic claims to the contrary) that will predict with certainty which biographical conditions will ensure that an anatomically normal boy or girl will become erotically homosexual, bisexual, or heterosexual. Once the pattern is established in the early development years, however, it is remarkably tenacious. The hormones of puberty bring it into full expression.[1]

[1]The most recent publication on hormonal and other biochemical studies in male homosexuality is by Ray B. Evans, "Physical and biochemical characteristics of homosexual men," *Journal of Consulting and Clinical Psychology* 39(1972): 140–47. There is also a recent report on gonadotropin levels in male homosexuals by R. C. Kolodny, L. S. Jacobs, W. H. Masters, G. Toro, and W. H. Daughaday, "Plasma gonadotrophins and prolactin in male homosexuals," *Lancet* 2 (1972): 18–12.

12

POSTPUBERTY AND EROTIC DIMORPHISM OF BRAIN AND BEHAVIOR

Sexual Programing in the Brain

In the final analysis, all of a person's experience and behavior of falling in love and mating belongs to a program in the brain. Some parts of the program may have been phyletically laid down. Some may be the individualized product of prenatal hormonal history, and some the product of individual social history and learning. Whatever its origin, there is no behavior if it is not represented in the functioning of the brain.

It is still too early in the history of brain-behavior research to specify homologous locations and circuits responsible for dimorphism of sexual behavior. It is also historically too early to specify accurately, from spinal cord to neocortex, the organization of mating behavior in either a male or female brain. An indication of where future research may lead comes from the work of Paul MacLean and his colleagues (see reviews by MacLean, 1967, 1969). Figure 12.1, reproduced from MacLean, shows schematically the three phyletic systems that comprise man's brain. The innermost and least complex—and presumably least evolved—of the systems is shared with the reptiles. With only this reptilian brain, man would be able, metaphorically speaking, to live and behave sexually like a lizard, snake, or turtle. With only a paleomammalian cortex or limbic system added to the reptilian core, man's sexual behavior would resemble that of a mammal

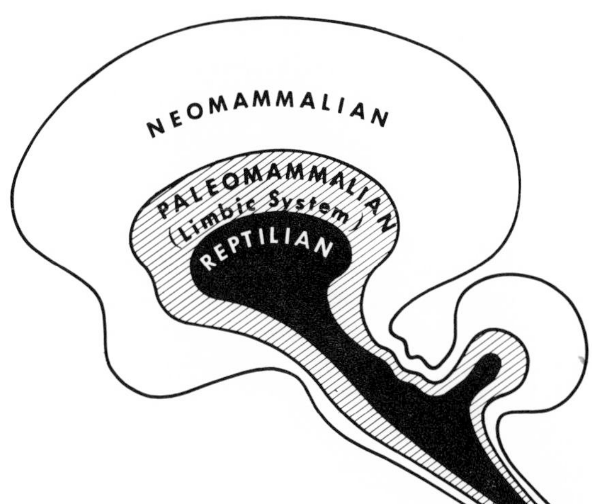

Figure 12.1. MacLean's diagrammatic representation of man's three brains. The innermost brain is shared with lower vertebrates, including reptiles. The paleocortex or limbic system is shared with other mammals. The neocortex, the outermost brain, is poorly developed in lower mammals, and most highly developed in man (reproduced by courtesy of Paul MacLean).

somewhat more lowly than the rabbit. The outermost of the three systems, that of the neomammalian cortex, is the one that differentiates most complexly in the primates, and maximally in man.

The neomammalian cortex—usually referred to as the neocortex, or simply as the cerebral cortex—is prerequisite to man's talking, writing, and symbolic thinking. Without his neocortex, in matters of sexual-behavior dimorphism man would have no love poetry, no erotic narratives, and no visual erotica. But he would probably be able to fall in love and have a relationship of long-term fidelity. Even a bird brain may prescribe lifetime pairing, as it does, for instance, in the jackdaw, the goose, and the penguin.

To a very significant extent, mating and procreative behavior in mammals is processed not by the neocortex, but by the paleocortex or limbic system, in conjunction with pathways of the innermost, reptilian brain. The mammalian female can copulate and procreate in the absence of the neocortex (see review by Lisk, 1967)—which is not to say that the neocortex does not contribute anything, but simply that its contribution is dispensable. Without it, there is not total disruption or loss of reproduction.

The mammalian male, by contrast, needs part of his neocortex in order to be able to carry out his role in copulation. The sensory-motor and motor-sensory projection cortical areas especially are needed. They are significant with respect to positioning in sexual activity. Smell, insofar as it plays a role in activating sexual arousal, presumably can be processed directly within the palecortex, without being dependent on support from the neocortex. Tactile stimulation which can by itself arouse the penis to erection, does not imperatively require processing in any part of the brain whatsoever: the penis is capable of engorging with blood and erecting in response to touch on the basis of a spinal reflex—which can be demonstrated when the lower part of the spinal cord is severed from all communication, sensory and motor, with the brain. The evidence in man comes from patients with the traumatic spinal injury that produces paraplegia (Money, 1960b).

In man and other primates, the neocortex is presumptively prerequisite not only to male positioning, but also to the imagery of visual signals and calls that might initiate a male's genitopelvic arousal. In human beings, it is only through the neocortex that spoken or written messages might induce genitopelvic arousal (erection) in the male, or erotic interest in either male or female.

Recent work of MacLean (1969; 1972) on the squirrel monkey suggests that some visual information is routed directly from the eyes to the limbic brain (paleocortex) without first being processed in the visual zone of the neocortex.

In the processing of information in the limbic system, the evidence so far available indicates that a gate or funnel for eroticism and mating behavior is situated in the proximity of the hypothalamus (see Figure 12.2), not far from where the optic nerves make their cross-over (the optic chiasm). Lisk (1967), in summarizing his review, remarks specifically that the preoptic region and the anterir hypothalamus must be intact for mating behavior. In experimental females, a small blob of estrogen implanted in this region can result in a complete mating response. A lesion in the same location will irreversibly delete the same behavior.

This hypothalamic region has plentiful communication with the septum (Figure 12.2), in the limbic system. MacLean (1969) specifies the septal region as particularly important for the organization of reproductive behavior. He characterizes the septal circuits as involved in "sociability, procreation and the preservation of the species," and contrasts them with the neighboring circuits of the amygdala "that are kept busy with the selfish demands of feeding, fighting and self-protection." Sexually, the septum is more the representative of the tail end of the body, and the amygdala of the snout end. Juxtaposition of both ends in the limbic

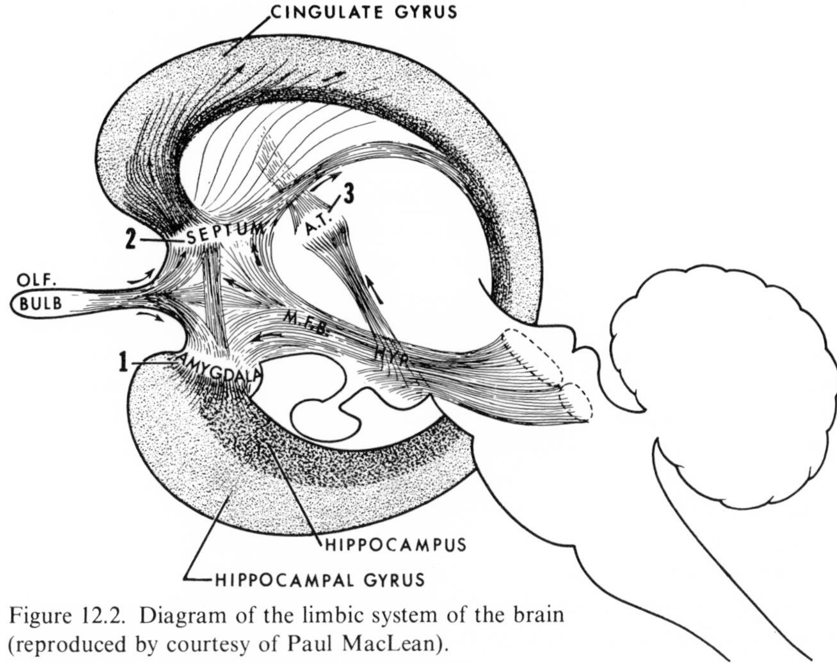

Figure 12.2. Diagram of the limbic system of the brain (reproduced by courtesy of Paul MacLean).

brain parallels their behavioral juxtaposition in most mammals for delivery of the young. It also reflects the interaction of snout end and tail end in those species that are dependent on genital odors as pheromones to signal readiness to breed.[1]

In Figure 12.2, there is shown a third major circuit system of the paleocortex that also, in addition to the systems of the septum and amygdala, transmits sexual programs. This is the circuit system of the anterior

[1]The mouse is a good example (Parkes and Bruce, 1961; Vandenbergh, Drickamer, and Colby, 1972; Bronson, 1971). If four female mice are kept in a small cage, without a male nearby, they are likely to become pseudopregnant (Lee-Boot effect). If thirty are crowded into small living quarters, they become anestrous. Then, if the odor of a male is introduced, they all go into synchronous estrus (Whitten effect), and are, of course, acceptable to a male partner, should one be provided. Having copulated, a female will be unable to conceive and become pregnant, if exposed to the interfering odor of a strange male (Bruce effect). Juvenile females will have an earlier estrus (on day 46 versus day 54) if living in contact with the odor of an intact male, or even of his fresh bedding (Vandenbergh effect). Similarly, in juvenile males, maturation of the testes is accelerated by the presence of an adult female, after the age of 21 days. By contrast, the presence of an overpopulation of adult males in a colony will retard the maturation of juveniles, male and female, doubling the length of the period of immaturity. Removal of all males, will allow the young females to develop earlier.

thalamic nuclei. It connects with the hypothalamus and the cingulate gyrus. It also connects with the medial dorsal nucleus of the thalamus (not in view in Figure 12.2), which projects to the orbitofrontal and prefrontal neocortex, a part of the brain involved in anticipation and planning ahead. Phylogenetically, the circuit system of the septal region in primates does not differ much between species, whereas that of the anterior thalamic nuclei becomes progressively larger in higher primates and reaches a maximum size in man. There is some evidence that this condition reflects a phylogenetic shift from olfactory toward visual influences in mating and sexual behavior (MacLean, 1972).

MacLean and his co-workers (MacLean and Ploog, 1962; MacLean, Denniston, and Dua, 1963; MacLean, Dua, and Denniston, 1963; Dua and MacLean, 1964) did an extensive series of stimulation and ablation studies on the male squirrel monkey. They traced the circuits of erection and ejaculation within the limbic system and hypothalamus, and downwards through the brain stem to the spinal cord, whence they eventually reach the genitalia.

There has not yet been any corresponding study of the female. The neurophysiology of sexual representation in the brain still is at the stage of exploring the sexes separately. Systematic exploration of the homologues of female functioning in the male, and of male functioning in the female, remains to be undertaken, for today's knowledge of sexual dimorphism of the brain after puberty is still on the basis of piecemeal evidence and inference.

Human Brain Dimorphism: Neurosurgical Observations

One source of direct information about sexual pathways in the human brain comes from an experimental form of psychosurgery performed on male sex offenders (Roeder and Müller, 1969). As of the present writing, eleven cases have been reported (Roeder, Orthner, and Müller, 1971). The operation takes advantage of what has been learned from animal studies, namely, that pathways important to the activation of sexual behavior are funneled through the anterior hypothalamus. Roeder's surgical technique is to implant a depth electrode in the region of the ventromedial nucleus of the hypothalamus, which is then partially destroyed by the passage of an electrical current through the electrode.

Roeder's case reports are in tabular form only, and do not give the detailed sexual histories that are needed. From the information available, it would appear that the operation obliterates or partially obliterates sexual behavior from the person's life. It does not selectively obliterate the legally offending behavior (homosexuality with younger men and adolescents, in the majority of cases reported) and leave heterosexual behavior fully intact—one would not expect otherwise, on the basis of animal evidence. The operation does not, therefore, throw light on sexual dimorphism in the organization of sexual behavior in the human brain.

The operation is a drastic procedure, and one hopes it will not become a fad. Nonetheless, it has a place in therapeutics, in the sense that it may prove to be preferable to the still more drastic procedure of the death sentence for a sex murderer, and perhaps preferable even to lifetime imprisonment.

Another source of direct information about sexual pathways in the human brain lies in the pathology of temporal lobe epilepsy (Gastaut and Collomb, 1954; Epstein, 1961; 1969), and its treatment by means of brain surgery (Blumer and Walker, 1967). Each temporal lobe is in part comprised of limbic system structures, namely the amygdala and the hippocampus. Epileptic foci in the temporal lobe may, therefore, have an effect on sexual functioning which is related to these limbic structures. Conversely, the surgical removal of these seizure foci may also affect sexual functioning.

The commonest sexual finding in temporal lobe epilepsy, before surgery, is hyposexuality. The lack of sexual drive may, in the male, include impotence (Hierons and Saunders, 1966). After surgery, if the focal defect is successfully removed and seizures no longer occur, then there is likely to be an increase in sexual desire and practice. In some few cases, gross and socially impolite hypersexuality was postsurgically reported (Blumer, 1970). Subsequently, if there was a relapse into more seizures, hypersexuality then also relapsed into hyposexuality.

The hypersexual effect resembles that obtained in monkeys (Klüver and Bucy, 1939) when both temporal lobes have been removed—the so-called Klüver-Bucy syndrome in which hypersexuality is associated with increased tameness, excessive taking notice of things, excessive mouthing of objects, and inability to recognize things.

There is some evidence, from temporal lobe epilepsy, of a rather close connection in the temporal lobes between visual memory and sexual response. The evidence comes from selected cases of fetishism closely bonded to temporal lobe abnormalities and seizures (Epstein, 1960). Mitchell, Falconer, and Hill (1954) reported a case of a bizarre safety-pin fetish, in which a seizure would be induced by gazing at the pin. Left temporal lobectomy relieved the patient of seizures and of the fetish-urge to gaze at the pin.

This same safety-pin fetishist had, prior to surgery, also experienced a confusional state, immediately after a seizure, when sometimes he would dress in his wife's clothing. Transvestism itself, in some instances, represents a form of fetishism, and it may be associated with temporal lobe seizures. Davies and Morgenstern (1960) reported such a case, both symptoms appearing together in middle life. Hunter, Logue, and McMenemy (1963) reported also a case of fetishism-transvestism and temporal lobe seizures, both of which were eliminated by left anterior temporal lobectomy.

In his followup report, Hunter (1967) also presented a case of long-term, compulsive transvestism which disappeared under the influence of anticonvulsive treatment at the age of thirty-eight. The EEG showed focal disturbance in the left fronto-temporal area. There was no history of actual convulsion, but temporal lobe dysfunction was indicated by reason of déjà vu experiences, vivid dreaming, and psychologic-test signs of minimal verbal impairment. There was a history of compulsive masturbation, but heterosexual impotence. Treatment was sought prior to marriage. Impotence was ameliorated along with disappearance of transvestite fantasies and practices. Medication was discontinued after six months, and two years later symptoms were still in remission.

In fetish and transvestite cases such as the foregoing, the relationship to sexual dimorphism of behavior is indirect: all reported cases are in males. Epilepsy affects both sexes; but fetishism and transvestism, as obligatory for sexual arousal, are apparently male disorders exclusively. There may possibly be some relationship here to the special importance of vision as a distance receptor in man's erotic, genitopelvic arousal. Otherwise nothing more has yet been uncovered concerning sexual dimorphism in the human brain, in this context.

Fetishism and transvestism do not exhaust the variety of sexual dysfunctions that may be associated with temporal lobe dysfunction. Kolářský, Freund, Machek, and Polák (1967) addressed themselves to the problem of differential etiology. In a well-designed statistical study, they demonstrated that many sexual behavior disorders may coexist with temporal lobe epilepsy. The dual disorder then tends to be associated with early exposure of the temporal lobes to harm or injury, retrospectively identified, before the age of three.

In this study, the authors made the inference that brain injury had occurred in cases for which they could document a history of protracted delivery, neonatal asphyxia, forceps delivery producing presumptive brain trauma, infantile head trauma producing unconsciousness, or severe infectious disease with signs of brain involvement.

The authors postulated a delayed interaction effect between the early insult to the brain and subsequent developmental anomaly: a brain rendered less than perfect at an early stage of development thenceforth has an increased risk of having its imperfection compounded in later development. One may say that it is more vulnerable to disorders of development in a general, rather than a specific way. Thus, in the case of sexual behavior disorders, one would not expect the symptoms to be identical from case to case, but to reflect personal developmental history superimposed on a brain somewhat impaired to begin with.

The human brain at birth is still, embryologically speaking, not finished. It does not have its full complement of neural cells, and its fibers are not all myelinated. Not until the eighteenth month of age is the brain anatomically complete. It requires twenty-seven months from the day of conception to reach perfection—twenty-seven months in which something could go wrong. The first chance for something to go wrong lies in the genes and chromosomes. Boys with Klinefelter's (XXY) syndrome, for example, have been shown to constitute a population at risk for developmental psychopathology, including psychosexual pathology (Hambert, 1966; Nielsen, 1969; Nielsen, Sørensen, Theilgaard, Anders, and Johnsen, 1969).

The second chance for something to go wrong lies in the intrauterine era, and could stem from sources as divergent as malnutrition and viral infection, drug toxicity, and radiation. The third era with its own dangers is the perinatal. There may then be too much or too little of many things: breathing oxygen, being handled, being nourished, and others. In the fourth era, that of infancy and later, many of the old dangers remain, and to them are added those that stem from social interaction in its various manifestations and degrees. The developmental process of imprinting, that type of learning that persists with special tenacity, requires that the brain encounter certain stimuli at a sensitive or critical developmental period. Otherwise its functioning with respect to that particular type of stimulus material may be forever impaired. Then one would attribute long-term brain impairment to lack of developmental opportunity. The other alternative is that a brain, already impaired in an earlier developmental phase, is unable to take advantage of stimulus materials with which it should exercise itself.

Brain Dimorphism and Gender Identity

A case like that reported by Mitchell, Falconer, and Hill (1954), in which safety-pin fetishism plus epileptic attacks both were "cut out" by the same surgical excision, is theoretically important because of its rarity. The same applies to the case of Hunter, Logue, and McMenemy (1963), in which fetishism-transvestism and seizures were simultaneously extirpated.

These cases indicate that imagery which is coded as nonerotic in the brain and the memory of the majority of the human race can, in special cases and for reasons still undiscovered, have its coding switched from erotically negative to positive. In consequence, individuals so afflicted appear peculiar because of their ability to be erotically turned on by imagery that to the majority of other people is nonerotic. For example, the ordinary man cannot get an erection and be erotically stimulated by a fantasy or by pictures of a man dressing to impersonate a woman. Such a portrayal is, by contrast, erotically stimulating to a transvestite dependent on the imagery of wearing of women's clothes for his own erectile potency (Epstein, 1960; Stoller, 1970).

Transvestism as a form of fetishism in the male is not too far removed from transexualism (Green and Money, 1969), a condition which dictates that a person, in the present instance a male, totally and continuously impersonate a female, in sexual anatomy as well as clothing and behavior. A male transexual may or may not have used his penis in penile orgasm. Either way, he despises the organ and wants, above all else, to be rid of it.

Some male transexuals have, when they first present themselves for sex-reassignment surgery, lived so long and so successfully in the female impersonating role, that they are unable to present themselves as males without appearing so effeminate as to attract widespread attention. Other male transexuals, however, and a great many male transvestite impersonators who do not desire a permanent sex reassignment, are uncannily expert at metamorphosing from one sex role and mode of dress to the other. Even the voice is changed in pitch and loudness. One has here a manifestation akin to the phenomenon of multiple personality, well known in R. L. Stevenson's story of Dr. Jekyll and Mr. Hyde.

Whereas some male transexuals can switch public sex roles from male to female, and whereas others have lived so long and intensively full-time in the female role that they cannot change, the vast majority of men are unable to impersonate a female without appearing clumsy and feeling awkward and embarrassed. These observations suggest what has already been mentioned in Chapter 8, namely that the brain's primary gender assignment in infancy and early childhood is to code into coherent and separate systems that which constitutes culturally prescribed masculinity versus femininity. This learning assignment is identical for boys and girls. The difference for each sex is the sign, positive or negative, with which each gender system is coded. It is as if a boy knows how to say and do boy things, because he has simultaneously assimilated the knowledge of how not to say and not to do girl things. For the ordinary boy, the feminine system becomes coded as negative. Cerebrally, its status is that of being subject to inhibition with respect to personal expression. It does, however, act as the boy's template of what to expect in the behavior of girls and women and, secondarily, of how to respond in order to reciprocate or complement their behavior. The same statements may be made, vice versa, for girls. In either sex, the negative system may be released under conditions of impaired or diseased brain function. Such release can be accounted for as yet another instance, hitherto unrecognized, of the Jacksonian Law of Release.

Children who fail in the task of dichotomizing their own gender development may do so for a variety of, as yet, presumptive causes. The new era of chromosome counting has shown that boys with 47, XXY or 47, XYY chromosomes, constitute a population at risk, as compared with normal 46, XY boys, with respect to imperfect differentiation of gender identity by teenage or later. Too many psychosexual and other behavioral anomalies are represented among them.

There is no clear and definitive human evidence yet as to whether the prenatal hormonal environment affects the incidence of subsequent bisexual or homosexual behavior with respect to the erotic use of the genitalia. Dominance behavior and academic achievement may, however, be affected positively in girls exposed to an excess of prenatal androgens, while maternalism is negatively affected (see Chapter 6). Boys exposed to an insufficiency of prenatal androgens are possibly rather placid, but the chief effect in them would seem to be after the age of adolescence. Then there is a deficit of male orgasm and male sexual initiative leading to arousal, for replacement androgen is usually needed. Even with replacement therapy, the effect on erotic functioning may be only partial and incomplete, at best. By contrast, boys exposed to an excess of fetal androgens, who subsequently undergo the precocious virilization of a too-early puberty, were found to be not excessive in heterosexual initiative, and also lacking in homosexual play and inclination (Money and Alexander, 1969).

On the basis of today's evidence—and here one must be judiciously tentative—it appears that the period of greatest risk for errors of gender-identity formation, of long-lasting effect in the brain, is after birth, and at around the time of acquiring the native language. The most convincing evidence is that obtained from matched pairs of hermaphrodites, disparately raised (Money, 1970a; see also Chapter 8).

Gender identity differentiation of the brain after birth is a process that one may surmise to resemble differentiation of the internal rather than the external genitalia. Neither the male nor the female system is totally and completely obliterated, but one becomes dominant over the other. A boy knows how to do and say boy things, because he simultaneously recognizes girl things as unfitting for him to express, though requiring complementarity or reciprocity of reaction on his part—and vice versa for girls. The parallel with bilingualism, when one language is used for talking and listening, and the other for listening only, has been presented in Chapter 8. The more one stops to think of it, the more remarkable does it seem that an infant brain can receive the sound waves of two languages spoken around him, and differentiate them as two nonoverlapping systems, vocally and linguistically. The task is facilitated if each language is spoken by different people. Then each language can be identified as belonging to the person or persons speaking it. There is less confusion than when the same speaker alternates between two languages. The parallel with gender-identity formation is obvious, for the masculine and feminine models in a child's environment are usually quite clearly differentiated, regardless of the amount of overlap that may be culturally permitted.

Autonomy of the brain relative to the peripheral organs and with respect to gender-appropriate erotic functioning is exemplified in cases of traumatic injury to the spinal cord that produced paraplegia or quadriplegia (Money, 1960b). In paraplegia, the body below the waist is deprived of all sensation and voluntary movement. In quadriplegia, all of the body below the neck is involved. Men with these grim disabilities may have an erection, and possibly even an ejaculation (Bors and Comarr, 1960; Tsuji, Nakajima, Morimato, and Nounaka, 1961; Comarr, 1970), on the basis of spinal reflexes. They will not feel anything, and will not know what is happening, unless they watch, and perceive it visually. Independently of genital functioning, however, they remain capable of erotic imagery in daydreams. When first disabled, a paraplegic may experience the imagery of intercourse culminating in orgasm in a sleeping dream. Such an orgasm is a purely cerebral event, with no genitopelvic concomitants.

Like her male counterpart, a woman paraplegic may also have a phantom orgasm in a dream. If she has a male partner to copulate with her, her vagina can receive the penis without feeling it. Pregnancy is not impossible, though unlikely.

Though severed from their reproductive organs, not metaphorically, but almost literally, paraplegic or quadriplegic men and women do not lose their gender identity. Rather, they feel the deprivation of their loss, and wish that the complete expression of their psychosexual function could be restored.

Neural disconnection of the peripheral genitalia from the brain and cognition is complete in paraplegia. Other lesions and injuries of the genitalia may impose a lesser degree of sensory or kinetic loss, as for example when parts of the organs are traumatically or surgically severed, or when specific functions, like erection, are permanently and irreversibly damaged (Money, 1961b; 1967b; Aronson and Cooper, 1968). Trauma or damage at the periphery inevitably impairs the overall performance of mating, but does not abolish the totality of that performance. Permanent loss of erectile tissue in the penis after an attack of priapism, for example, does not abolish orgasm and ejaculation; and amputation of the penis leaves intact sexual desire and the capacity for orgasm (Money, 1961b; Money and Hirsch, 1965). Since the capacity to satisfy the partner is lost, the blow to the man's morale is severe. A woman who undergoes radical loss of sexual tissue, as in surgical cancer therapy, may be somewhat better off in this respect. Provided her vaginal cavity has been spared, she will be able to receive the penis, as well as experiencing some erotic pleasure herself.

These examples, like that of paraplegia, indicate that gender identity, once it has differentiated, is capable of sustaining itself independently of the integrity of the peripheral genitalia—despite the hardship imposed on the individual concerned.

Postpubertal Hormones and the Brain

In the early 1960s, demonstration of cellular uptake of radioactively labeled estrogen in individual brain cells (Michael and Glascock, 1963) justified speculation that sexually dimorphic behavior after puberty might be a function of brain-hormone interaction. Subsequent studies have shown that there is no neat and simple, sexually dimorphic relationship between brain cells, sex-hormone uptake, and behavior. It is, however, clear that the rate and amount of hormone uptake varies regionally in the brain and according to the test hormone employed, especially estradiol versus testosterone or progesterone (Stumpf, 1968; Zigmond and McEwen, 1970; Stern and Eisenfeld, 1971).

McGuire and Lisk (1969) found an increased uptake of radioactively labeled estradiol in the hypothalamus of female rats that had been injected at birth with estradiol instead of androgen. Green, Luttge, and Whalen (1969) found that males, females, and females androgenized at birth do not differ from one another in the rate at which different parts of the brain accumulate radioactive estradiol. The same authors (1970) found also no difference between normal females and neonatally androgenized females in the rate of brain uptake of radioactive testosterone. Luttge and Whalen (1970), found regional variation in the brain's uptake of estradiol and estrone, with no difference between males and females; they also found that most brain tissues maintained the same level of estradiol uptake, regardless of the phase of the estrous cycle, which did influence uptake in the uterus and the pituitary (see also McGuire and Lisk, 1968; Kato, Inaba, and Kobayashi, 1969).

Just as the male's brain cells can take up estrogen, conversely the female's brain can take up androgen (Pfaff, 1968). By implanting minute amounts of testosterone directly into the hypothalamus of rabbits, Palka and Sawyer (1966b) induced estrous behavior. Whalen and Hardy (1970) also induced estrous behavior in rats and cats with testosterone, not implanted but given simply by intramuscular injections. The results paralleled those produced when estradiol benzoate was injected instead of testosterone. The counterpart of Whalen and Hardy's experiment would be to induce mounting in males by injection of either estradiol or testosterone. In the hamster, Swanson (1971) showed that this effect could be produced by injecting estradiol in the place of testosterone, but only if the males had been ultramasculinized by an injection of testosterone at birth. Normal, neonatally untreated male hamsters respond to estradiol with lordosis, allowing themselves to be mounted by another male. The mounting effect could be produced in females given an injection of testosterone at birth, their mounting being in response to either estradiol or testosterone injected in adulthood. Normal, neonatally untreated females were unable to respond to testosterone by showing mounting behavior, and likewise, of course, to estradiol.

Another action of sex hormone on the brain was found by Fisher (1956, 1966, 1969) in relation to the release, by testosterone, of both mating and parental behavior in the male rat (see below).

Another form of behavior response to direct brain stimulation by testosterone propionate is territorial marking (Thiessen and Yahr, 1969). Mongolian gerbils are one species that mark objects in their environment with the secretion of a sebaceous scent gland on the underside of the body. Such behavior is androgen dependent. It may be induced or increased by injecting androgen intramuscularly. In castrated male gerbils, Thiessen and Yahr demonstrated that marking could be reestablished if minute amounts of testosterone were injected directly into the fluid of the lateral ventricles of the brain, or implanted through microcannulae into neighboring tissue of the hypothalamus. The effect could be blocked by combining testosterone with the investigative antibiotic, actinomycin-D.

Thiessen and Yahr performed their experiment only on male gerbils. It is known, however, that female gerbils also manifest territorial marking behavior, and that it increases in frequency if females are given intramuscular injections of testosterone (Thiessen and Lindzey, 1970). Marking is, therefore, yet another example of bisexual behavior that is monosexually—in this case, male—predominant.

Though not all the permutations, combinations, and variations of brain region, hormonal chemistry, and behavioral entity have been worked out, it is already quite clear from the foregoing experiments alone that, in addition to eliciting bisexually shared behavior, an androgen can elicit some predominantly feminine behavior, and an estrogen some predominantly masculine behavior. Under certain test conditions, it is less important whether the adult hormone is androgenic or estrogenic, than whether the brain has had a history of prenatal or neonatal history of exposure to an excess of either hormone, or deprivation of both.

Nonetheless, after maturity, there are some circumstances under which estradiol and testosterone cannot be used interchangeably. Estradiol given to a normal man, for instance, has a functional castrating effect, quite the opposite of the effect of testosterone. The site of action may be the peripheral organs rather than solely the brain, since testicular androgen secretion becomes suppressed.

The two hormones conventionally used in experiments, estradiol benzoate and testosterone propionate may turn out to be in some way unique. Other androgens and estrogens may behave differently. Conversely, other nonhormones may be found to mimic estradiol and testosterone. Fisher (1969; see also Beach, 1965) found that he could replicate the effect of testosterone (see above) by injecting into the hypothalamus the commercial compound, Versene, a chelating agent that removes metallic ions. Ionic change on the surface of a neural cell may perhaps be in part the mechanism whereby the sex hormones generally work in the brain (see references to other compounds in Chapters 4 and 5).

There is, of course, the possibility that, within the brain, the release or inhibition of programs for sexual behavior is only secondarily or tertiarily related to the uptake of sex hormones by brain cells. Conceivably, sex hormones might be necessary only as a relatively nonspecific component of the cellular environment, enabling a triggering stimulus, which might be visual, olfactory, or tactile, to take effect in behavior.

Dimorphism of Erotic Arousal and Imagery

Before the penis can be of any use to the vagina, a stimulus of some sort must have initiated an erection response. In its regular, flaccid state, the penis is a urinary and not a copulatory organ. The vagina, by contrast, has nothing to do with urination at any time. In its regular state, it is not able to perform its expulsional function of childbirth, which requires the activation of its maximum muscular stretch; but it is able to perform its implosional function of receiving the penis. Refusal of the penis requires activation of the vagina's maximum muscular constriction or clamping. Ideally, the vagina should be erotically stimulated and actively ready to fill itself with the penis, though in its regular resting state it can be forcefully entered by the penis. As a simple exercise in copulatory mechanics, the penis can make its way into even an anesthetized vagina.

Mechanically speaking, therefore, nature could have ordained a coital scheme whereby the vagina would be noncontributory, with respect to the timing of when it would receive a penis. According to this scheme, the vagina would accommodate the penis at any time that the penis would be ready with an erection according to its own coital program. Whether or not coitus coincided with ovulation and thus with the optimal chance of conception would be a matter of chance.

The antithesis of such a coital scheme would be the one already mentioned in Chapter 8, in which the penis would be in a constant state of erectile readiness, and the time-table of its use would be set by the vagina's own program, perhaps to coincide with ovulation. Instead of being constantly ready, the penis could become erectile in response to a signal transmitted from the vagina, at the time of the female's ovulatory readiness to conceive. This is the scheme, with the signal being odiferous (pheromonal), that governs the timing of coitus in many of the lower species.

Among the primates, there is evidence from the rhesus monkey (see Chapter 11) that the male's arousal is partly in response to vaginal odor at the ovulatory phase of the menstrual cycle. The rhesus male also favors one partner over others, quite apart from odors, if the others are at the same phase of her menstrual cycle. Her favored status as a lover may last for years.

In the human species, there is no convincing evidence as yet of a consistent pheromonal odor by which the female communicates with the male and stimulates his arousal—or vice versa. There is, however, some evidence of a relationship between the sex hormones and smell acuity. Le Magnen (1952) reported that, after puberty, women have greater sensitivity than men or children to the smell of synthetic musk and certain urinary steroids. They lose their acuity after ovariectomy, but regain it if given estrogen replacement therapy. Schneider and Wolf (1955) found that in most women smell acuity diminishes during the progestinic (menstrual) phase of the cycle, and peaks during the estrogenic (ovulatory) phase.

The timing or frequency of coitus in human beings is not known to be pheromonally regulated, nor to be regulated solely on the basis of some other, either feminine or masculine, vaginal or penile, copulatory rhythm. There is a coital signaling system between the sexes, and it appears to be primarily visual and imagistic, when the couple are beyond arm's length, and haptic when they are closer. Either type of signal may be transmitted at second hand by means of language.

In a male, a visual perception or visual image may, without tactile stimulation, be sufficient to initiate erotic arousal and erection. Continued arousal may, under special conditions of fantasy and with masturbatory stimulation, build up to orgasm without two-person contact. Typically, however, the visual stimulus is augmented by communicating with the partner, in signs, or words, or both, through which an expectancy of intimate body contact, now or later, is established. Habitual partners may shorten the process by beginning with touch and body contact, perhaps quite explicitly genital.

When established partners are close enough to touch each other—a married couple in bed, for instance—it is equally feasible for the man or the woman to make the first move, for each is responsive to the eroticism of touch. If the man happens to be apathetic, perhaps because of fatigue, then the performance is canceled. By contrast, when the man is ready and makes the first move, the woman can go through with a perfunctory performance, even if she does feel too tired and apathetic.

Of course, it is possible for a woman as well as a man to respond to the visual stimulus of a lover or potential partner in sex (Sigusch, Schmidt, Reinfeld, and Wiedemann-Sutor, 1970; Schmidt and Sigusch, 1970). Her imagery of arousal will, however, tend to be different, as though geared to the premise that he, the man, will be coitally useless to her, except that the stimulus of her receptive body is capable of erecting his penis. Her arousal fantasy tends to build itself around the sentiment and romance of his reacting to her and wanting her—of wanting to hold, caress, and kiss her. If he wants her enough, then his penis will erect and want her too, and perhaps not only once, but again and again for a lasting love affair, and even an entire lifetime.

There has been a great deal of misunderstanding of female and male differences concerning visual erotic imagery and arousal. A chief source of misunderstanding has been a confusion between the question of whether women do or don't get aroused by visual images, and the question of how imagery is programed, allowing it to bring about erotic arousal. The comparison of projection versus objectification in the deployment of imagery, presented in the following paragraphs, resolves the confusion. There is good empirical support for this imagistic difference between the sexes, even in the absence of systematic experimental design. The reader can test this hypothesis on the basis of his or her own experience.

The man's arousal fantasy is not the exact reciprocal of the woman's, for it is much less focused on her wanting him, than on his wanting her, which is precisely the same focus as that of her fantasy. There is here a difference between the sexes which shows itself also in their differential response to pictorial erotica.

When he reacts to a sexy pinup picture of a female, a man sees the figure as a sexual object. In imagery, he takes her out of the picture and has a sexual relationship. He may masturbate. It is not unheard of that he may make a genital aperture in the picture and put his penis through it, and then masturbate.

The very same picture may be sexually appealing to a woman, but that would not mean she is a lesbian. Far from it. She is not in imagery bringing the figure toward herself as a sexual object, as does the man. She is projecting herself into the picture and identifying herself with the female to whom men respond. She herself becomes the sexual object.

What if the picture portrays a sexy male? The basic sex difference still manifests itself. Men are typically inattentive. If they are homosexual or bisexual, they may see the figure homosexually as a sexual object, but they do not project themselves into the picture and identify with the man there represented. Women, unable to identify with the male figure, also do not respond to it as a sexual object. An exception may be an erotic pose of a male with a flaccid penis, especially if the picture includes also a female partner. Then a woman viewer may identify herself with the female figure and see, in imagination, the male's nonerect penis as a challenge to her.

Depictions of sexual intercourse, especially in a movie, are erotically stimulating to women as well as men, but the same basic difference of identification versus objectification applies once again. The woman viewer is likely to build her erotic excitement into a fantasy of enlarging her repertory of sexual skills, learning something from the female in the movie, with the intention of utilizing it on the next available occasion with her lover or sexual partner. The man viewer builds up a level of erotic excitement, imagining that the woman on the screen is having intercourse with him on the spot. It would not, in fact, be difficult for him to copulate with any live surrogate for the female in the movie.

Whether in a movie or any other form of erotica, the romantic story leading up to the embrace of the penis in intercourse is important to a woman's erotic fantasy. There is evidence of this in the circulation, among adolescent girls and women, of magazines and stories of the true romance, true confession type. These narratives are, indeed, woman's pornography (Stoller, 1970). They are so different from the carnal pictures and narratives that constitute man's pornography, that the law, made by men, does not even recognize them as such.

The direct focus of the man's imagery of erotic arousal in his sexual organs is exemplified in the developmental fact that a boy at puberty may have his first orgasm, as many do, unsolicited in his sleep, accompanied by an erotic dream. In the dream he may be presented with images of a would-be sexual partner, her body partly or fully exposed, or engaging sexually in intercourse with either the dreamer himself or another partner. It is a rare girl who has such an experience of an "illustrated" orgasm, while alone, in sleep, as her first introduction to the phenomenon. The dreaming of orgasm in the female usually follows masturbatory or coital orgasmic experience. It may not begin in teenage at all, but only later, in the twenties or thirties (see also Chapter 8).

In the boy's sleeping orgasm, the timing of the event is scheduled by the individual's own erotic rhythms. Such scheduling is extremely variable, both within a person over time, and between persons. The sources of variation are largely unknown. The imagery and theme of a sexual dream is historically determined and reflects personal experience. It reveals also the type of actual-life stimulus to which the boy could be erotically attuned, and to which he could respond with an erection in an erotic relationship.

There is a good possibility that the occurrence of erotic dreams is in some way related to the level of androgen circulating in the bloodstream. High androgen levels were characteristic of women with the congenital female andrenogenital syndrome in the era prior to the discovery of cortisone treatment of the condition in 1950. They tended to report a history of eroticism in dreams paralleling that characteristic of normal males, though the content of the dream imagery would be appropriate for a female.

A similar parallel may be observed also in teenaged genetic male hermaphrodites who, lacking an adequate phallus are reared as girls. If the gonads happen not to have been earlier removed, and if they initiate an androgenizing puberty, until they finally are removed, then dreams, the equivalent of so-called wet dreams, though with suitably feminine imagery, are likely to occur. They tend to fade after gonadectomy and replacement hormonal therapy with estrogen.

In the case of genetic male hermaphrodites with the androgen-insensitivity syndrome there is no erotic dreaming corresponding to the wet dream of the ordinary adolescent boy. This is true not only when the affected individual has the external body morphology of a perfect female and has lived all her life as one, but also when, because of a very small phallus and palpable (feminizing) testes, the baby was assigned and reared as a boy. In teenage, this boy feminizes instead of masculinizing. His lack of dreaming, despite a primarily masculine gender identity, parallels the incapacity of the body to respond to its own testicular adrogen.

Sexual dimorphism in erotic response to imagery may possibly be related to dimorphism in erotic assertiveness. In primate troops it does seem to be the case that the male asserts himself sexually over the female who stimulates him, though there is no a priori reason why the female, having stimulated a male to be sexually aroused, should not then be assertive over him. One may conjecture that the sexual assertiveness of the male is phyletically related to dominance assertiveness, and that both are related to defense of the troop against predators and territorial competitors and intruders. The higher a male's position in the dominance hierarchy, the greater his sexual assertiveness and the larger the number of females, and their young, whom he must ultimately protect. The distribution of many females among a few males frees some of the adult males to die in defense of the troop without risking extermination of the troop itself. In the human species, this phyletic formula does not need to be conceptualized as having the same stereotypic validity as in the lower primates. There are intelligent alternatives, but our primate heritage seems to be all too much with us, still, and we do not, as a society, utilize them.

It is self-evident that the only erotic imagery to which an observer has direct access is his own. The solipsism of imagery keeps it forever private and unknown to others except through verbal report or, to a lesser extent, through other behavioral or somatic signs. In animals other than man, imagery can be studied only by inference from behavioral signs.

In work with animals, it is fashionable to evade the concept of imagery as having too much subjective implication, in favor of a more simple and mechanistic stimulus-response conception. A model of the latter is the response to light (Wurtman, 1967; Hardy, 1970), as a stimulus to the hormonal activation of breeding, particularly in some seasonal species. Another model is the ovulation of the cat and the rabbit in response to the stimulus of vaginal coitus (Clegg and Doyle, 1967).

Evading an issue does not solve it, however. The real challenge of imagery in animals is to find nonverbal methods of assessing it. Some work with birds points the way.

Schein and Hale (1965) investigated the importance of the visual image to mating in the turkey by using taxidermic models of varying degrees of completion (Figures 12.3 and 12.4). They showed that the male's correct copulatory orientation is dependent on the signal image of the head of the female. Without the head, a male cannot correctly orient himself. A head alone elicits copulatory behavior, but the more complete the model the greater the frequency of elicited sexual behavior.

In a similar investigation, Carbaugh and Schein (1961) showed that white leghorn roosters are sexually aroused by a headless model of the female body, but they cannot correctly orient themselves for copulation unless the head is added to the model. Sexual response is most effective when the stimulus model is morphologically complete and is in the appropriate, fully crouched position. Partial models, as with turkeys, produce a less effective response.

Minimal cues for eliciting sexual response have been demonstrated also in another species, the Brewer blackbird, in California. In this species, the sexes are highly differentiated in color. Howell and Bartholomew (1952) found that:

> To obtain a mating response from the male, a dummy must meet certain minimum conditions. The wings are not necessary. Either a head or a tail must be present, but one or the other may be removed without eliminating the response. Further removal of parts inhibits the mating reaction. If the tail is present, it should be at an angle above horizontal. Eye color is not important. The plumage color should be predominantly that of a female, but a female head and neck on an otherwise male-colored dummy may be effective when the male is in a stage of high excitement. When the dummy presents any one of the appropriate combinations of characteristics, the response of the male may be virtually instantaneous.

A female dummy with a male head, neck and breast evoked mounting behavior, but not copulation. The mating responses of the males to this dummy were inhibited by the male characteristics of the head and neck. In fact, one male was so infuriated that when he "alighted directly on the back of the dummy (and) started to copulate, (he) looked down and seemed suddenly disturbed, hopped into the air, and thereby knocked over the dummy. He looked at it from the side and gave it an aggressive peck on the head." With a male dummy having a female neck and head, the male birds made initial overtures and showed sexual arousal, but quickly lost interest.

An example in human beings paralleling the sexual response of birds to a visual image, or part thereof, can be found in the partners of sex-reassigned transexuals (Money and Brennan, 1970). Most partners respond initially to what they see. Even before the transexual's genitalia have been reconstructed, some partners are so strongly influenced by clothed appearance and behavior, that they regard the incongruity as an anomaly needing to be corrected. Others, like the blackbirds above, are turned off by the discrepancy.

The contour and color of the visual image to which a male bird responds with mating behavior is to a very large degree set by phylogeny. Ontogenetic learning—the product of an individual bird's own life history—is minimally important. In man, the equation is the other way round, witness those individuals whose development decrees that they will be sexually aroused by bizarre images that signify pathology, psychosexually.

The story of the regions and circuits of dimorphic sexual imagery in the brain is one that has not yet been uncovered. It is important that eventually it be uncovered, for in the human being, imagery is related not only to the more rare bizarreries of sexual arousal and behavior, but also to the very common problems of sexual apathy, impotence, and frigidity. Men and women so affected are unable to respond to contact arousal alone, and the images that might, perhaps, once have induced some arousal have lessened in power. Such people may be too inhibited to pursue the other, elusive image that, though socially condemned, has always secretly been the one to arouse them. They become erotically apathetic instead. Others may embark on an obsessive round of sexual encounters, seeking always to find the elusive image with maximal power to turn them on. Sisyphus-like, they too are condemned not to achieve what they so desperately pursue.

Gender Dimorphism and Parentalism

The experiments of Fisher on brain stimulation of male rats, already mentioned in this chapter, indicate that many elements of behavior usually referred to as maternal are programed in the brain of males as well as females, even though the males do not normally display maternal behavior. Fisher injected minute amounts of testosterone directly into the preoptic area of the brains of male rats, and obtained maternal and mating behavior. Maternal behavior included nest building and persistent retrieving and grooming of litters of young. All aspects of mating behavior were seen, sometimes accentuated. One male continuously retrieved his tail when stimulated, and then repeatedly retrieved a female in heat. When pups and paper were supplied, however, the animal built a nest and retrieved and groomed the young, neglecting the objects to which he had previously reacted. In another male, maternal and sexual behavior were activated simultaneously. When presented with a female (not in heat) and with newborn rat pups, the male attempted copulation twice, while a pup he was retrieving to a nest was still in his mouth. Variations in response to injected androgen appeared to depend on small variations in placement of the cannulae in the brain.

Fisher's experiment clearly demonstrates not only that testosterone might release parental behavior of the type usually designated as maternal, but also that males carry in their brains the capacity for this behavior.

Maternalism should, therefore, more accurately be designated parentalism. It is a bisexual trait. Among some species of rodents, the male does not need testosterone to be injected into the hypothalamus in order to display retrieving, nesting, cleaning and grooming the young, assuming a hovering posture, or even eating the placenta and gnawing the umbilical cord. Such caretaking behavior is part of the regular repertoire of male behavior in the mouse, according to the pooled observations of several investigators (Newton, Peeler, and Rawlins, 1968). The lactating female, however, has more single-mindedness of purpose and will overcome more obstacles in order to be near to and take care of the young. Rosenblatt (1967), already referred to in Chapter 5, showed that even the relatively nonmaternal male rat will, if exposed to helpless neonates for five or six days, begin to show retrieving and licking behavior.

Neumann, in the experiments outlined in Chapter 5, was able to show that feminization of the unborn male rat by the use of antiandrogen included also feminization of the mammary glands and of the brain mechanisms responsible for the control of lactation and feeding of the young. It was necessary to supply the appropriate female hormones in adulthood, and also to remove the feminized males' testes and their androgens in order to obtain lactation and suckling behavior. The amount of milk produced was insufficient to allow the foster pups to survive, however.

Secretion of milk from the breast is dependent in part on the neural stimulation of suckling (which also is erotically stimulating), and in part on hormones released from the pituitary (Cowie and Folley, 1961). In lower species, the manifestation of parental behavior is also hormone regulated (Lehrman, 1961), in connection with the hormone changes of nesting or parturition.

The parentalism of males in some species of birds is well known. Male penguins, for instance, share in keeping the egg warm to hatch it, and when it is hatched, share in feeding the young. The male kiwi is fully responsible for incubating the egg, a ninety-day task.

In mammalian species, one may infer that the release of maternal or caretaking behavior in adulthood is to some degree a function of prenatal hormonal history. Regardless of genetic sex, prenatal or neonatal presence of male hormones, whether endogenous or exogenous, has an inhibiting effect on the neural mechanisms that otherwise would later mediate maternal behavior. There is probably a timing and a dose-response factor involved. The prenatal masculinization of human genetic females with the adrenogenital syndrome, as severe as it may be, has not prevented breast feeding in the few known cases where it was attempted (Chapter 6), even though the prenatal masculinization may have inhibited the play-rehearsal of maternalism in childhood and dampened the desire to be a mother in young adulthood.

Primate males living in troops in the wild show varying degrees of parental behavior. In human beings, the stimulus of the small infant or child, quite apart from hormone levels in the adult, itself is a powerful evoker of parental behavior. Men are responsive to this stimulus as well as women. Except for lactation, maternal and paternal responses to the helpless young are similar. Human parental or caretaking behavior is not, therefore, a gender-dimorphic aspect of behavior, even though the threshold for its activation may be lower for women than men.

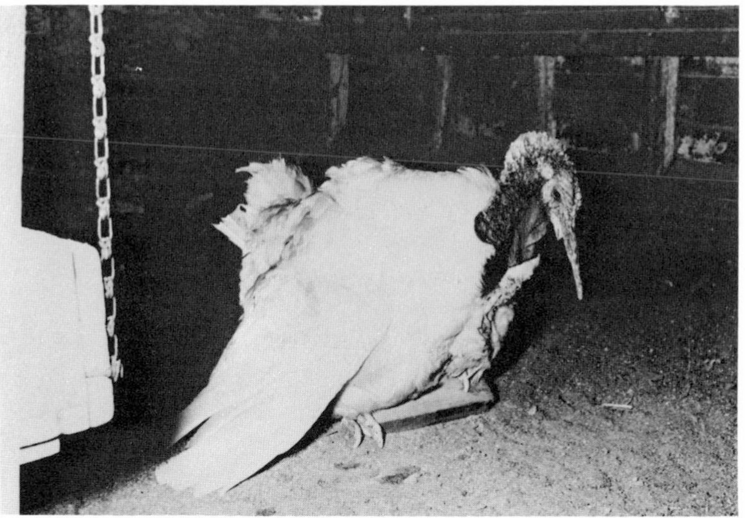

Figure 12.3. The head of the turkey hen is the signal which evokes mating in the male (photo courtesy of M. W. Schein and E. B. Hale).

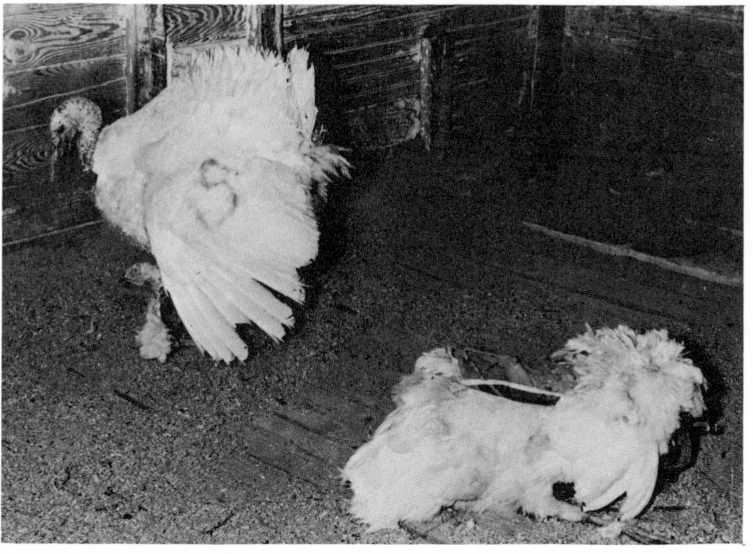

Figure 12.4. The hen turkey's head also directs the orientation of the male's mounting, so that he neglects the stuffed model of the headless body in favor of an isolated head supported on wire (photo courtesy of M. W. Schein and E. B. Hale).

EPILOGUE

Parents are caretakers not only of their offspring, but also—in a more primordial, phyletic sense—of the germ plasm and the genetic code. They are caretakers without authority or power to make decisions as to how their own full complement of forty-six chromosomes will be halved, so that the sperm conjoins only twenty-three with the twenty-three of the egg. Likewise parents make no decision as to whether, in the swimming race of the sperms, the winner will bear a Y chromosome to seal the genetic fate of the egg as a male, or an X, to seal its fate as a female. They have the same status of bystanders who watch while fate makes decisions about chromosome errors and about fetal hormones and the embryonic differentiation of sexual morphology. After the baby is born, parental powerlessness gives way to an august feeling of authority to make decisions about how well the child will be reared, and how normal he or she will be in sexual life. If the truth be known, parents have much less power over their child's destiny than they think. All the words in all twelve chapters of this book do not add up to give the power of prophecy as to how any given individual child will grow up sexually and psychosexually. There are many intervening variables still to be ascertained, and many opportunities for fate to let chance make decisions. Impressive as may be the growing body of knowledge on human psychosexual differentiation, no one concerned with research need feel like Alexander, crying for lack of new worlds to conquer.

BIBLIOGRAPHY

Anderson, C. O.; Zarrow, M. X.; and Denenberg, V. H. 1970. Maternal behavior in the rabbit: Effect of androgen treatment during gestation upon the nest-building behavior of the mother and her offspring. *Hormones and Behavior* 1:337–45.

Anon. 1970. Effects of sexual activity on beard growth in man. *Nature* 226:869–70.

Arai, Y., and Gorski, R. A. 1968. Critical exposure time for androgenization of the rat hypothalamus determined by antiandrogen injection. *Proceedings of the Society for Experimental Biology and Medicine* 127:590–93.

Aronson, L. R., and Cooper, M. L. 1968. Desensitization of the glans penis and sexual behavior in cats. In M. Diamond (ed.), *Reproduction and Sexual Behavior*. Bloomington, Indiana University Press.

Baal, J. van. 1966. *Déma. Description and Analysis of Marind Anim Culture, South New Guinea*. The Hague, Martinus Nijhoff.

Baird, D.; Horton, R.; Longcope, C.; and Tait, J. F. 1968. Steroid prehormones. *Perspectives in Biology and Medicine* 11:384–421.

Bardwick, J. M. 1971. *Psychology of Women: A Study of Bio-Cultural Conflicts*. New York, Harper and Row.

______(ed.). 1972. *Readings on the Psychology of Women*. New York: Harper and Row.

Barr, M. L., and Bertram, E. G. 1949. A morphological distinction between neurones of the male and female, and the behavior of the nucleolar satellite during accelerated nucleoprotein synthesis. *Nature* 163:676–77.

Barraclough, C. A. 1967. Modifications in reproductive function after exposure to hormones during the prenatal and early postnatal period. In L. Martini and W. F. Ganong (eds.), *Neuroendocrinology*, vol. II. New York, Academic Press.

Barraclough, C. A., and Gorski, R. A. 1962. Studies on mating behaviour in the androgen-sterilized female rat in relation to the hypothalamic regulation of sexual behaviour. *Journal of Endocrinology* 25:175–82.

Bartalos, M., and Baramki, T. A. 1967. *Medical Cytogenetics*. Baltimore, Williams and Wilkins.

Beach, F. A. 1947. A review of physiological and psychological studies of sexual behavior in mammals. *Physiological Reviews* 27:240–307.

——— . 1965. Experimental studies of mating behavior in animals. In J. Money (ed.), *Sex Research: New Developments*. New York, Holt, Rinehart and Winston.

——— . 1968. Factors involved in the control of mounting behavior by female mammals. In M. Diamond (ed.), *Perspectives in Reproduction and Sexual Behavior*. Bloomington, Indiana University Press.

——— . 1970. Hormonal effects on socio-sexual behavior in dogs. In H. Gibian and E. J. Plotz (eds.), *21. Colloquium der Gesellschaft fur Biologische Chemie*. New York, Springer.

Beach, F. A.; Noble, R. G.; and Orndoff, R. K. 1969. Effects of perinatal androgen treatment on responses of male rats to gonadal hormones in adulthood. *Journal of Comparative and Physiological Psychology* 68:490–97.

Blumer, D. 1970. Hypersexual episodes in temporal lobe epilepsy. *American Journal of Psychiatry* 126:83–90.

——— , and Walker, A. E. 1967. Sexual behavior in temporal lobe epilepsy. *Archives of Neurology* 16:31–43.

Bobrow, N. A.; Money, J.; and Lewis, V. G. 1971. Delayed puberty, eroticism, and sense of smell: a psychological study of hypogonadotropinism, osmatic and anosmatic (Kallmann's syndrome). *Archives of Sexual Behavior* 1:329–43.

Bogdanove, E. M. 1964. The role of the brain in the regulation of pituitary gonadotropin secretion. *Vitamins and Hormones* 22:205–60.

Bors, E., and Comarr, A. E. 1960. Neurological disturbances of sexual function with special reference to 529 patients with spinal cord injury. *Urological Survey* 10:191–222.

Bremer, J. 1959. *Asexualization. A follow-up study of 244 cases*. New York, Macmillan.

Bronson, F. H. 1971. Rodent pheromones. *Biology of Reproduction* 4:344–57.

Brown, D. G. 1957. Masculinity-femininity development in children. *Journal of Consulting Psychology* 21:197–202.

Burns, R. K. 1955. Experimental reversal of sex in the gonads of the opossum, Didelphys virginiana. *Proceedings of the National Academy of Sciences of the United States of America* 41:669–76.

——— . 1961. Role of hormones in the differentiation of sex. In W. C. Young (ed.), *Sex and Internal Secretions*, 3rd ed. Baltimore, Williams and Wilkins.

Calhoun, J. B. 1962. Population density and social pathology. *Scientific American* 206: 139–48.

Cappon, D.; Ezrin, C.; and Lynes, P. 1959. Psychosexual identification (psychogender) in the intersexed. *Canadian Psychiatric Association Journal* 4:90–106.

Carbaugh, B. T., and Schein, M. W. 1961. Sexual response of roosters to full and partial models. *American Zoologist* 1:62–63.

Chan, S. T. H. 1970. Natural sex reversal in vertebrates. *Philosophical Transactions of the Royal Society, London* B.259:59–71.

Clegg, M. T., and Doyle, L. L. 1967. Role in reproductive physiology of afferent impulses from the genitalia and other regions. In L. Martini and W. F. Ganong (eds.), *Neuroendocrinology*, vol. II. New York, Academic Press.

Clemens, L. G.; Hiroi, M.; and Gorski, R. A. 1969. Induction and facilitation of female mating behavior in rats treated neonatally with low doses of testosterone propionate. *Endocrinology* 84: 1430–38.

Clemens, L. G.; Shryne, J.; and Gorski, R. A. 1970. Androgen and development of progesterone responsiveness in male and female rats. *Physiology and Behavior* 5:673–78.

Comarr, A. E. 1970. Sexual function among patients with spinal cord injury. *Urologia Internationalis* 25:134–68.

Conn, J. H. 1940. Children's reactions to the discovery of genital differences. *American Journal of Orthopsychiatry* 10:747–54.

Conner, R. L., and Levine, S. 1969. Hormonal influences on aggressive behavior. In S. Garattini and E. B. Sigg (eds.), *Aggressive Behavior*. Amsterdam, Excerpta Medica Foundation.

Cowie, A. T., and Folley, S. J. 1961. The mammary gland and lactation. In W. C. Young (ed.), *Sex and Internal Secretions*, 3rd ed. Baltimore, Williams and Wilkins.

Dantchakoff, V. 1936. Sur les facteurs de l'histogenèse chez des hermaphrodites. *Comptes Rendus des Séances de la Société de Biologie et de ses Filiales (Paris)* 123:856–58.

______. 1937. Réalisation du sexe à volonté par inductions hormonales II. Inversions et déviations de l'histogenèse sexuelle chez l'embryon des Mammifères génétiquement femelle. *Bulletin Biologique de la France et de la Belgique* 71:269–321.

Davenport, W. 1965. Sexual patterns and their regulations in a society of the Southwest Pacific. In F. Beach (ed.), *Sex and Behavior*. New York, Wiley and Sons, Inc.

Davies, B. M., and Morgenstern, F. S. 1960. A case of cysticercosis, temporal lobe epilepsy, and transvestism. *Journal of Neurological and Neurosurgical Psychiatry* 23:247–49.

Davis, A. J. 1969. *Report on Sexual Assaults in the Prison System and Sheriff's Vans*. Philadelphia, District Attorney's Office and Police Department.

Dewhurst, C. J., and Gordon, R. R. 1969. *The Intersexual Disorders*. London, Baillière, Tindall and Cassell.

Diamond, M. 1965. A critical evaluation of the ontogeny of human sexual behavior. *Quarterly Review of Biology* 40:147–75.

____ . 1966. Progestagen inhibition of normal sexual behavior in the male guinea-pig. *Nature* 209:1322–24.

Dörner, G. 1968. Hormonal induction and prevention of female homosexuality. *Journal of Endocrinology* 42:163–64.

____ . 1969. Zur Frage einer neuroendokrinen Pathogenese, Prophylaxe und Therapie angeborener Sexualdeviationen. *Deutsche Medizinische Wochenschrift* 94:390–96.

Dua, S., and MacLean, P. D. 1964. Location for penile erection in medial frontal lobe. *American Journal of Physiology* 207:1425–34.

Eaton, G. 1970. Effect of a single prepubertal injection of testerone propionate on adult bisexual behavior of male hamsters castrated at birth. *Endocrinology* 87:934–40.

Edwards, D. A. 1968. Mice: fighting by neonatally androgenized females. *Science* 161:1027–28.

____ . 1969. Early androgen stimulation and aggressive behavior in male and female mice. *Physiology and Behavior* 4:333–38.

____ . 1970. Post-neonatal androgenization and adult aggressive behavior in female mice. *Physiology and Behavior* 5:465–67.

Ehrhardt, A. A. 1969. Zur Wirkung fötaler Hormone auf Intelligenz und geschlechtsspezifisches Verhalten. Unpublished doctoral dissertation, University of Düsseldorf.

____ . Epstein, R., and Money, J. 1968. Fetal androgens and female gender identity in the early treated adrenogenital syndrome. *Johns Hopkins Medical Journal* 122:160–67.

Ehrhardt, A. A.; Evers, K.; and Money, J. 1968. Influence of androgen and some aspects of sexually dimorphic behavior in women with the late-treated adrenogenital syndrome. *Johns Hopkins Medical Journal* 123:115–22.

Ehrhardt, A. A.; Greenberg, N.; and Money, J. 1970. Female gender identity and absence of fetal hormones: Turner's syndrome. *Johns Hopkins Medical Journal* 126:237–48.

Ehrhardt, A. A., and Money, J. 1967. Progestin-induced hermaphroditism: IQ and psychosexual identity in a study of ten girls. *Journal of Sex Research* 3:83–100.

Elger, W. 1966. Die Rolle der fötalen Androgene in der Sexualdifferenzierung des Kaninchens und ihre Abgrenzung gegen andere hormonale und somatische Faktoren durch Anwendung eines starken Antiandrogens. *Archives d'Anatomie Microscopique et de Morphologie Expérimentale* 55:658–743.

Elger, W.; von Berswordt-Wallrabe, R.; and Neumann, F. 1967. Der Einfluss von Antiandrogenen auf androgenabhaengige Vorgaenge im Organismus. *Die Naturwissenschaften* 54:549–52.

Epstein, A. W. 1960. Fetishism: A study of its psychopathology with particular reference to a proposed disorder in brain mechanisms as an etiological factor. *Journal of Nervous and Mental Disease* 130:107–19.

——— . 1961. Relationship of fetishism and transvestism to brain and particularly to temporal lobe dysfunction. *Journal of Nervous and Mental Disease* 133:247–53.

——— . 1969. Fetishism, a comprehensive view. *Science and Psychoanalysis* 15:81–87.

Everett, J. W. 1964. Central neural control of reproductive functions of the adenohypophysis. *Physiological Reviews* 44:373–431.

——— . 1969. Neuroendocrine aspects of mammalian reproduction. *Annual Review of Physiology* 31:383–416.

Everitt, B. J., and Herbert, J. 1969. Adrenal glands and sexual receptivity in female rhesus monkeys. *Nature* 222:1065–66.

——— . 1970. The maintenance of sexual receptivity by adrenal androgens in female rhesus monkeys. *Journal of Endocrinology* 48:xxxviii.

——— . 1971. The effects of dexamethasone and androgens on sexual receptivity of female Rhesus monkeys. *Journal of Endocrinology* 51:575–88.

Federman, D. D. 1967. *Abnormal Sexual Development*. Philadelphia, W. B. Saunders.

Filler, W., and Drezner, N. 1944. Results of surgical castration in women over forty. *American Journal of Obstetrics and Gynecology* 47:122–24.

Fisher, A. E. 1956. Maternal and sexual behavior induced by intracranial chemical stimulation. *Science* 124:228–29.

——— . 1966. Chemical and electrical stimulation of the brain in the male cat. In R. A. Gorski and R. E. Whalen (eds.), *The Brain and Gonadal Function*, Brain and Behavior, vol. III. Berkeley, University of California Press.

——— . 1969. Chemical stimulation of the brain. In P. Black (ed.), *Drugs and the Brain; Papers on the Action, Use, and Abuse of Psychotropic Drugs*. Baltimore, Johns Hopkins Press.

Flerkó, B. 1967. Brain mechanisms controlling gonadotrophin secretion and their sexual differentiation. In K. Lissar (ed.), *Symposium on Reproduction. Congress of the Hungarian Society for Endocrinology and Metabolism*. Budapest, Akademiai Kiado.

Frisch, R. E., and Revelle, R. 1970. Height and weight at menarche and a hypothesis of critical body weights and adolescent events. *Science* 169:397–98.

Gallien, L. 1956. Inversion expérimentale du sexe chez un anoure inférieur Xenopus laevis Daudin. Analyse des consequences génétique. *Bulletin Biologique de la France et de la Belgique* 90:163–83.

Garai, J. E. 1970. Sex Differences in Mental Health. *Genetic Psychology Monographs* 81:123–42.

Garai, J. E., and Scheinfeld, A. 1968. Sex differences in mental and behavioral traits. *Genetic Psychology Monographs* 77:169–299.

Gastaut, H., and Collomb, H. 1954. Étude du comportement sexuel chez les épileptiques psychomoteurs. *Annales Médico-psychologiques* 112:657–96.

Glascock, R. F., and Michael, R. P. 1962. The localization of oestrogen in a neurological system in the brain of the female cat. *Journal of Physiology* 163:38–39P.

Goldberg, S., and Lewis, M. 1969. Play behavior in the year-old infant: early sex differences. *Child Development* 40:21–31.

Goldfoot, D. A.; Feder, H. H.; and Goy, R. W. 1969. Development of bisexuality in the male rat treated neonatally with androstenedione. *Journal of Comparative and Physiological Psychology* 67:41–45.

Gorski, R. A. 1963. Modification of ovulatory mechanisms by postnatal administration of estrogen to the rat. *American Journal of Physiology* 205:842–44.

____ . 1966. Localization and sexual differentiation of the nervous structures which regulate ovulation. *Journal of Reproduction and Sterility (Supplement)* 1:67–68.

____ . 1968. Influence of age on the response to paranatal administration of a low dose of androgen. *Endocrinology* 82:1001–4.

____ . 1971. Gonadal hormones and the perinatal development of neuroendocrine function. In L. Martini and W. F. Ganong (eds.), *Frontiers in Neuroendocrinology, 1971*. New York, Oxford University Press.

Goy, R. W. 1970. Experimental control of psychosexuality. In G. W. Harris and R. G. Edwards (eds.), *A Discussion on the Determination of Sex*. London, Philosophical Transactions of the Royal Society, series B., vol. 259:149–62.

____ ; Bridson, W. E.; and Young, W. C. 1964. The period of maximal susceptibility of the prenatal female guinea pig to masculinizing actions of testosterone propionate. *Journal of Comparative and Physiological Psychology* 57:166–74.

Goy, R. W.; Phoenix, C. H.; and Young, W. C. 1962. A critical period for the suppression of behavioral receptivity in adult female rats by early treatment with androgen. *Anatomical Record* 142:307.

Grady, K. L., and Phoenix, C. H. 1963. Hormonal determinants of mating behavior; the display of feminine behavior by adult male rats castrated neonatally. *American Zoologist* 3:482–83.

____ , and Young, W. C. 1965. Role of the developing rat testis in differentiation of the neural tissues mediating mating behavior. *Journal of Comparative and Physiological Psychology* 59:176–82.

Green, R.; Luttge, W. G.; and Whalen, R. E. 1969. Uptake and retention of tritiated estradiol in brain and peripheral tissues of male, female and neonatally androgenized female rats. *Endocrinology* 85:373–78.

____ . 1970. Induction of receptivity in ovariectomized female rats by a single intravenous injection of estradiol-17β . *Physiology and Behavior* 5:137–41.

Green, R., and Money, J. (eds.), 1969. *Transsexualism and Sex Reassignment*. Baltimore, Johns Hopkins Press.

Greene, R. R.; Burrill, M. W.; and Ivy, A. C. 1940. The effects of estrogens on the antenatal sexual development of the rat. *American Journal of Anatomy* 67: 305–45.

Hambert, G. 1966. *Males with Positive Sex Chromatin: An Epidemiologic Investigation Followed by Psychiatric Study of Seventy-Five Cases*. Göteberg: Elanders Boktryckeri Aktiebolag.

Hamilton, J. B.; Walter, R. O.; Daniel, R. M.; and Mestler, G. E. 1969. Competition for mating between ordinary and supermale Japanese medaka fish. *Animal Behavior* 17:168–76.

Hampson, J. L., and Hampson, J. G. 1961. The ontogenesis of sexual behavior in man. In W. C. Young (ed.), *Sex and Internal Secretions*, 3rd ed. Baltimore, Williams and Wilkins.

Hardy, D. F. 1970. The effect of constant light on the estrous cycle and behavior of the female rat. *Physiology and Behavior* 5:421–25.

Harlow, H. F., and Harlow, M. K. 1965. The effect of rearing conditions on behavior. In J. Money (ed.), *Sex Research: New Developments*. New York, Holt, Rinehart and Winston.

Harlow, H. F.; Joslyn, W. D.; Senko, M. G.; and Dopp, A. 1966. Behavioral aspects of reproduction in primates. *Journal of Animal Science* 25:49–67.

Harris, G. W. 1964. Sex hormones, brain development and brain function. *Endocrinology* 75:627–48.

———, and Jacobsohn, D. 1952. Functional grafts of the anterior pituitary gland. *Proceedings of the Royal Society of London, Series B* (Biological Sciences) 139:263–76.

Harris, G. W., and Levine, S. 1965. Sexual differentiation of the brain and its experimental control. *Journal of Physiology* 181:379–400.

Harris, G. W., and Michael, R. P. 1964. The activation of sexual behavior by hypothalamic implants of estrogen. *Journal of Physiology* 171:275–301.

———, and Scott, P. P. 1958. Neurological site of action of stilboestrol in eliciting sexual behavior. In G. E. W. Wolstenholme and C. M. O'Connor (eds.), *Ciba Foundation Symposium on the Neurological Basis of Behavior*. Boston, Little, Brown.

Heinrichs, W. L., Gellert, R. J., Bakke, J. L., and Lawrence, N. L. 1971. DDT administered to neonatal rats induces persistent estrus syndrome. *Science* 173:642–43.

Henry, J., and Henry, Z. 1944. *Doll Play of Pilagá Indian Children* (Research Monographs No. 4). New York, American Orthopsychiatric Association, Inc.

Herbert, J. 1967. The social modification of sexual and other behavior in the rhesus monkey. In *Progress in Primatology*. First Congress of the International Primatological Society, Stuttgart, Gustav Fischer.

———. 1968. Sexual preference in the rhesus monkey Macaca mulatta in the laboratory. *Animal Behaviour* 16:120–28.

———. 1970. Hormones and reproductive behaviour in rhesus and talapoin monkeys. *Journal of Reproduction and Fertility (Supplement)* 11:119–40.

Hierons, R., and Saunders, M. 1966. Impotence in patients with temporal lobe lesions. *Lancet* 2:761–64.

Hoffet, H. 1968. Ueber die Anwendung des Testoseronblockers Cyproteronazetat (SH 714) bei Sexualdelinquenten und psychiatrischen Anstaltspatienten. *Praxis* 7:221–30.

Howell, T. R., and Bartholomew, G. A. 1952. Experiments on the mating behavior of the Brewer blackbird. *The Condor* 54:140–51.

Hunter, R. 1967. Transvestism, impotence and temporal lobe dysfunction. *Journal of the Neurological Sciences* 4:357–60.

Hunter, R.; Logue, V.; and McMenemy, W. H. 1963. Temporal lobe epilepsy supervening on longstanding transvestism and fetishism. *Epilepsia* 4:60–65.

Jacobsohn, D. 1965. Some effects of sex hormones on the fetus and newborn in relation to later reproductive functions. *Acta Universitatis Lundensis* vol. II., no. 17, pp. 1–19.

Jean, C. 1968a. Malformations génitales induites chez la souris adulte par une action oestrogène prénatale. I. Le mâle (pseudo-hermaphrodisme mâle). *Archives d'Anatomie Microscopique et de Morphologie Expérimentale* 57:121–66.

——. 1968b. Malformations génitales induites chez la souris adulte par une action oestrogène prénatale. II. La femelle. *Archives d'Anatomie Microscopique et de Morphologie Expérimentale* 57:191–226.

Johanson, A. J.; Guyda, H.; Light, C.; Migeon, C.; and Blizzard, R. M. 1969. Serum luteinizing hormone by radioimmunoassay in normal children. *Journal of Pediatrics* 74:416–24.

Jones, H. W., Jr., and Verkauf, B. S. 1971. Congenital adrenal hyperplasia: age at menarche and related events at puberty. *American Journal of Obstetrics and Gynecology* 109:292–98.

Jones, J. R. 1972. Plasma testosterone concentrations in female transexuals. *Archives of Sexual Behavior*, in press.

Jost, A. 1947. Recherches sur la différenciation sexuelle de l' embryon de Lapin. I. Introduction et embryologie génitale normale. *Archives d'Anatomie Microscopique et de Morphologie Expérimentale* 36:151–200.

——. 1958. Embryonic sexual differentiation. In H. W. Jones and W. W. Scott (eds.), *Hermaphroditism, Genital Anomalies and Related Endocrine Disorders.* Baltimore, Williams and Wilkins.

——. 1972. A new look at the mechanisms controlling sex differentiation in mammals. *Johns Hopkins Medical Journal* 130:38–53.

Kagan, J., and Lewis, M. 1965. Studies in attention in the human infant. *Merrill-Palmer Quarterly* 11:95–127.

Kane, F. T.; Lipton, M. A.; and Ewing, J. A. 1969. Hormonal infuences in female sexual response. *Archives of General Psychiatry* 20:202–9.

Katcher, A. 1955. The discrimination of sex differences by young children. *Journal of Genetic Psychology* 87:131–43.

Kato, J.; Inaba, M.; and Kobayashi, T. 1969. Variable uptake of tritiated oestradiol by the anterior hypothalamus in the postpubertal female rat. *Acta Endocrinologica* 61:585–92.

Kincl, F. A., and Maqueo, M. 1965. Prevention by progesterone of steroid-induced sterility in neonatal male and female rats. *Endocrinology* 77:859–62.

Kinsey, A. C.; Pomeroy, W. B.; Martin, C. E.; and Gebhard, P. H. 1953. *Sexual Behavior in the Human Female.* Philadelphia, Saunders.

Klüver, H., and Bucy, P. C. 1939. Preliminary analysis of the functions of the temporal lobes in monkeys. *Archives of Neurology and Psychiatry* 42:979–1000.

Kobayashi, F., and Gorski, R. A. 1970. Effects of antibiotics on androgenization of the neonatal female rat. *Endocrinology* 86:285–89.

Koch, H. L. 1944. A study of some factors conditioning the social distance between the sexes. *Journal of Social Psychology* 20:79–107.

Kolářský, A.; Freund, K.; Machek, J.; and Polák, O. 1967. Male sexual deviation. Association with early temporal lobe damage. *Archives of General Psychiatry* 17:735–43.

Kollar, E. J.; Beckwith, W. C.; and Edgerton, R. B. 1968. Sexual behavior of the ARL colony chimpanzees. *Journal of Nervous and Mental Disease* 147:444–59.

Kolodny, R. C.; Masters, W. H.; Hendryx, J.; and Toro, G. 1971. Plasma testosterone and semen analysis in male homosexuals. *The New England Journal of Medicine* 285:1170–74.

Korenman, S. G.; Perrin, L. E.; and McCallum, T. P. 1969. A radio-ligand binding assay system for estradiol measurement on human plasma. *Journal of Clinical Endocrinology and Metabolism* 28:879–83.

Kurcz, M.; Kovács, K.; Tiboldi, T.; and Orosz, A. 1967. Effect of androgenisation on adenohypophysial prolactin content in rats. *Acta Endocrinologica* 54:663–67.

Laschet, U. 1969. Die Anwendbarkeit von Antiandrogenen in der Humanmedizin. *Saarlaendisches Aerzteblatt* 22:370–71.

——, and Laschet, L. 1968. Die Behandlung der pathologisch gesteigerten und abartigen Sexualität des Mannes mit dem Antiandrogen Cyproteronacetat. In *Das Testosteron. Die Struma. 13. Symposion der Deutschen Gesellschaft für Endokrinologie.* Berlin, Springer.

Lehrman, D. S. 1961. Gonadal hormones and parental behavior in birds and infrahuman mammals. In W. C. Young (ed.), *Sex and Internal Secretions*, 3rd ed. Baltimore, Williams and Wilkins.

Le Magnen, J. 1952. Les phénomènes olfactosexuels chez l'homme. *Archives des Sciences Physiologiques* 6:125–60.

Levine, S., and Mullins, R. 1964. Estrogen administered neonatally affects adult sexual behavior in male and female rats. *Science* 144:185–87.

Lewis, V. G.; Money, J.; and Epstein, R. 1968. Concordance of verbal and nonverbal ability in the adrenogenital syndrome. *Johns Hopkins Medical Journal* 122:192–95.

Lillie, F. R. 1917. The freemartin: a study of the action of sex hormones in the fetal life of cattle. *Journal of Experimental Zoology* 23:371–452.

Lisk, R. D. 1962. Diencephalic placement of estradiol and sexual receptivity in the female rat. *American Journal of Physiology* 203:493–96.

——. 1967. Sexual Behavior: hormonal control. In L. Martini and W. F. Ganong (eds.), *Neuroendocrinology*, vol. 2. New York, Academic Press.

——. 1969. Progesterone: role in limitation of ovulation and sex behavior in mammals. *Transactions of the New York Academy of Sciences* 31:593–601.

——; Pretlow, R. A., 3rd; and Friedman, S. M. 1969. Hormonal stimulation necessary for elicitation of maternal nest-building in the mouse (Mus musculus). *Animal Behaviour* 17:730–37.

Loraine, J. A.; Ismail, A. A. A.; Adamopoulos, D. A.; and Dove, G. A. 1970. Endocrine function in male and female homosexuals. *British Medical Journal* 4:406–9.

Lorenz, K. Z. 1952. *King Solomon's Ring.* New York, Thomas Y. Crowell.

Loy, J. 1970. Perimenstrual sexual behavior among rhesus monkeys. *Folia Primatologica* 13:286–97.

Luttge, W. G., and Whalen, R. E. 1969a. Fluctuations in 6,7-^{3}H-estradiol-17 β uptake by the rat as a function of the estrous cycle. *American Zoologist* 9:100.

——, and Whalen, R. E. 1969b. Partial defeminization by administration of androstenedione to neonatal female rats. *Life Sciences* 8:1003–8.

——. 1970. Regional localization of estrogenic metabolites in the brain of male and female rats. *Steroids* 15:605–12.

Maccoby, E. E. 1963. Woman's intellect. In S. M. Farber and H. L. Wilson (eds.), *Man and Civilization: The Potential of Woman.* New York, McGraw-Hill.

——, (ed.). 1966. *The Development of Sex Differences.* Stanford, Stanford University Press.

MacLean, P. D. 1967. The brain in relation to empathy and medical education. *Journal of Nervous and Mental Disease* 144:374–82.

——. 1969. The paranoid streak in man. In A. Koestler and J. Smythies (eds.), *Beyond Reductionism.* London, Hutchinson.

——. 1972. *A Triune Concept of the Brain and Behavior.* The Hincks Memorial Lectures (T. Boag, ed.). Toronto, Toronto University Press. In press.

——; Denniston, R. H.; and Dua, S. 1963. Further studies on cerebral representation of penile erection: caudal thalamus, midbrain and pons. *Journal of Neurophysiology* 26:273–93.

MacLean, P. D.; Dua, S., and Denniston, R. H. 1963. Cerebral localization for scratching and seminal discharge. *Archives of Neurology* 9:485–97.

MacLean, P. D., and Ploog, D. W. 1962. Cerebral representation of penile erection. *Journal of Neurophysiology* 25:29–55.

Margolese, M. 1970. Homosexuality: a new endocrine correlate. *Hormones and Behavior* 1:151–55.

Marshall, W. A., and Tanner, J. M. 1968. Growth and physiological development during adolescence. In A. C. De Graff (ed.), *Annual Review of Medicine* 19:283–300. Palo Alto, California, Annual Reviews, Inc.

_____ . 1969. Variations in pattern of pubertal changes in girls. *Archives of Disease in Childhood* 44:291–303.

_____ . 1970. Variations in the pattern of pubertal changes in boys. *Archives of Disease in Childhood* 45:13–23.

Martinez, C., and Bittner, J. J. 1956. A non-hypophyseal sex difference in estrous behavior of mice bearing pituitary grafts. *Proceedings of the Society for Experimental Biology and Medicine* 91:506–9.

Masica, D. N.; Money, J.; and Ehrhardt, A. A. 1971. Fetal feminization and female gender identity in the testicular feminizing syndrome of androgen insensitivity. *Archives of Sexual Behavior* 1:131–42.

_____ ; and Lewis, V. G. 1969. IQ, fetal sex hormones and cognitive patterns: Studies in the testicular feminizing syndrome of androgen insensitivity. *Johns Hopkins Medical Journal* 123:105–14.

Masters, W. H., and Johnson, V. E. 1966. *Human Sexual Response.* Boston, Little, Brown.

McClintock, M. K. 1971. Menstrual synchrony and suppression. *Nature* 229:244–45.

McGuire, J. L., and Lisk, R. D. 1968. Estrogen receptors in the intact rat. *Proceedings of the National Academy of Sciences* 61:497–503.

_____ . 1969. Oestrogen receptors in androgen or oestrogen sterilized female rats. *Nature* 221:1068–69.

Meites, J., and Nicoll, C. S. 1966. Adenohypophysis: prolactin. *Annual Review of Physiology* 28:57–88.

Michael, R. P. 1962. Estrogen sensitive neurons and sexual behavior in female cats. *Science* 136:322–23.

_____ . 1968. Gonadal hormones and the control of primate behaviour. In R. P. Michael (ed.), *Endocrinology and Human Behaviour.* London, Oxford University Press.

_____ . 1971. Neuroendocrine factors regulating primate behavior. In L. Martini and W. F. Ganong (eds.), *Frontiers in Neuroendocrinology, 1971.* New York, Oxford University Press.

_____ , and Glascock, R. F. 1963. The distribution of C^{14}- and H^{3}-labelled oestrogens in brain. *Proceedings. 5th (1961) International Congress Biochemistry* 9,11.37.

Michael, R. P., and Herbert, J. 1963. Menstrual cycle influences grooming behavior and sexual activity in the rhesus monkey. *Science* 140:500–1.

Michael, R. P., and Keverne, E. B. 1968. Pheromones in the communication of sexual status in primates. *Nature* 218:746–49.

_____ . 1970. Primate sex pheromones of vaginal origin. *Nature* 225:84–85.

Michael, R. P.; Keverne, E. B.; and Bonsall, R. W. 1971. Pheromones: isolation of a male sex attractant from a female primate. *Science* 172:964–66.

Migeon, C. J.; Rivarola, M. A.; and Forest, M. G. 1968. Studies of androgens in transsexual subjects. Effects of estrogen therapy. *Johns Hopkins Medical Journal* 123:128–33.

Mikamo, K., and Witschi, E. 1963. Functional sex-reversal in genetic females of Xenopus laevis induced by implanted testes. *Genetics* 48:1411–21.

——. 1964. Masculinization and breeding of the WW Xenopus. *Experientia* 20:622–23.

Miller, P. 1946. An experimental study of the development of sex roles. Unpublished honors project, Psychology Laboratory, Connecticut College. See G. Seward (ed.), *Sex and Social Order*. New York, McGraw-Hill.

Mitchell, W.; Falconer, M. A.; and Hill, D. 1954. Epilepsy with fetishism relieved by temporal lobectomy. *Lancet* 2:626–30.

Money, J. 1952. *Hermaphroditism: An Inquiry Into the Nature of a Human Paradox*. Doctoral Dissertation, Harvard University Library. University Microfilms Library Services, Xerox Corporation, Ann Arbor, Michigan, 1967.

——. 1960a. Components of eroticism in man: cognitional rehearsals. In J. Wortis (ed.), *Recent Advances in Biological Psychiatry*. New York, Grune and Stratton.

——. 1960b. Phantom orgasm in the dreams of paraplegic men and women. *Archives of General Psychiatry* 3:373–82.

——. 1961a. Components of eroticism in man: I. The hormones in relation to sexual morphology and sexual desire. *Journal of Nervous and Mental Disease* 132:239–48.

——. 1961b. Components of eroticism in man: II. The orgasm and genital somesthesia. *Journal of Nervous and Mental Disease* 132:289–97.

——. 1961c. Sex hormones and other variables in human eroticism. In W. C. Young (ed.), *Sex and Internal Secretions*, 3rd ed. Baltimore, Williams and Wilkins.

——. 1965a. Influence of hormones on sexual behavior. *Annual Review of Medicine* 16:67–82.

——. 1965b. Negro illegitimacy: An antebellum legacy in obstetrical sociology. *Pacific Medicine and Surgery* 79:350–52.

——. 1967a. Cytogenetic and other aspects of transvestism and transexualism. *Journal of Sex Research* 3:141–43.

——. 1967b. Sexual problems of the chronically ill. In C. H. Wahl (ed.), *Sexual Problems; Diagnosis and Treatment in Medical Practice*. New York, Free Press.

——. 1968a. Psychologic approach to psychosexual misidentity with elective mutism: sex reassignment in two cases of hyperadrenocortical hermaphroditism. *Clinical Pediatrics* 7:331–39.

——. 1968b. *Sex Errors of the Body*. Baltimore, Johns Hopkins Press.

——. 1969. Sex reassignment as related to hermaphroditism and transsexualism. In R. Green and J. Money (eds.), *Transsexualism and Sex Reassignment*. Baltimore, Johns Hopkins Press.

——. 1970a. Matched pairs of hermaphrodites: behavioral biology of sexual differentiation from chromosomes to gender identity. *Engineering and Science* (California Institute of Technology, Special Issue: Biological Bases of Human Behavior) 33:34–39.

——. 1970b. Sexual dimorphism and homosexual gender identity. *Psychological Bulletin* 74:425–40.

——. 1970c. Use of an androgen-depleting hormone in the treatment of male sex offenders. *Journal of Sex Research* 6:165–72.

——. 1971. Prenatal hormones and intelligence: a possible relationship. *Impact of Science on Society* 21:285–90.

——, and Alexander, D. 1967. Eroticism and sexual function in developmental anorchia and hyporchia with pubertal failure. *Journal of Sex Research* 3:31–47.

_____ . 1969. Psychosexual development and absence of homosexuality in males with precocious puberty: review of 18 cases. *Journal of Nervous and Mental Disease* 148:111–23.

Money, J., and Brennan, J. G. 1970. Heterosexual vs. homosexual attitudes: male partners' perception of the feminine image of male transexuals. *Journal of Sex Research* 6:193–209.

Money, J.; Cawte, J. E.; Bianchi, G. N.; and Nurcombe, B. 1970. Sex training and traditions in Arnhem Land. *British Journal of Medical Psychology* 47:383–99.

Money, J.; Ehrhardt, A. A.; and Masica, D.N. 1968. Fetal feminization induced by androgen insensitivity in the testicular feminizing syndrome: effect on marriage and maternalism. *Johns Hopkins Medical Journal* 123:160–67.

Money, J., and Hirsch, S. 1965. After priapism: orgasm retained, erection lost. *Journal of Urology* 94:152–57.

Money, J., and Lewis, V. 1966. IQ, genetics and accelerated growth: adrenogenital syndrome. *Bulletin of The Johns Hopkins Hospital* 118:365–73.

Money, J.; Potter, R.; and Stoll, C. S. 1969. Sex reannouncement in hereditary sex deformity: psychology and sociology of habilitation. *Social Science and Medicine* 3:207–16.

Money, J., and Raiti, S. 1967. Breasts in intersexuality and transexualism: I. Mammary growth. *Journal of the American Medical Women's Association* 22:865–69.

Money, J., and Walker, P. 1971. Psychosexual development, maternalism, nonpromiscuity and body image in 15 females with precocious puberty. *Archives of Sexual Behavior* 1:45–60.

Money, J., and Wang, C. 1966. Human figure drawing. I: Sex of first choice in gender-identity anomalies, Klinefelter's syndrome and precocious puberty. *Journal of Nervous and Mental Disease* 143:157–62.

Moore, K. L. (ed.). 1966. *The Sex Chromatin.* Philadelphia, Saunders.

Murphy, L. 1947. Social factors in child development. In T. M. Newcomb and E. R. Hartley (eds.), *Readings in Social Psychology.* New York, Holt.

Nadler, R. D. 1968. Masculinization of female rats by intracranial implantation of androgen in infancy. *Journal of Comparative and Physiological Psychology* 66:157–67.

_____ . 1969. Differentiation of the capacity for male sexual behavior in the rat. *Hormones and Behavior* 1:53–63.

_____ . 1971. Sexual differentiation following intrahypothalamic implantation of steroids. In D. H. Ford (ed.), *The Influence of Hormones on the Nervous System.* New York, S. Karger.

Napoli, A. M., and Gerall, A. A. 1970. Effect of estrogen and anti-estrogen on reproductive function in neonatally androgenized female rats. *Endocrinology* 87:1330–37.

Neumann, F. 1970. Antiandrogens. *Research in Reproduction* 2(#3):3–4.

_____ , and Elger, W. 1965. Proof of the activity of androgenic agents on the differentiation of the external genitalia, the mammary gland and the hypothalamic-pituitary system in rats. In *Androgens in Normal and Pathological Conditions, International Congress Series No. 101, Proceedings of the Second Symposium on Steroid Hormones.* Amsterdam, Excerpta Medica.

_____ . 1966. Permanent changes in gonadal function and sexual behaviour as a result of early feminization of male rats by treatment with an antiandrogenic steroid. *Endokrinologie* 50:209–25.

Neumann, F., and Hamada, H. 1964. Intrauterine Feminisierung maennlicher Rattenfeten durch das stark gestagen wirksame 6-chlor- Δ^6-1,2-methylen-17α-hydroxy-progesteronacetat. In *10. Symposion der Deutschen Gesellschaft fuer Endokrinologie in Wien, 1963.* Berlin, Springer-Verlag.

Neumann, F.; Steinbeck, H.; and Hahn, J. D. 1970. Hormones and brain differentiation. In L. Martini, M. Motta, and F. Fraschini (eds.), *The Hypothalamus*. New York, Academic Press. Pp. 569–603.

New, M. I., and Suvannkul, L. 1970. Male pseudohermaphroditism due to 17α-hydroxylase deficiency. *Journal of Clinical Investigation* 49:1930–41.

Newton, N.; Peeler, D.; and Rawlins, C. 1968. Effect of lactation on maternal behavior in mice with comparative data on humans. *Lying-in: The Journal of Reproductive Medicine* 1:257–62.

Nielsen, J. 1969. Klinefelter's syndrome and the XYY syndrome: A genetical, endocrinological and psychiatric-psychological study of thirty-three severely hypogonadal male patients and two patients with karyotype 47,XXY. *Acta Psychiatrica Scandinavica*, vol. 45, supplementum 209. Copenhagen, Munksgaard.

Nielsen, J.; Sørensen, A.; Theilgaard, A.; Anders, F.; and Johnsen, S. G. 1969. A psychiatric-psychological study of 50 severely hypogonadal male patients, including 34 with Klinefelter's syndrome, 47,XXY. *Acta Jutlandica* XLI:3. Universitetsforlaget i Aarhus. Copenhagen, Munksgaard.

Palka, Y. S., and Sawyer, C. H. 1966a. The effects of hypothalamic implants of ovarian steroids on estrous behavior in rabbits. *Journal of Physiology* 185:251–69.

———. 1966b. Induction of estrous behavior in rabbits by hypothalamic implants of testosterone. *American Journal of Physiology* 211:225–28.

Parkes, A. S., and Bruce, H. M. 1961. Olfactory stimuli in mammalian reproduction; odor excites neurohumoral responses affecting oestrus, pseudopregnancy, and pregnancy, in the mouse. *Science* 134:1049–54.

Patton, R. G., and Gardner, L. I. 1969. Short stature associated with maternal deprivation syndrome: disordered family environment as a cause of so-called idiopathic hypopituitarism. In L. I. Gardner (ed.), *Endocrine and Genetic Diseases of Childhood*. Philadelphia, Saunders.

Payne, A. , and Swanson, H. H. 1971. Hormonal control of aggressive dominance in the female hamster. *Physiology and Behavior* 6:355–57.

Pearson, P. L.; Bobrow, M.; and Vosa, C. G. 1970. Technique for identifying Y chromosomes in human interphase nuclei. *Nature* 226:78–80.

Pfaff, D. W. 1968. Autoradiographic localization of radioactivity in rat brain after injection of tritiated sex hormones. *Science* 161:1355–56.

———, and Zigmond, R. E. 1971. Neonatal androgen effects on sexual and non-sexual behavior of adult rats tested under various hormone regimes. *Neuroendocrinology* 7:129–45.

Pfeiffer, C. A. 1936. Sexual differences of the hypophyses and their determination by the gonads. *American Journal of Anatomy* 58:195–226.

Phoenix, C. H., Goy, R. W.; Gerall, A. A.; and Young, W. C. 1959. Organizing action of prenatally administered testosterone propionate on the tissues mediating mating behavior in the female guinea pig. *Endocrinology* 65:369–82.

Phoenix, C. H.; Goy, R. W.; and Young, W. C. 1967. Sexual behavior: general aspects. In L. Martini and W. F. Ganong (eds.), *Neuroendocrinology*, vol. II. New York, Academic Press.

Powell, G. F.; Brasel, J. A.; and Blizzard, R. M. 1967. Emotional deprivation and growth retardation simulating idiopathic hypopituitarism: I. Clinical evaluation of the syndrome. *New England Journal of Medicine* 276:1271–78.

Powell, G. F.; Brasel, J. A.; Raiti, S.; and Blizzard, R. M. 1967. Emotional deprivation and growth retardation simulating idiopathic hypopituitarism. II. Endocrinologic evaluation of the syndrome. *New England Journal of Medicine* 276:1279–83.

Rabban, M. 1950. Sex-role identification in young children in two diverse social groups. *Genetic Psychology Monographs* 42:81–158.

Raiti, S.; Johanson, A.; Light, C.; Migeon, C. J.; and Blizzard, R. M. 1969. Measurement of immunologically reactive follicle stimulating hormone in serum of normal male children and adults. *Metabolism* 18:234–40.

Raiti, S.; Light, C.; and Blizzard, R. M. 1969. Urinary follicle stimulating hormone excretion in boys and adult males as measured by radioimmunoassay. *Journal of Clinical Endocrinology and Metabolism* 29:884–90.

Ramaley, J. A., and Gorski, R. A. 1967. The effect of hypothalamic deafferentation upon puberty in the female rat. *Acta Endocrinologica* 56:661–74.

Revesz, C. D.; Kernaghan, D.; and Bindra, D. 1963. Sexual drive of female rats "masculinized" by testosterone during gestation. *Journal of Endocrinology* 25:549–50.

Richter, C. P. 1965. *Biological Clocks in Medicine and Psychiatry*. Springfield, Illinois, Charles C Thomas.

Roeder, F., and Müller, D. 1969. The stereotaxic treatment of paedophilic homosexuality. *German Medical Monthly* (English Language Edition) 14:265–71.

_____, and Orthner, H. 1971. Weitere Erfahrungen mit der stereotaktischen Behandlung sexueller Perversionen. In H. Orthner (ed.), *Zentralnervöse Sexualsteuerung, Journal of Neuro-Visceral Relations*, Supplementum X, pp. 317–24, Wien and New York, Springer-Verlag.

Rose, R. M.; Holaday, J. W.; and Bernstein, I. S. 1971. Plasma testosterone, dominance rank and aggressive behaviour in male rhesus monkeys. *Nature* 231:366–68.

Rosenblatt, J. S. 1967. Nonhormonal basis of maternal behavior in the rat. *Science* 156:1512–14.

Ross, S.; Sawin, P. B.; Zarrow, M. X.; and Denenberg, V. H. 1963. In H. L. Rheingold (ed.), *Maternal Behavior in Mammals*. New York, John Wiley and Sons, Inc.

Saunders, F. J. 1968. Effects of sex steroids and related compounds on pregnancy and on development of the young. *Physiological Reviews* 48:601–43.

Sawyer, C. H. and Gorski, R. A. (eds.), 1972. *Steroid Hormones and Brain Function*. Berkeley, Los Angeles, University of California Press.

Schein, M. W., and Hale, E. B. 1965. Stimuli eliciting sexual behavior. In F. A. Beach (ed.), *Sex and Behavior*. New York, John Wiley and Sons.

Schmidt, G., and Sigusch, V. 1970. Sex differences in responses to psychosexual stimulation by films and slides. *Journal of Sex Research* 6:268–83.

Schneider, R. A., and Wolf, S. 1955. Olfactory perception thresholds for citral utilizing a new type olfactorium. *Journal of Applied Physiology* 8:337–42.

Schutz, F. 1965. Homosexualitaet und Praegung. Eine experimentelle Untersuchung an Enten. *Psychologische Forschung* 28:439–63.

_____. 1968. Sexuelle Praegungserscheinungen bei Tieren. In *Die Sexualitaet des Menschen. Handbuch der medizinischen Sexualforschung*. Stuttgart, Ferdinand Enke Verlag.

Seebandt, G. 1968. Gedanken und Überlegungen zur Behandlung sexualtriebabartiger Psychopathen mit Antiandrogenen. *Das oeffentliche Gesundheitswesen: Monatsschrift für Gesundheitsverwaltung und Sozialhygiene* 30:66–71.

Segal, S. J., and Johnson, D. 1959. Inductive influence of steroid hormones on the neural system. Ovulation controlling mechanisms. *Archives d' Anatomie Microscopique et de Morphologie Expérimentale 48:261–74.*

Shepher, J. 1971a. Self-imposed incest avoidance and exogamy in second generation kibbutz adults. Unpublished doctoral Dissertation. Brunswick, N. J., Rutgers University.

———. 1971b. Mate selection among second generation Kibbutz adolescents and adults: Incest avoidance and negative imprinting. *Archives of Sexual Behavior* 1:293–307.

Sigusch, V.; Schmidt, G.; Reinfeld, A.; and Wiedemann-Sutor, I., 1970. Psychosexual stimulation: sex differences. *Journal of Sex Research* 6:10–24.

Southam, A. L., and Gonzaga, F. P. 1965. Systemic changes during the menstrual cycle. *American Journal of Obstetrics and Gynecology* 91:142–65.

Stern, J. J. 1969. Neonatal castration, androstenedione, and the mating behavior of the male rat. *Journal of Comparative and Physiological Psychology* 69:608–12.

Stern, J. M., and Eisenfeld, A. J. 1971. Distribution and metabolism of ^{3}H-testosterone in castrated male rats; effects of cyproterone, progesterone and unlabeled testosterone. *Endocrinology* 88:1117–25.

Stoller, R. J. 1968. *Sex and Gender. On the Development of Masculinity and Femininity.* New York, Science House.

———. 1970. Pornography and perversion. *Archives of General Psychiatry* 22:490–99.

Stumpf, W. E. 1968. Estradiol-concentrating neurons: topography in the hypothalamus by dry-mount autoradiography. *Science* 162:1001–3.

Swanson, H. E., and van der Werff ten Bosch, J. J. 1964. The "early-androgen" syndrome: differences in response to prenatal and postnatal administration of various doses of testosterone propionate in female and male rats. *Acta Endocrinologica* 47:37–50.

Swanson, H. H. 1967. Alteration of sex-typical behaviour in hamsters in open field and emergence tests by neonatal administration of androgen or oestrogen. *Animal Behaviour* 15:209–16.

———. 1969. Interaction of experience with adrenal and sex hormones on the behaviour of hamsters in the open field test. *Animal Behaviour* 17:148–54.

———. 1970. Effects of castration at birth in hamsters of both sexes on luteinization of ovarian implants, oestrous cycles and sexual behavior. *Journal of Reproduction and Fertility* 21:183–86.

———. 1971. Determination of the sex role in hamsters by the action of sex hormones in infancy. In D. H. Ford (ed.), *The Influence of Hormones on the Nervous System.* New York, S. Karger.

———, and Crossley, D. A. 1971. Sexual behaviour in the golden hamster and its modification by neonatal administration of testosterone propionate. In M. Hamburgh and E. J. W. Barrington (eds.), *Hormones in Development.* New York, Appleton-Century-Crofts.

Tanner, J. M. 1962. *Growth at Adolescence* (2nd ed.). Oxford, Blackwell Scientific Publications.

———. 1969. Growth and endocrinology of the adolescent. In L. I. Gardner (ed.), *Endocrine and Genetic Diseases of Childhood.* Philadelphia, W. B. Saunders.

Thiessen, D. D., and Lindzey, G. 1970. Territorial marking in the female mongolian gerbil: short term reaction to hormones. *Hormones and Behavior* 1:157–60.

Thiessen, D. D., and Yahr, P. 1969. Central control of territorial marking in the mongolian gerbil. *Physiology and Behavior* 5:275–78.

Tjio, J. H., and Levan, A. 1956. The chromosome number of man. *Hereditas* 42:1–6.

Tsuji, I.; Nakajima, F.; Morimato, J.; and Nounaka, Y. 1961. The sexual function in patients with spinal cord injury. *Urologica Internationalis* 12:270–80.

Turner, C. D., and Asakawa, H. 1964. Experimental reversal of germ cells in ovaries of fetal mice. *Science* 143:1344–45.

Turner, C. H.; Davenport, R. K.; and Rogers, C. M. 1969. The effect of early deprivation on the social behavior of adolescent chimpanzees. *American Journal of Psychiatry* 125: 85–90.

Udry, J. R., and Morris, H. M. 1968. Distribution of coitus in the menstrual cycle. *Nature* 220:593–96.

Vandenbergh, J. G.; Drickamer, L. C.; and Colby, D. R. 1972. Social and dietary factors in the sexual maturation of female mice. *Journal of Reproduction and Fertility* 28:397–405.

Ward, I. 1972. Prenatal stress feminizes and demasculinizes the behavior of males. *Science* 175:82–84.

Waxenberg, S. E. 1963. Some biologic correlates of sexual behavior. In G. Winokur (ed.), *Determinants of Sexual Behavior*. Springfield, Ill., Charles C Thomas.

Wehmer, F.; Porter, R. H.; and Scales, B. 1970. Pre-mating and pregnancy stress in rats affects behaviour of grandpups. *Nature* 227:622.

Whalen, R. E. 1964. Hormone-induced changes in the organization of sexual behavior in the male rat. *Journal of Comparative and Physiological Psychology* 57:175–82.

_____ . 1968. Differentiation of the neural mechanisms which control gonadotropin secretion and sexual behavior. In M. Diamond (ed.), *Perspectives in Reproduction and Sexual Behavior*. Bloomington, Indiana University Press.

_____ , and Edwards, D. A. 1966. Sexual reversibility in neonatally castrated male rats. *Journal of Comparative and Physiological Psychology* 62:307–10.

_____ . 1967. Hormonal determinants of the development of masculine and feminine behavior in male and female rats. *Anatomical Record* 157:173–80.

Whalen, R. E., and Hardy, D. F. 1970. Induction of receptivity in female rats and cats with estrogen and testosterone. *Physiology and Behavior* 5:529–33.

Whalen, R. E., and Maurer, R. A. 1969. Estrogen "receptors" in brain: an unsolved problem. *Proceedings of the National Academy of Sciences* 63:681–85.

Whalen, R. E., Peck, C. K., and LoPiccolo, J. 1966. Virilization of female rats by prenatally administered progestin. *Endocrinology* 78:965–70.

Wiener, H. 1966. External chemical messengers. I. Emission and reception in man. *New York State Journal of Medicine* 66:3153–70.

Williams, R. H. (ed.) 1968. *Textbook of Endocrinology*, 4th ed. Philadelphia, W. B. Saunders.

Witschi, E. 1950. Génétique et physiologie de la différenciation du sexe. *Archives d'Anatomie Microscopique et de Morphologie Expérimentale* 39:215–46.

_____ . 1965. Hormones and embryonic induction. *Archives d'Anatomie Microscopique et de Morphologie Expérimentale* 54:601–11.

_____ , and Dale, E. 1962. Steroid hormones at early developmental stages of vertebrates. *General and Comparative Endocrinology (Supplement)* 1:356–61.

Wolf, T. P. 1968. Geschlechtswechsel bei Hermaphroditen. Unpublished doctoral dissertation. Heidelberg, Ruprecht-Karl-Universitaet.

Wolff, G., and Money, J. 1972. Relationship between sleep and growth in patients with reversible somatotropin deficiency (psychosocial dwarfism). *Psychological Medicine*, in press.

Wurtman, R. J. 1967. Effects of light and visual stimuli on endocrine function. In L. Martini and W. F. Ganong (eds.), *Neuroendocrinology*, vol. II. New York, Academic Press. Press.

_____ , Axelrod, J., and Kelly, D. E. 1968. *The Pineal*. New York and London, Academic Press.

Yamamoto, T. 1955. Progeny of artificially induced sex-reversals of male genotype (XY) in the medaka (Oryzias latipes) with special reference to YY-male. *Genetics* 40:406–19.

——. 1962. Hormonic factors affecting gonadal differentiation in fish. *General and Comparative Endocrinology (Supplement)* 1:341–45.

Young, W. C. 1961. The hormones and mating behavior. In W. C. Young (ed.), *Sex and Internal Secretions*, 3rd ed. Baltimore, Williams and Wilkins.

——, Goy, R. W., and Phoenix, C. H. 1964. Hormones and sexual behavior. *Science* 143:212–18.

Zarrow, M. X.; Farooq, A.; Denenberg, V. H.; Sawin, P. B.; and Ross, S. 1963. Maternal behaviour in the rabbit: Endocrine control of maternal-nest building. *Journal of Reproduction and Fertility* 6:375–83.

Zigmond, R. E., and McEwen, B. S. 1970. Selective retention of oestradiol by cell nuclei in specific brain regions of the ovariectomized rat. *Journal of Neurochemistry* 17:889–99.

Zilboorg, G. 1944. Masculine and feminine; some biological and cultural aspects. *Psychiatry* 7:257–96.

Zuger, B. 1970. Gender role determination; a critical review of the evidence from hermaphroditism. *Psychosomatic Medicine* 32:449–63.

GLOSSARY

Addison's disease: a chronic condition of adrenocortical insufficiency in children or adults in which production of the adrenocortical hormones cortisol, aldosterone, and androgen is variably affected. The clinical manifestations include, in the severe form, shock and death from mild infections; in the less severe form, marked dehydration from minimal fluid deprivation; and in the mild form, fatigue and hyperpigmentation. Long-term treatment includes replacement of adrenocortical hormones.

adrenal cortex: the outer three layers of the adrenal gland, as contrasted with the innermost part, the medulla. The cortex produces steroidal hormones, among them the glucocorticoid, cortisol, and nonpotent sex hormones. The medulla produces adrenalin (epinephrine), a catecholamine; *see also* **cortex**.

adrenogenital syndrome: a condition produced by a genetically transmitted enzymatic defect in the functioning of the adrenal cortices of males or females, which induces varying degrees of insufficiency of cortisol and aldosterone and excesses of adrenal androgen and pituitary adrenocorticotropin. Abnormal function of the adrenal cortex starts in fetal life and, unless treated, continues chronically after birth. Females born with the syndrome have ambiguous genitalia and, if they survive without salt loss and dehydration, undergo severe virilization. Males are usually not recognized at birth, but if they survive, will prematurely develop sexually during the first years of life. In the severe form of the disease, untreated, mortality rate is almost 100 percent for both sexes. Treatment with glucocorticoids and in some cases also with salt-retaining hormone is life-saving and prevents postnatal virilization. Plastic surgery is needed on the female genitalia. With appropriate therapy, prognosis for survival and good physical and mental health is excellent.

agenesis (*adjective*, **agenetic**): partial or complete failure of an organ or part of the body to form or develop.

amazon: a tall, strong, masculine woman who might be also a lesbian—named after the Amazons, a race of woman warriors in Greek mythology; *synonym*, virago.

amenorrhea: absence or failure of the menstrual periods.

amygdala: a structure of the old cortex (paleocortex), or limbic system of the brain, situated close to the temporal lobe of the neocortex.

androgen: male sex hormone, produced chiefly by the testis, but also by the adrenal cortex and, in small amounts, by the ovary. In biochemical structure, there are several different but related steroid hormones that qualify as androgens. They differ in biological strength and effectiveness.

androgen-insensitivity syndrome (also called testicular-feminizing syndrome): a congenital condition identified by a 46,XY male karyotype in girls or women who appear externally to be not sexually different from normal females, except in some cases for a swelling or lump in each groin, or for the absence of pubic hair after puberty. The cells of the body are unable to respond to the male sex hormone which is made in the testes in normal amounts for a male. They respond instead to the small amount of female sex hormone, estrogen, which is normally made in the testes. The effect before birth is that masculine internal development commences but does not get completed. It goes far enough, however, to prevent internal female development. Externally, the genitalia differentiate as female, except for a blind vagina which is usually not deep enough for satisfactory intercourse and needs surgical lengthening in or after middle teenage. There is no menstruation and no fertility. Breasts develop normally.

androgyny: condition of showing some male and some female characteristics in body build.

androstenedione: one of the natural androgens, measurable in the blood of men and women. It is produced mainly by the adrenal cortices, and in lesser degree by the gonads. It has low biological potency as an androgen, but is the direct precursor of testosterone, a very powerful androgen.

anlage (*plural,* **anlagen**): in embryology, the initial element or structure that develops and differentiates into a more complex structure.

anorchia: a condition in the male in which the fetal gonads differentiate as testes and subsequently degenerate. Treatment includes hormonal replacement with testosterone at puberty, and surgical implantation of artificial testes; *see also* **hyporchia**.

anosmia: lack of acuity in the sense of smell, as contrasted with hyposmia which means diminished smell acuity. In the strictest sense anosmia means total inability to smell anything. More loosely, it may be used to mean inability to discriminate odors one from another.

anovulatory: without ovulation, as when an estrous or menstrual cycle occurs without the release of an egg from the ovary. Anovulatory cycles are infertile cycles. Until ovulation resumes, a female is said to manifest anovulatory sterility.

areola (*plural,* **areolae**): the area of pigmented skin immediately surrounding the nipple of the breast.

arrhenoblastoma: an infrequent tumor of the ovary in women, malignant, which may sometimes secrete a male sex hormone which has a masculinizing effect on the woman's body or, if she is pregnant, on her unborn daughter.

atrophy (*adjective,* **atrophied, atrophic**): a defect or failure of cell nutrition manifested as decrease in size and healthiness of an organ or tissue; *see also* **dystrophy.**

autoradiography: the technique of making an autoradiograph, a type of photograph resembling an X-ray, in which a very thin slice of tissue is developed as if it were a photographic film. Radioactive test material that has found its way into any of the cells shows up as darkly colored.

barbiturate: one of several pharmaceutical products used medicinally for sleeping pills or elixirs.

Barr body: the color-staining spot (the sex chromatin) located at the edge of the nucleus of cells taken from individuals with more than one X chromosome. It is normally found in female cells, and so is used as a sign of female genetic sex. It is also found in men with the 47,XXY (Klinefelter's) syndrome. It is missing in girls with the 45,X (Turner's) syndrome. The Barr-body test is rapid and inexpensive as compared with actual chromosome counting, and so is used as a method of preliminary X chromosome screening.

bestiality: *see* **zoophilia**

bicornate uterus: a condition in which the arms of the fallopian tubes branch off wrongly, like the arms of a Y instead of a T.

cachexia: weakness or emaciation or, in children, failure to thrive and grow strong, as a result of disease or a metabolic or endocrine deficiency condition.

cannula (pl. **cannulae**): a small tube inserted into body tissue through which fluid may be passed.

cingulate gyrus: a structure in the old cortex (paleocortex) or limbic system of the brain.

clitoris: the small, hooded organ at the top of the cleft of the female sex organs, which is the counterpart of the penis in the male. In the rat, mouse, and hamster, the clitoris is not hooded but its covering is fused as in the male's penis to form a urinary tube.

coprophilia (*adjective,* **coprophiliac**): the condition of being responsive to, or dependent on, the smell or taste of feces for erotic arousal and the facilitation or achievement of orgasm. From the point of view of the species, it probably has its origins in mammalian hygiene whereby infants are licked clean. In individual biography, the correlation between feces and eroticism is varied in origin. It may be related to masochism and self-deprecation. Coprophilia may involve also the sight and sound of a person defecating.

copulin: the odiferous substance or pheromone from the vagina that attracts the male to copulate at the time of the female's ovulation. The name was first proposed by Richard Michael and coworkers in connection with experimental studies of mating in the rhesus monkey. In 1971 they isolated the substance and defined it chemically as being composed of short-chain aliphatic acids.

core gender identity: a term newly introduced into psychoanalytic theory to refer to a infant's developing sense of self as a boy or girl in the second year of life, well in advance of the classic oedipal phase to which the origin of differences in the psychology of sex is attributed in traditional theory.

corpora cavernosa: the pair of "cavernous" or spongy columns of erectile tissue in the penis below which is the urethra and corpus spongiosum. Pumped full of blood, these spongy bodies hold the penis erect.

corpus luteum (*plural,* **corpora lutea**): "yellow body"; a yellow mass in the ovary formed from the graafian follicle after the egg is released. It produces progesterone, the pregnancy hormone, and grows and lasts for several months if the egg is fertilized and pregnancy occurs.

cortex (*plural,* **cortices**): literally, the bark or outer layer; in anatomy, the outer layer or section of an organ, as the cortex of the brain and the cortex of the adrenal gland; *see also* **adrenal cortex, neocortex, paleocortex**.

cortisol: the main glucocorticoid hormone in man produced by the adrenal cortices; also known as hydrocortisone. It is essential to the maintenance of life. It is available in synthetic form.

cortisone: one of the glucocorticoid hormones, a metabolite of cortisol. In synthetic form it is used therapeutically, and is converted in the body into the biologically more potent hormone, cortisol. Historically, the term "cortisone" has also been used generically to refer to all the synthetic glucocorticoids used therapeutically.

cryptorchidism: the condition of having one testis (unilateral) or both (bilateral) undescended.

cunnilingus: erotic stimulation of the female sex organs with the tongue and mouth by a partner of either sex. It is considered a normal part of love play.

Cushing's syndrome: a condition of chronically increased cortisol secretion from the adrenal cortices, either associated with adrenal hyperplasia of postnatal onset or due to an adrenal cortical neoplasm. Clinical manifestations include, in children, marked decrease in linear growth, the development of flabby obesity, a moon face, and occasionally demineralization of the bones; in adults, women are affected by hirsutism and menstrual irregularities, males experience impotence. Treatment is aimed at removal or irradiation of the primary lesion, which may be in the pituitary or the adrenal.

cyproterone: a synthetic, hormonal steroid substance, related to progesterone, which is highly potent as an antiandrogen. A variant form is cyproterone acetate, which is more powerful in its antiandrogenic effect.

cytogenetic syndromes: those conditions of development marked by various bodily and behavioral symptoms which stem from a deficiency, excess, or other gross defect in the number, size, and shape of the chromosomes in each of the body's cells. For example, in most girls with Turner's syndrome, one sex chromosome is missing (45,X); in most boys with Klinefelter's syndrome, the male's one X chromosome is duplicated (47,XXY); and in most boys with the YY syndrome, the male's Y chromosome is duplicated (47,XYY).

cytogenetics: that branch of the science of heredity that deals with the chromosomes and genes (carriers of the genetic code) within the cell nucleus.

dehydroisoandrosterone: one of the natural androgens measurable in the blood of men and women. It is produced almost entirely by the adrenal cortices. It has extremely low biological potency as an androgen.

dexamethasone: a biologically very active, synthetic adrenocortical hormone, a glucocorticoid, (i.e., resembling cortisol). It is used in a test to suppress the pituitary's release of ACTH (adrenocorticotrophic hormone).

diethylstilbestrol: a synthetic drug that acts as a female sex hormone. Structural variants include dipropionate, dilaurate, and dibutyrate esters, and C^{14}-diethylstilbestrol dibutyrate, the radioactive form used only for special investigative procedures.

dimorphism: having two forms or manifestations, though of the same species, as in a juvenile and adult form, or a male and a female form. Though usually used to refer to bodily form and appearance, in this book the meaning of the term is extended by analogy to apply to sex differences in behavior and language.

dwarfism, hypopituitary: short stature, at least four standard deviations below the mean of the age group, due to failure of the pituitary gland to produce growth hormone. Treatment with human growth hormone may result in normal growth rate. Other pituitary hormones may be also missing, in particular gonadotropins, so that sexual infantilism persists into adult life. Treatment with sex hormones will induce reasonable sexual maturity, though the beard cannot be induced to grow in males.

dysgenesis (*adjective,* **dysgenetic**)**:** abnormal or incomplete differentiation of tissue or an organ, with resultant deformity or malfunction; *see also* **agenesis**.

dystrophy (*adjective,* **dystrophic**)**:** partial atrophy of tissue or an organ as a result of imperfect cell nutrition; *see also* **atrophy**.

epiphysis (*adjective,* **epiphysial** or **epiphyseal**)**:** a piece of bone separated from a long bone by cartilage in the juvenile years of life, but later fusing with the larger bone. After epiphysial fusion or closure is complete in late teenage, no further growth in height is possible.

estradiol: the most biologically potent of the naturally occurring estrogens. It is produced chiefly by the ovary. Commercially it is prepared in various compounds, such as estradiol benzoate and ethinyl estradiol.

estrogen: female sex hormone, produced chiefly by the ovary, but also by the adrenal cortex and, in some amount , by the testis. Named so because, in lower animals, it brings the female into estrus (heat). In biochemical structure there are several different but related steroid hormones that qualify as estrogens. They differ in biological strength and effectiveness; *see also* **progesterone**.

estrus (*adjective,* **estrous**)**:** the phenomenon of being sexually receptive, or in heat, as found in the sexual cycle of the females of some species. A condition or syndrome of persistent estrus can be produced in some animals (for example, the rat) by hormonal injection of the newborn, notably with androgen; *see also* **TSR.**

exhibitionism (*noun*, **exhibitionist**): the condition of being responsive to, or dependent on the debasement, shock, and outcry of a stranger (usually female), unexpectedly exposed to the sight of the penis, in order to maintain one's erotic arousal and facilitate or achieve orgasm.

fallopian tubes: the left and right tubes of the uterus which connect the uppermost part of the uterine cavity with the ovarian region. They are so positioned as to be able to transport the egg released from the ovary to the uterine cavity for implanting. They are named for the Italian anatomist Gabriello Fallopius (1523–62).

fellatio: stimulation of the penis by taking it into the mouth, possibly to the point of orgasm. The partner may be of either sex. It is considered a normal part of love play.

forme fruste (*plural*, **formes frustes**): an incomplete, defective or abortive form, version or manifestation of a process, condition or disease.

freemartin: a male calf's twin sister which is born partially hermaphroditic and sterile, as a result of having been fetally influenced by the male twin's testicular secretions transferred by way of connecting blood vessels.

frotteur: a person for whom the most effective stimulus to erotic arousal is the act of rubbing up against another person's body, especially when crowded together with strangers in a public place or conveyance. The act of rubbing is an end in itself and may be sufficient to produce orgasm.

FSH: follicle-stimulating hormone. It is produced by the pituitary gland and stimulates the formation of the ovarian follicle on the ovary, and the production of estrogen. When the follicle ripens, lutenizing hormone takes over, and the progestinic phase of the menstrual cycle appears.

fugue state: Latin *fuga*, a fleeing, flight. A condition resembling sleep walking in which a person, though awake, flees from familiar surroundings and has a large part of his own past history dissociated or unrecallable. When the fugue state ends, the history of what happened during it will, in turn, be largely unrecallable or dissociated.

gender identity: the sameness, unity, and persistence of one's individuality as male or female (or ambivalent), in greater or lesser degree, especially as it is experienced in self-awareness and behavior. Gender identity is the private experience of gender role, and gender role is the public expression of gender identity.

gender role: everything that a person says and does, to indicate to others or to the self the degree in which one is male or female or ambivalent. It includes but is not restricted to sexual arousal and response. Gender role is the public expression of gender identity, and gender identity is the private experience of gender role.

gestagen: an alternative term for progestin.

glucocorticoid: a type of hormone which has its main metabolic effect on carbohydrate. The chief natural glucocorticoid is cortisol, produced by the adrenal cortices.

gonadal dysgenesis: imperfect formation or genesis of the gonads or sex glands. There is a syndrome of gonadal dysgenesis in phenotypic females, also known as Turner's syndrome.

gonadotropin: one of the hormones released by the anterior lobe of the pituitary gland, which programs the activity of the ovary in the female and the testis in the male.

graafian follicle: the follicle on the ovary in which the egg grows. After the egg is released, the graafian follicle become the corpus luteum. Named for R. de Graaf, Dutch anatomist (1641–73).

gynandromorphy: a term of Greek etymology meaning woman-man-shape. Thus, literally, the term means having some of the body morphology and measurements of an average woman, and some of an average man, or being at neither extreme.

gynecomastia: the development of breasts on a male, spontaneously or as a result of hormonal treatment.

haptic: having to do with touch and the sense of touch.

hermaphroditism: a congenital condition of ambiguity of the reproductive structures so that the sex of the individual is not clearly defined as exclusively male or exclusively female. The condition is named for Hermes and Aphrodite, the Greek god and godess of love.

hippocampus: a structure of the limbic system of the brain named for the resemblance of its curved shape to a sea horse. It is situated in the region of the temporal lobe of the cerebral cortex and is important, among other things, in the processing of short-term memory. *Synonym*, Ammon's horn.

hirsutism: hairiness, especially excessive hairiness.

homosexuality, facultative: optional homosexuality. It presents itself in a person's awareness in such a way as to not exclude heterosexuality. The person is in effect bisexual. Facultative homosexuality may be situationally elicited under conditions of sex-segregation, as when a person is in jail.

homosexuality, obligative: compelling or exclusive homosexuality. It presents itself in a person's awareness in such a way as to leave no bisexual or heterosexual option to that person.

hydroxycorticosteroids: *see* **17-hydroxycorticosteroids**.

hyperplasia (*adjective*, **hyperplastic**)**:** an increase in the number of cells in an organ, and thus of the size of the organ; *see* **hypertrophy**; *antonym*, **hypoplasia**.

hypertrophy (*adjective*, **hypertrophied, hypertrophic**)**:** over-development in size of an organ or of its constituent cells; *see* **hyperplasia**; *antonym*, **atrophy**.

hypopituitarism: a generalized endocrine deficiency condition produced by failure, either partial or complete, of the pituitary gland to secrete its proper hormones. Failure after surgery for a pituitary tumor is usually complete. Idiopathic failure may be either complete or partial. In some instances, partial failure may involve chiefly the secretion of pituitary gonadotrophins, the hormones that stimulate the ovaries or the testes to produce their own hormones.

hypoplasia (*adjective*, **hypoplastic**): structural smallness, as in the case of genitalia that are too small to function as expected in adulthood. Hypoplasia of an organ may result from failure of embryonic tissue growth and differentiation, or from subsequent unresponsiveness and failure of growth; *antonym*, **hyperplasia**.

hyporchia: a condition in the male marked by partial degeneration of gonads which have differentiated fetally as testes. Treatment with testosterone replacement at puberty is necessary in severe cases; *see also* **anorchia**.

hypospadias (*adjective*, **hypospadiac**): a birth defect in the positioning of the urinary opening on the penis. In mild hypospadias, the opening is only slightly removed from the tip of the penis. In severe hypospadias, the opening is in the female position, and the penis has an open gutter on its underside, instead of a covered urinary canal. A hypospadiac penis may be normal-sized or small; *see* **microphallus**. A small penis with a severe degree of hypospadias is identical in appearance with an enlarged clitoris below which is a single opening or urogenital sinus leading to both the urethra and the vagina; *see* **hermaphroditism**.

hypothalamus: a structure of the diencephalon, a portion of the brain of special importance in regulating vital functions, including sex, by means of the release of neurohumoral substances from nerve cells. These substances in turn regulate the nearby pituitary gland.

iatrogenic: a condition that results as a side-effect or by-product of a program of therapy. An iatrogenic symptom or condition may be inadvertent and undesirable, or predicted and desirable.

ICSH: interstitial cell stimulating hormone; *see* **lutenizing hormone**.

idiopathic: possessing the quality of being pathologically self-generated or spontaneous in origin. It is commonly applied to developmental disorders or conditions for which no antecedent or cause has been found or postulated, as in idiopathic hypopituitarism.

imprimatur: in publishing, permission or sanction to print and publish something. In this book (Chapter 1) the term is used, by analogy, to mean that a permitted or sanctioned part of the program of development expresses itself and leaves permanent sequelae.

imprinting: developmental learning of a type first brought to scientific attention in studies of animal behavior by ethologists. Imprinting takes place in a given species when behavior programed into the nervous system of that species requires a matching social-environmental stimulus to release it, when the matching must take place during a critical or sensitive developmental period (not before or after), and when, having occurred, the resultant behavioral pattern is unusually resistant to extinction. In human beings, language learning is a manifestation of imprinting.

intersexuality: an alternative term for hermaphroditism. In past usage, a genetic etiology was sometimes assumed for intersexuality, and a hormonal etiology for hermaphroditism, but the distinction is now known to be untenable.

Kallmann's syndrome: a rare condition of deficient maturation characterized by insufficient release of gonadotropic hormones from the pituitary to stimulate the testes or ovaries, infertility, and lack or severe impairment of the sense of smell.

ketosteroids: *see* **17-ketosteroids**.

Klinefelter's syndrome: a condition identified by a chromosomal anomaly in phenotypic males with the pathognomonic symptoms of a small penis, small testes, and sterility. The basic genetic defect is an extra sex chromosome with a total count of 47,XXY. Variants of the syndrome are characterized by more than one extra X chromosome, e.g., 48,XXXY. The secondary sex characteristics are usually weakly developed and do not respond well to treatment with male sex hormone.

Klüver-Bucy syndrome: a pattern of changed behavior, experimentally produced in animals by surgical removal of the amygdala from the brain, and first demonstrated by H. Klüver and P.C. Bucy in the late 1930s. Among other things, this syndrome includes change from aggressiveness to docility in undomesticated monkeys, indiscriminant food choice, and changes in the regulation of sexual behavior.

lactogenic: stimulating the production of milk from the mammary glands.

lesbian (*adjective*, **lesbian**)**:** female homosexual; named after the Aegean island, Lesbos, whence came the homosexual woman poet, Sappho, of ancient Greece. There is no corresponding word for a male homosexual.

LH: *see* **luteinizing hormone**.

limbic system: the old cortex or paleocortex, as contrasted with the neocortex of the brain. Its functions pertain to those aspects of the human mind and behavior that are shared by lower species.

lordosis: the position of arching the back and elevating the haunches so as to receive the male in intercourse, typical of most mammals.

LTH: *see* **luteotropic hormone**.

luteinizing hormone (LH): one of the gonadotropic hormones of the pituitary gland. It induces release of the egg from the graafian follicle and transformation of the latter into a corpus luteum. LH in the female is the same as ICSH (interstitial cell stimulating hormone) which stimulates testosterone production in the male.

luteotropic hormone (LTH): the hormone from the pituitary gland that in the nonpregnant woman maintains the corpus luteum for about two weeks and causes the release of progesterone from it. LTH is the same as lactogenic hormone or prolactin and is responsible for the initiation of milk production at the end of pregnancy.

masochism (*adjective*, **masochistic**)**:** the condition of being responsive to or dependent on being the recipient of punishment and humiliation in order to maintain erotic arousal and facilitate or achieve orgasm. As the partner of a sadist, a person may impersonate a masochist for commercial gain, within the limits set by the pain threshold.

mastectomy: surgery for removal of the glandular tissue of the breasts. It applies to females or to those few males whose breasts enlarge with glandular mammary tissue; *synonym*, mammectomy.

median eminence: a small structure of the brain at the base of the hypothalamus in which the neurovascular link with the pituitary gland is situated.

medroxyprogesterone acetate: a pharmaceutical hormonal product marketed under the name of Provera®. It has many of the physiological properties of progesterone, and so is known as a synthetic progestin, though in chemical structure it is actually an androgen, like testosterone, which is closely related to progesterone. Therapeutically, medroxyprogesterone acetate has varied uses: to suppress ovulation (in the birth-control pill); to prevent threatened miscarriage; and to suppress androgen release and libido, reversibly, in male sex offenders. In preventing miscarriage, it may have a rare, paradoxical, and unexplained masculinizing effect on the female fetus, causing the birth of a daughter with a masculinized clitoris.

menopause: in a female, the change of life, cessation of menstrual functioning. It does not bring about cessation of sex life.

metabolite: a biological substance which is a by-product or waste product produced by metabolism of another substance in the body. For example, after a hormone has been secreted into the bloodstream and used by target tissues or organs, its metabolites may be measured in the urine.

microphallus: an exceptionally small penis that resembles a clitoris in size. A microphallus may carry the urethral tube or may be hypospadiac. Typically it is formed mostly of skin, the body (corpora cavernosa) of the penis being hypoplastic. The condition is also known as penile agenesis and micropenis.

mosaicism, chromosomal: an abnormality in the number of chromosomes in which different karyotypes exist in different cells from the same individual. It can involve both autosomes and sex chromosomes. An example is the 45,X/46,XX mosaicism found in some girls with Turner's syndrome, instead of the expected 45,X count.

mullerian ducts: the structures in the fetus that will, in the female, develop into the uterus and fallopian tubes; named for Johannes P. Müller, German physiologist (1801–58); *see also* **wolffian ducts**.

myelination: in nerve cells, those fibers which are sheathed in myelin (a mucoprotein substance). In the brain, the white matter is made up of myelinated fibers.

narratophilia (*adjective*, **narratophiliac**): the condition of being responsive to, or dependent on reading or listening to erotic narratives in order to maintain erotic arousal and facilitate or achieve orgasm.

necrophilia (*adjective*, **necrophiliac**): the condition of being responsive to or dependent on sexual activity with a cadaver in order to maintain erotic arousal and facilitate or achieve orgasm. In necrophilia there is an obsession with death, not with killing, as there is in sexual homicide.

necrosis (*adjective*, **necrotic**): loss of life in tissue which degenerates, as at the site of a wound, while still in contact with the living body.

neocortex: the outermost layer or cortex of the brain which in the evolutionary sense is new and is most highly developed in man. It is contrasted with the paleocortex (the old cortex or limbic system) which it encapsulates.

nidation: the implantation of the fertilized egg in the endometrial wall of the uterus in pregnancy.

Norlutin:® trade name for a preparation of norethindrone. Norethindrone is 17α-ethinyl-19-nortestosterone, used as a synthetic progestin.

ovotestis: an abnormally developed sex gland of which the cell structure partially resembles an ovary and partially a testis.

paleocortex: *see* **limbic system**.

paraphilia (*adjective*, **paraphiliac**): a psychosexual condition of being obsessively responsive to, and dependent on an unusual or unacceptable stimulus in order to have a state of sexual arousal initiated or maintained, and in order to achieve or facilitate orgasm. The majority of paraphilias are believed to occur significantly more frequently in males than females. For examples, *see* **coprophilia**, **exhibitionism**, **masochism**, **narratophilia**, **necrophilia**, **pederasty**, **pictophilia**, **sadism**, **scatology**, **urophilia**, **voyeurism**.

pederasty: literally, boy love; *see* **pedophilia**. Pederasty is usually used in the restricted sense to refer to anal intercourse performed by an older man on a prepubertal or early pubertal boy. It is not applied to the relationship between an older woman and a boy.

pedophilia (*adjective*, **pedophiliac**): the condition of being responsive to or dependent on sexual activity with a prepubertal or early pubertal boy, in order to maintain erotic arousal and facilitate or achieve orgasm. A pedophiliac may be a male or a female, though typically a man.

phallus: a synonym for penis which is also used to refer to the enlarged clitoris or penis-like structure of a female hermaphrodite.

pheromone: an odiferous substance which acts as a chemical messenger between individuals. By contrast, a hormone acts as a chemical messenger within the bloodstream of a single individual. In mammals, pheromones serve as foe repellants, boundary markers, child-parent attractants, and sex attractants.

phyletic: of or pertaining to a race. Phyletic components or aspects of behavior in human beings are those shared by all members of the human race, as compared with behavior which is individual and biographically idiosyncratic. Phyletic behavior is the product of both prenatal and postnatal determinants, as is personal biographic behavior. Both are the end product of both innate and experiential determinants.

pictophilia (*adjective*, **pictophiliac**): the condition of being responsive to or dependent on erotic pictures in order to maintain erotic arousal and facilitate or achieve orgasm.

pineal (Latin, *pinus*, pine cone) **gland:** a small cone-shaped body, also known as the epiphysis cerebri, located in the midline of the midbrain in the region of the thalamus.

pituitary gland: an endocrine gland situated deep in the brain in the midline behind the eyes. The hormones of the anterior pituitary regulate many functions of the other endocrine glands of the body. The pituitary is also known as the hypophysis.

pituitary-gonadal axis: an hypothetical construct called upon to explain the two-way, reciprocal regulatory effect that exists between the hormonal output of the pituitary gland and the gonads (ovaries or testes).

polycystic: containing or made up of many cysts, as in polycystic ovaries.

pregnanediol: a urinary metabolite of progesterone which itself is one of the two main female sex hormones.

pregnanetriol: a urinary metabolite of 17-hydroxyprogesterone which itself is the precursor of all biologically active steroid hormones, including cortisol and the sex hormones.

preoptic region: a part of the hypothalamus, closely related to the pituitary gland, and situated near the transverse crossing of the optic nerves, the optic chiasma. It is believed that the cells of the preoptic area secrete neurohumoral substances.

priapism: persistent abnormal and painful erection of the penis, usually without sexual desire. The cause is often unknown. It almost always results in destruction of the spongy tissues of the penis as a result of coagulation of blood in them, with resultant chronic impotence.

progesterone: pregnancy hormone, one of the two sex hormones chiefly characteristic of the female. It is produced by the ovary in the corpus luteum, following ovulation, and also by the placenta during pregnancy. The metabolic pathway of hormone production in the body leads from progesterone to androgen to estrogen.

progestin: any one of the class of synthetic sex-hormonal steroids that has a physiologic action resembling progesterone; also known as gestagen.

prolactin: the milk-stimulating hormone secreted from the pituitary gland. It is the same as luteotropin; *see also* **LTH**.

pseudocyesis: spurious or false pregnancy, marked by some of the hormonal changes of genuine pregnancy and possible abdominal enlargement, but without a fetus: also known as pseudopregnancy.

pseudohermaphroditism: hermaphroditism. The prefix was once used to denote the fact that the gonads were not hermaphroditically mixed (ovarian plus testicular tissue) as in true hermaphroditism, but were either testicular (male pseudohermaphroditism) or ovarian (female pseudohermaphroditism). In modern usage, the preferred terms are male, female, and true hermaphroditism. Agonadal hermaphroditism is a fourth form.

pseudopregnancy: *see* **pseudocyesis**.

radioimmunoassay: a method of assaying or measuring the uptake or rejection of hormones or other biological substances by body tissues after injection of radioactive forms of those hormones or substances.

rubella: German measles.

sadism (*adjective*, **sadistic**): the condition of being responsive to or dependent on punishing or humiliating one's partner in order to maintain erotic arousal and facilitate orgasm. A person, especially a woman, may impersonate a sadist to oblige masochistic partners for commercial gain.

scatology (*adjective*, **scatological**): literally, the study of excrement; metaphorically, the study of verbal or graphic material legally defined as filthy or obscene, and pertaining to sexual rather than excremental activity. A scatological telephone caller talks sexually in a manner that he expects will be offensive or shocking to a female listener who does not know him. He is dependent on this maneuver to maintain erotic arousal and facilitate or achieve orgasm.

septum: a dividing wall or partition. In the brain, the septum or septal area is part of the limbic system.

17-hydroxycorticosteroids: a group of metabolites of cortisol measurable in the urine.

17-hydroxylase: an adrenal cortical enzyme necessary in the synthesis of most steroids, in particular cortisol.

17-ketosteroids: a group of metabolites of androgens measurable in the urine of both men and women.

Stein-Leventhal syndrome: a condition in females marked by failure to ovulate, secondary amenorrhea, and hirsutism, associated with abnormal ovarian function. The ovaries are usually polycystic with a thickened capsule and are believed to produce an excess of androgen. Treatment includes usually removal of a pie-shaped piece of the enlarged ovaries, and is often, but not always, successful in relieving symptoms.

stilbestrol: same as **diethylstilbestrol**.

testosterone: the most biologically potent of the naturally occurring androgens, measurable in blood plasma and in urine. It is produed chiefly by the testis.

transexual (*adjective,* **transexual**): a person manifesting the phenomena of transexualism.

transexualism: behaviorally, the act of living and passing in the role of the opposite sex, before or after having attained hormonal, surgical, and legal sex reassignment; psychically, the condition of people who have the conviction that they belong to the opposite sex and are driven by a compulsion to have the body, appearance, and social status of the opposite sex.

transsexual: transexual

transvestism (*adjective*, **transvestic, transvestitic**): behaviorally, the act of dressing in the clothes of the opposite sex; psychically, the condition of feeling compelled to cross-dress, often in relation to sexual arousal and attainment of orgasm.

TSR: an acronym from the words Testosterone Sterilized (female) Rat. A TSR manifests the persistent estrus syndrome. Lacking ovulatory estrous cycles, she is sterile. The condition is induced experimentally by injections of testosterone prior to the age of eleven days. The first five days of life are the most sensitive or critical ones. Smaller doses are then effective. The effect is lifelong.

Turner's syndrome: a condition marked by a chromosomal anomaly in phenotypic females with the chief pathognomonic symptoms of absence of ovaries (gonadal agenesis or dysgenesis) and short stature. The basic genetic defect is a missing sex chromosome, so that the total count is 45,X. There are several variants of this syndrome. For example, in some cases, the second X may, though present, be partially deleted. In others, the so-called mosaics, some cells of the body are 45,X, and some 46,XX. Treatment includes administration of female sex hormone at the age of puberty to induce adult appearance and menstruation. Girls with Turner's syndrome are almost invariably sterile.

undinism (*adjective*, **undinist):** urophilia; derived from undine (*German*) or ondine (*French*), a fabled female water spirit; *see* **urophilia**.

urophilia (*adjective*, **urophiliac):** the condition of being responsive to or dependent on the smell or taste of urine, or the sight and sound of someone urinating, in order to maintain erotic arousal and facilitate or achieve orgasm; *see* **undinism.**

vaginal atresia: a congenital condition in which the vagina is missing or malformed. Typically, it is a shallow dimple rather than a canal connecting with a uterus, and the uterus itself is likely to be malformed and cordlike in structure.

vas deferens (*plural*, **vasa deferentia):** literally the vessel that carries away the sperms from the testicle (or strictly from the epididymis of the testicle) to the ejaculatory duct. Cutting of the vasa, surgically known as vasectomy, is the operation performed on men as a permanent form of infertility for purposes of birth control.

ventromedial: situated in the middle of the ventral (belly or anterior) side of a region or structure, for example, the ventromedial region of the hypothalamus, on the floor of the third ventricle of the brain.

ventromedial nucleus: in the hypothalamus, a cluster or knot of cell bodies in the ventromedial region. It is important in the regulation of vital functions, especially appetite.

Versene: a trade name for various synthetic amino acids and their salts which are used as chelating or sequestering agents, that is to bind divalent metallic ions, such as calcium and magnesium; Versene is used as a cleaning and degreasing agent, as a textile processing assistant, as a decontaminating agent for radioactive materials, and as a dissolving agent for proteins.

voyeurism (*noun*, **voyeur):** the condition of being responsive to, or dependent on the risk of being apprehended while illicitly peering at an individual (usually female) or a couple undressing or engaged in sexual activity, in order to maintain one's own erotic arousal and facilitate or achieve orgasm. A voyeur is also known as a Peeping Tom.

wolffian ducts: the embryonic structures which develop into the internal reproductive anatomy of the male, attached to the testicles; named for Kaspar F. Wolff, German embryologist (1733–94); *see also* **mullerian ducts**.

zoophilia (*adjective*, **zoophiliac):** the condition of being responsive to, or dependent on sexual activity with an animal in order to maintain erotic arousal and facilitate orgasm; also known as bestiality. Sexual contact (oral or genital) with an animal may also occur sporadically in the course of human development without leading to long-term zoophilia.

NAME INDEX

SUBJECT INDEX

Library of Congress Cataloging in Publication Data

Money, John.
Man and woman, boy and girl.

Bibliography: p.
1. Sex—Cause and determination. 2. Sex differences (Psychology).
I. Ehrhardt, Anke A., joint author. II. Title.
QP251.M56 612.6 72-4012
ISBN 0-8018-1405-7
ISBN 0-8018-1406-5 (pbk)